MEDICAL LIBRARY
ASSOCIATION *Guides*

The Medical Library Association Guide *to* Cancer Information

**Authoritative, Patient-Friendly
Print and Electronic Resources**

RUTI MALIS VOLK

NEAL-SCHUMAN PUBLISHERS, INC.
NEW YORK   LONDON

The information in this book is intended to help the reader locate information about cancer. It is not intended to replace the advice of a qualified health care professional. While every effort has been made to ensure accuracy and currency of the facts presented, this information should not be used to make decisions about medical care. Please consult with your physician before making any decisions regarding medical treatment.

Contact information and Web addresses listed in this book were accurate at the time the manuscript went to print.

Published by Neal-Schuman Publishers, Inc.
100 William Street, Suite 2004
New York, NY 10038-4512

The information in this book is presented for educational purposes only, and is not intended to replace the advice of a qualified healthcare professional. Please consult with your physician before making any decisions regarding medical treatment.

Printed and bound in the United States of America.

Published in cooperation with the Medical Library Association.

The paper used in this publication meets the minimum requirements of American National Standard for Information Sciences—Permanence of Paper for Printed Library Materials, ANSI Z39.48-1992.

CIP 13: 978-1-55570-585-5 (alk. paper)
CIP 10: 1-55570-585-5 (alk. paper)

Library of Congress Cataloging-in-Publication Data

The Medical Library Association guide to cancer information : authoritative, patient-friendly print and electronic resources / Ruti Malis Volk.
    p. cm.
  ISBN-13: 978-1-55570-585-5 (alk paper)
  ISBN-10: 1-55570-585-5 (alk paper)
1. Cancer—Information services—Directories. I. Volk, Ruti Malis. II. Medical Library Association.
RC262.M427 2007
616.99'40025-dc22

2006101677

To my wonderful daughters,

Maia and Ella,

and in loving memory of

my eldest child, Shelly.

She lights my path, marks my way,

and leads me in everything I do.

Table of Contents

Part III: Best Information Resources about Cancer Prevention, Treatment, and Quality-of-Life Concerns

Foreword

A cancer diagnosis creates many unknowns. Patients, family, and friends soon discover a bewildering array of information, some useful and accurate and some inaccurate and misleading. The ever-expanding Internet only makes this avalanche of information grow bigger each year. There are tens of thousands of sites related to cancer, so it is more important than ever for librarians to have a reliable resource to help them to assist patients and their families. *The Medical Library Association Guide to Cancer Information: Authoritative, Patient-Friendly Print and Electronic Sources* is the new standard against which all others will be judged.

When the author, Ruti Volk, a librarian, lost a daughter to cancer, she realized the critical importance of accurate cancer information. Ruti turned her information-gathering experiences into a sound system that could lead the public toward dependable advice. She helped establish and direct the Patient Education Resource Center at the University of Michigan Comprehensive Cancer Center. As the center's founding director, responsible for coordinating all cancer activities related to research and patient care, I know her guide will find an eager audience.

The Medical Library Association Guide to Cancer Information draws on Volk's experiences with thousands of cancer patients and their families. This is a comprehensive guide to sources of information on cancer in general as well as the most common forms of cancer. It is an important resource for librarians as well as other healthcare workers who are responsible for ensuring that patients have access to accurate and understandable information about their disease. Use of this resource will help ensure that cancer patients and their families can obtain critical and timely information to help guide them through their cancer journey.

Max S. Wicha, M.D.

Director, Comprehensive Cancer Center,
University of Michigan, Ann Arbor, Michigan

Review Board and Advisory Panel

The Medical Library Association Guide to Cancer Information: Authoritative, Patient-Friendly Print and Electronic Sources

Merav Ben-David, M.D., is the chief medical reviewer of the book. An oncologist practicing at the Chaim Sheba Medical Center, Tel-Hashomer, Israel, Ben-David earned her M.D. degree from Ben-Gurion University Medical School in 1995 and completed her residency at the Sheba Medical Center in 2003. In 2006, she completed a three-year fellowship in radiation oncology at the University of Michigan, Department of Radiation Oncology.

Nancy Burke, R.D., is a pediatric and adult oncology dietitian at the University of Michigan Comprehensive Cancer Center in Ann Arbor, Michigan. Burke reviewed the sections on nutrition during cancer treatment and nutrition for cancer prevention.

Lorrie Carbone, L.M.S.W., is a clinical social worker at the University of Michigan Comprehensive Cancer Center in Ann Arbor, Michigan. Carbone reviewed the sections on appearance and body image, emotional distress, end-of-life, pain control, parenting through cancer, practical issues of survivorship, and sexuality.

Avraham Eisbruch, M.D., is Professor and Associate Chair of Clinical Research at the Department of Radiation Oncology, University of Michigan Health System in Ann Arbor, Michigan. Eisbruch reviewed the section on head and neck cancer.

Karen Hammelef, M.S., is Director of Patient and Family Support Services and Patient Education at the University of Michigan Comprehensive Cancer Center in Ann Arbor, Michigan. Hammelef reviewed the section on cancer supportive care.

Marcia Leonard, R.N., P.N.P., is a pediatric nurse practitioner and Coordinator of the Fertility Counseling & Gamete Cryopreservation Program and the Long Term Follow-Up clinic for childhood cancer survivors at the

University of Michigan Comprehensive Cancer Center in Ann Arbor, Michigan. Leonard reviewed all the childhood cancer types, childhood cancer survivors, and fertility sections.

Sheila Morris, B.S., C.C.L.S., is a child life specialist at the University of Michigan Comprehensive Cancer Center in Ann Arbor, Michigan. Morris reviewed the section on key concepts in childhood cancer.

Rivka Siden, M.Sc., Pharm.D., is a clinical pharmacist with the Investigational Drug Service at the University of Michigan Health System, Ann Arbor, Michigan. Siden reviewed the section on drug therapy.

Preface

ancer recently surpassed heart disease as the top killer of Americans under the age of 85. Each year over one and a quarter million people in the United States receive a diagnosis of cancer, and slightly over half-a-million die. Fortunately, death rates are falling: the percentage of patients surviving more than five years after being diagnosed with cancer has increased over the past two decades. Experts are hoping that the improvements in cancer prevention, detection and treatment may be helping to reduce mortality rates and improve survival. It is estimated that more than 10 million Americans living today have a history of cancer. Some of these survivors are free of the disease while others are still undergoing treatment.

Knowledge plays a significant role in determining the cancer experience. Patients and families who are knowledgeable about their disease feel empowered and are able to make informed decisions. I know this from personal experience. My daughter Shelly died from a brain tumor at age seven. I still remember the intense panic and fear, and the thousands of unanswered questions I had right after Shelly was diagnosed. To find the answers I spent hours on the computer, surfing the Internet, looking for authoritative information in understandable language. I resented the fact that information seeking was taking me away from my daughter and my family, but I desperately needed to educate myself about the disease. I needed information in order to make decisions about treatment and about managing our lives, rearranging priorities and organizing logistics so that I can care for Shelly and my family. Becoming knowledgeable about Shelly's illness marked a turning point in my ability to cope with the situation. I felt empowered to take control over the aspects in my life I could control, make decisions and parent my sick child and her sister.

The Medical Library Association Guide to Cancer Information is based on bibliographies I developed as the librarian in charge of the Patient Education Resource Center at the University of Michigan Comprehensive Cancer Center (UMCCC). I started working at the UMCCC in August of 1999, eight months after Shelly's death.

My experience as a parent of a child with cancer led to my decision to create short concise information guides that include a few carefully selected quality information sources that serve as starting points for information seeking. My goal then was—and is now—to enable patients and caregivers to quickly locate quality information sources and reduce time spent on information seeking. Knowledge has a positive impact on quality-of-life and even outcomes of people affected by cancer. It helps patients and families establish a productive and meaningful dialog with clinicians, and have a collaborative, rather than a passive role in the management of their health.

The challenge in answering questions about cancer lays with the fact that cancer is not one disease; cancer is a general name for a group of more than a hundred distinct diseases that affect people in very different ways. Some cancers progress rapidly, some are slow growers, some cancers respond very well to treatment while others are resistant. The effects of cancer encompass the entire spectrum of a person's life including family relationships, friendships, self-image, sexuality, fertility, mental health, employment and financial situation. The person with cancer or family members may have questions about any of these topics in the context of cancer.

In addition, patients require different types of information depending on their educational level and personality. Beyond the differences in literacy levels, people affected by cancer cope differently with information about disease. Some, overwhelmed by the challenges of a life-threatening illness may want only basic, general overviews, while others feel that having the most comprehensive, in-depth, detailed information about their condition helps them to take charge of their lives.

The great variety of cancer diseases and diversity of patients and situations means that there is no one-stop-shop for cancer information. The information on cancer is spread across hundreds of resources in a great variety of media. Finding the right information source to answer a patron's question can be a daunting, time-consuming task. This book is designed to enable the reader to quickly identify the most authoritative, unbiased, quality information sources in lay language to match a specific information request. The second objective of the book is to help librarians in collection development. The compilation of the resources listed in the chapters is in fact the cancer consumer health core bibliography.

Savvy cancer information seekers: patients, caregivers or supporters who want to familiarize themselves with key information sources on their disease can use this book as a guide to locate the resources in public libraries, hospital libraries, bookstores and the Internet.

How to use this book

The book is divided into three parts:

➤ Part I provides a foundation of knowledge required for providing cancer information to the public; it explains key concepts and terminology and describes the most important cancer information sources for both adult and childhood cancer.

➤ Part II focuses on 25 adult cancer types and ten childhood cancer types. Each topic has a similar structure:

➢ A short, concise introduction that explains the anatomy, terminology and special characteristics and information needs typical to the specific patient population. The number of annual diagnoses per year referenced in the introductions is based on the American Cancer Society's projections for 2007.

➢ An annotated list of information sources arranged by format from print to electronic. The list includes brochures, books, audiovisual and Web resources.

➢ A list of patient support organizations (when applicable). The listing enables the librarian to direct patients to support-services specific to the diagnosis.

➤ Part III covers topics that are common to all cancer types. They include topics in prevention, treatment methods and quality-of-life issues. Each topic has a similar structure with an introduction, an annotated list of information sources and a list of patient support organizations (when applicable).

The *Guide* ends with full references and a subject index.

In order to get the most benefit from the book, I recommended that users read and master the key concepts outlined in part one of the book. This knowledge is prerequisite to understanding the chapters in parts two and three of the book. The chapters focusing on specific types and topics may be read as the need arises, not in sequence. This independent structure is the reason for some redundancy and repetition of sources listed under different topics. The topic introductions enable the librarian to conduct an effective reference interview to pinpoint the information needs and formulate questions. After the questions have been identified it is possible to start the information seeking process by consulting the information sources listed in the annotated bibliography.

This book does not contain a glossary. Most terms are explained in the body of the text. The National Cancer Institute's *Dictionary of Cancer Terms*, accessible online at www.cancer.gov, can be used to clarify terms and vocabulary not included in the text. To facilitate access to illustrations I included

URLs for relevant graphics and images on the Web. These electronic versions are, in most cases, full color illustrations in printer-friendly format.

Topic selection

The adult cancer types were selected because they have an incidence of over 5000 diagnoses per year in the United States. The childhood types selected have an incidence of over 250 annual diagnoses in the United States. The topics in Part III of the book were selected because they have dedicated print or electronic materials that focus on the topic in their entirety.

As a general rule, research on topics that do not have a specific section should start in the primary information sources listing described in part one. The resources listed in Chapter 3 apply to both adult and childhood cancer types and topics.

Resource selection

The principle guideline in selecting resources for this book was to include authoritative sources in patient-friendly language. The goal was to offer a variety of high-quality sources that cover the topic in many levels of breadth and depth. The great majority of materials were published in English in the United States. A few resources from the United Kingdom and Canada are also included, mostly resources that offer unique content, not covered by U.S. resources.

The following considerations guided the selection of materials:

➤ *Relevancy*—Materials that are directly related to the topic. Preference was given to materials that relate to the topic in their entirety.
➤ Educational Level—Materials written in lay language and are intended for non-professionals.
➤ *Accuracy*—Materials authored or reviewed by credentialed medical professionals. Exceptions were made for unique resources that contain accurate and useful information and were recommended by professionals.
➤ *Quality*—Materials that received favorable reviews in professional review sources, or were favorably reviewed and recommended by University of Michigan specialists.
➤ *Timeliness*—Print and audiovisual materials that were published within the previous five years, or contain information that is still current and Web sites that update frequently and post revision dates.
➤ *Format*—Print, audiovisual and Web resources are included, as well as patient advocacy organizations that offer support services to patient and families.

Almost all audiovisuals listed are available in DVD format or may be viewed online. A few VHS videos that offer unique and still current content are included, as they are likely to be reissued in DVD format. At this point the number of cancer-related DVDs is quite limited, but this will probably change by the next edition.

Readers may notice that some resources they are familiar with are not included in the book. Some resources were not included because they focus on a sub-topic and do not address the full range of the subject. Some materials were omitted in order to avoid redundancy. Preference was given to materials that are accessible on the Internet in the form of Adobe Acrobat (.pdf) files, audio or video file. Non-inclusion of materials does not imply negative judgment on my part—the goal of the book was not to list every single resource on the topic, but rather to provide starting points for efficient information seeking.

References

American Cancer Society. (2006). *Cancer facts & figures 2007*. Atlanta, Ga: American Cancer Society.

American Cancer Society. (2005). *Detailed guide: Cancer (general information)*. Retrieved 1/11/06 from the American Cancer Society site at:http://www.cancer.org/docroot/CRI/CRI_2_3x.asp?dt=72

Jemal, Ahmedin, Siegel, Rebecca, Ward, Elizabeth, Murray, Taylor, Xu, Jiaquan, Thun, (2007). Cancer statistics, 2007. *CA Cancer J Clin, 57*, 43–66.

National Coalition for Cancer Survivorship (2006). *Facts and Statistics*. Retrieved 10/18/06 from the National Coalition for Cancer Survivorship site at: http://www.canceradvocacy.org/news/facts.aspx

Volk, Ruti. (In Press). Expert searching in consumer health: an important role for librarians in the age of the Internet and the Web. *J Med Libr Assoc., 95*(2)

Acknowledgments

First and foremost I would like to give special thanks and recognition to Merav Ben-David M.D., the medical reviewer of this book, who meticulously analyzed the text to ensure the accuracy of the medical information.

This book would not have come about without the support and encouragement I received at my place of work, the University of Michigan Comprehensive Cancer Center. Dr. Max Wicha, the founding director, and Marcy Waldinger, M.H.S.A., chief administrative officer, create an environment that promotes new ideas, stimulates excellence, and places compassion and caring for patients as a top goal. I am especially grateful for the constant help, support, and guidance I received over the years from Karen Hammelef, director of patient support services and the patient education program. Karen's leadership, innovation, and drive have been instrumental to my accomplishments and this book.

Roli Hasson Nesher, Barbara H. Kramer, and Emily Eisbruch deserve acknowledgment for their guidance and advice with the practical aspects of writing. I am also grateful to my friend and colleague Gale Oren, MILS, AHIP, who suggested that I write a bibkit for the Medical Library Association (MLA), an idea that eventually grew into this book.

Lastly, I would like to thank Dr. Max Wicha for writing the foreword and my coworkers at the University of Michigan Health System who reviewed sections of the text that pertain to their specific expertise: Nancy Burke, Lorrie Carbone, Dr. Avraham Eisbruch, Karen Hammelef, Marcia Leonard, Sheila Morris, and Rivka Siden.

Part I

Key Resources for Finding Cancer Information

Chapter 1

Cancer 101(a): Cancer Essentials

M any people describe their experience with cancer as a journey. Librarians encounter people at different points in this journey. Healthy people may inquire about cancer prevention, early detection, or genetic testing. People who have a suspicion of a cancer diagnosis may seek information on various diagnostic procedures. People who already have a confirmed diagnosis want to learn about their specific cancer type and treatment, and may also benefit from information about support and coping for the patient and family. During treatment people ask for information on supportive care issues, side effects, and practical matters of cancer survivorship. A relapse may bring about questions about novel therapies and/or clinical trials. Patients with advanced disease and their caregivers may need information on palliative care, hospice, and end-of-life issues.

Despite the commonalities, every person's journey in the cancer world is unique. The cancer experience is shaped by the patient's value system, family status, social environment, spiritual beliefs, personality and financial position. Even people who are of the same sex and age, and have the identical diagnosis, will have a completely different experience. Similarly, the information needs and wants of people with cancer vary dramatically. Some people see information as a source of empowerment and see obtaining information as the first step in the healing process, while others are overwhelmed by it and avoid information seeking. The same person may exhibit different behaviors of information seeking and avoidance in different stages of the cancer journey. All information seeking behaviors are equality legitimate.

This chapter presents the basics for those seeking information, those helping others to seek it, and for professionals providing cancer information to the public. An understanding of the process of cancer and the medical terminology used to describe it is essential in order to engage the information seeker in an effective dialogue that will produce a clearly defined question or questions. A successful reference interview is primary to providing relevant information in patient-friendly language.

Key Concepts in Cancer

Cancer is a general term that includes more than a hundred different diseases that start when the normal life cycle of cells goes out of control. Normal cells grow, divide, and die. New cells are produced only to replace old cells or to repair injury. If this cycle gets damaged, cells lose the ability to control their growth rate. Damaged cells divide and multiply at an accelerated rate and produce more abnormal cells that will outlive normal ones. The excess cells form a lump that is called a tumor. Tumors can be either benign or malignant. Benign tumors may grow and damage neighboring structures, but they do not spread to other parts of the body. Cancer is the name given to malignant tumors that have the capability to spread beyond the organ in which they had started and invade and destroy other tissues or organs. Cancers that start in the blood or in blood-forming organs produce damaged cells that circulate in the bloodstream and prevent healthy blood cells and blood-forming organs from functioning properly.

Even though all cancers start because of damage to the cell life cycle, these diseases are very different from one another. Different cancers produce different symptoms, progress at different rates, and respond differently to treatment.

Cancer Prevention and Early Detection

The cancer process starts when deoxyribonucleic acid (DNA), a substance that holds the genetic information in every cell in the body, gets damaged and is not able to repair itself. This results in a mutation, a mistake in the genetic code of the DNA. If a mutation occurs in the area of the DNA that controls the cell's growth rate, the cell life cycle goes out of control and the cancer process starts as described above. Some people inherit damaged DNA that may cause them to develop cancer, but in many cases the DNA becomes damaged by exposure to a cancer-causing substance (carcinogen) such as smoking, radiation, or some chemicals. Many factors that increase a person's risk to develop a specific type of cancer have been identified. By eliminating risk factors from a person's environment or lifestyle, it is possible to prevent many cancers. The American Cancer Society estimates that more then 75% of cancer cases in the United States are caused by environmental or lifestyle factors. It is important to note, however, that DNA mutations may also occur sporadically, not just via inherited and environmental means. As people age, cells continue to replicate and the possibility for DNA damage increases. This is the reason why even people who do not carry DNA mutations, and make healthy lifestyle choices, may still develop cancer.

Screening tests that enable the early detection of some cancer types are available, and make it possible to discover these cancers in early stages, while they are still treatable and curable.

Nomenclature

Cancer tumors are classified by the body part in which they began and are named after the type of cell they originated from (Eyre, Lange, and Morris, 2002).

➤ Carcinomas are tumors that start in the epithelial tissue that is found in many organs throughout the body. Eighty to ninety percent of cancers are carcinomas, which are divided into two main subtypes:
  ➤ Adenocarcinomas, which start in gland cells that secrete a substance (for example, breast, stomach, and colon cancers are of the adenocarcinoma type)
  ➤ Squamous cell carcinomas, which start in the flat cell that covers the surface of the skin and other organs (for example, most tumors in the head and neck region are squamous cell carcinomas)

Carcinomas may occur in different parts of the body and are considered completely different disease entities in different organs.

➤ Sarcoma tumors originate in the body's connective tissue, such as muscle, fat, cartilage, or bone. Sarcomas' names have a prefix that identifies the tissue the tumor arose from. For example, osteosarcoma starts in the bone tissue, liposarcoma starts in the fatty tissue, and leiyomyosarcoma starts in the involuntary muscles.

➤ Lymphomas start in the lymphoid tissue located mainly in the lymph nodes, spleen, tonsils, and thymus. There are two types of lymphomas, Hodgkin's and non-Hodgkin's, which are further divided into other subtypes.

➤ Leukemias are cancers that originate in blood cells. Malignant blood cells circulate in the bloodstream; therefore, leukemia affects the entire body, and not just a specific body part like other cancers. Leukemias are divided into subtypes according to the specific blood cell they developed from.

➤ Multiple myeloma is a cancer that starts in the plasma cells of the bone marrow located in bones.

➤ Nervous system tumors are named after the specific type of cell they started from. For example, astrocytoma is a tumor that arises from astrocyte cells, and ependymoma is a tumor that arises from ependymal cells. Some nervous system tumors names include the location of the tumor, for example, a brain stem glioma or a spinal cord ependymoma.

➤ Germ cell tumors arise in the reproductive system cells in the testicles and ovaries.

➤ Some cancers are named for the person who first discovered or described them, such as Wilms' tumor, which is a childhood kidney tumor.

Metastasis

The body part in which the cancer started to develop is called the primary site. Many cancers are capable of spreading beyond the primary site to other locations in the body. This is a process called "metastasis." It starts when cancer cells break off from the primary tumor and travel through the bloodstream or the lymphatic system to other organs and tissues and create new tumors. These tumors are called "metastatic tumors" or "secondary tumors." It is important to understand that secondary tumors are not new cancers but rather a metastatic form of the primary cancer. The most common sites for metastatic tumors are the lungs, liver, bones, and brain.

Metastasis is a process that affects solid tumors only. Leukemia, multiple myeloma and lymphoma cells may be found in different parts of the body, but this type of spread is not referred to as metastasis.

Diagnosis

The diagnosis of cancer is a complex process of analyzing symptoms, findings from a physical examination, and results from diagnostic tests. Many cancers are difficult to diagnose because their symptoms resemble symptoms of other diseases and conditions. Three main types of diagnostic tests are used in cancer:

➤ Biopsy techniques are used to retrieve suspected cells so they can be examined under a microscope. The examination of tissue under a microscope is called histology or histopathology. The location of the suspected mass in the body determines the type of biopsy that will be used. It is possible to obtain tissue through a needle, an endoscope, or surgery.

➤ Imaging examinations detect changes in normal anatomy and physiology and reveal suspected masses or changes in normal tissue. A mass may be benign or malignant. The most common imaging tests are ultrasound, mammography computerized tomography (CT scans), magnetic resonance imaging (MRI), and positron emission tomography (PET).

➤ Blood tests may detect substances produced by cancer cells called "tumor markers." Blood tests may also reveal that a particular organ is not functioning normally. A cancer process in the organ may be the cause of these abnormalities. With the exception of leukemia, which can be diagnosed based on abnormal blood count results, tumor markers or abnormal blood tests do not provide a definitive cancer diagnosis; they just point to a suspicion. They are mostly used for follow-up during and after treatment.

A cancer diagnosis can be made only after a histologic examination confirms that the cells composing the suspected tissue are indeed malignant. Imaging exams and blood tests cannot serve as the only basis for a cancer diagnosis, except in very rare cases when a biopsy is not possible.

Tumor Grade

Tumor grade is a system used to classify cancer cells according to how abnormal they look under a microscope and how quickly the tumor is likely to grow and spread. Cancer cells that resemble normal cells are called "well differentiated" or "low grade." Cancer cells that look very different from the normal cells they originated from are called "undifferentiated," "poorly undifferentiated," or "high-grade." Higher-grade tumors grow and spread more quickly than lower-grade tumors. Different cancers have different grading systems.

Tumor Stage

Staging is a system used to describe the extent of the disease in the body. Most cancers are classified into five stages from 0 to IV. As a rule of thumb, stage 0 defines a tumor that is confined to the place where it started and has not spread to neighboring tissue. These are also called "carcinoma in situ." Stage 1 tumors are small and confined to the primary organ; stage 2 tumors are still confined to the primary site but may have a minimal invasion to the closest lymph nodes; stage 3 tumors have spread into regional lymph nodes, and stage 4 cancers are tumors that have spread to other organs. Each cancer has its own staging system with specific parameters for the tumor's size and spread. In layperson's literature the term *early stage* is used to describe stages 1 and 2 and the term *advanced cancers* is used for larger tumors that have invaded lymph nodes or other organs and tissues. The tumor stage is a primary factor in deciding on a treatment plan.

Cancer Treatment

Treatment for cancer is determined by the tumor's specific pathology and stage. Other factors that influence treatment decisions are the patient's overall health, age, lifestyle, family status, logistical considerations, and personal preferences. The four main treatment modalities for cancer are surgery, radiation therapy, chemotherapy, and biological therapies. Over 90% of cancer patients undergo surgery at some stage during the illness. Removing cancerous tissue holds the most potential for cure in most cancers. Some surgeries are performed for diagnostic purposes. Adding other treatment modalities to surgery may further improve disease control and survival. The term *adjuvant therapy* refers to adding chemotherapy, radiation therapy, or biological therapies after surgery. Neoadjuvant therapy is treatment given before surgery in order to shrink the tumor and hopefully decrease the extent of the surgery. Many cancer patients receive a combination of therapies, mostly in sequence but sometimes simultaneously. If the cancer is diagnosed after the disease has already spread to other organs, the goal of therapy changes from trying to achieve a cure or remission to trying to alleviate symptoms and improve quality of life. This is called palliative care.

Remission

The term *remission* is used to describe a period of time in which the cancer has responded to treatment and the signs and symptoms it produced have disappeared partially or completely. Remission periods can last weeks, months, or years. It is possible to achieve complete remissions that continue for years and may be considered cures.

Recurrence

If the disease recurs after remission, the patient and the doctor will have to make decisions about starting treatment again or moving on to palliative care. Chances of achieving a cure when the disease recurs are lower; therefore a recurrence is very difficult emotionally for the patient and family, sometimes more than the initial diagnosis.

The Cancer Reference Interview

A good reference interview is primary to the librarian's ability to provide relevant and useful information. In her article "The Consumer Health Reference Interview," Deborah A. Thomas, director of library and community information at the Greater Baltimore Medical Center, makes the point that the consumer health reference interview presents unique challenges and difficulties (Thomas, 2005). With health issues the initial question a patron asks is not always what the patron really wants to know. There are several barriers to the patron's ability to articulate questions precisely. The librarian should be aware of these pitfalls and take action to ensure that the true information need is uncovered.

1. Privacy: Issues of health are confidential, and some people need to ask for information about a medical condition they wish to keep private. If their

privacy is threatened they may not be able to express their concerns. Thomas suggests that the interview be conducted in an area that affords some privacy and is free from interruptions.

2. Emotional turmoil: A diagnosis of a life-threatening or chronic illness is a life-altering event that strongly impacts one's emotions—and one's mental and cognitive functioning ability. The diagnosis invokes strong emotions of fear, anger, and sadness that may bring about difficulties in expression and communication for the patient and family. Patrons may have difficulties just verbalizing the name of the disease they have, let alone articulating exactly what they need to know about it. In the realm of cancer there are a few topics that may be embarrassing for some patrons to verbalize such as sexual dysfunction, gastrointestinal side effects, and depression. It is important to be approachable and show empathy by maintaining eye contact and letting the patron speak without interruption.

3. Unfamiliarity with medical terminology: Laypeople have difficulties talking about complex medical topics. Sometimes people pronounce terms incorrectly or provide wrong spelling. Patients may also lack important details about their diagnosis either because they forgot the exact term their clinician used, or because they simply were not informed of the exact sub-type and stage of their cancer. To avoid miscommunication and misinterpretation, librarians should work with a dictionary or encyclopedia together with the patron to select the correct terms and discover the correct spelling. If it is still impossible to identify the topic, or a patron does not know specific details, then the patron should be sent back to his health care provider for clarification of the condition and spelling.

Another challenge in working with health consumers is providing information in a reading level suitable for the client's abilities. Cancer information comes in different levels, but the basic texts, which may be easily readable and understandable, lack details and depth. On the other hand, more detailed and comprehensive texts are at a higher reading level. At the Patient Education Resource Center (PERC) at the University of Michigan Comprehensive Cancer Center, we ask patrons if they want basic level information (sixth-grade level), advanced layperson information (tenth-grade reading level and above), or professional technical information.

Code of Conduct

Working with people affected by a life-threatening illness requires special consideration, sensitivity, and tact. The librarian should provide information only on topics requested by the patron and avoid providing negative information if it was not specifically asked for. On the other hand, if a patron is requesting information that may be negative (for example, prognosis or survival rates of a hard-to-treat cancer), the librarian should respond to the question asked without making judgment about how the information will impact the patron. While empathy and understanding are primary to facilitate a successful interaction, the librarian should remain professional and adhere to the Medical Library Association's policy of providing health information to the public. The librarian's role is to help a patron formulate the question and provide access to a range of authoritative materials. Librarians should never give advice, suggest diagnosis, or recommend particular clinicians. It is not appropriate to share personal anecdotes concerning someone else's health situation. Librarians should not engage in active teaching and should not attempt to explain a condition. Patrons should be guided to other sources, such as dictionaries or encyclopedias, to explain terminology.

Librarians should explain to patrons, verbally and through disclaimers, that every patient has a unique situation with a different set of circumstances. Even if the information found is accurate and current, it may not be applicable to a specific patient. In order to evaluate how the information applies to one's specific situation, the patron must consult with a health care provider. One of the goals of providing health information to the public is the promotion of a good clinician-patient relationship. Librarians should take every opportunity to encourage this dialogue and remind patrons to seek their physician's input to the information provided.

Cancer-Specific Talking Points

In the context of cancer it is especially challenging to find out the exact cancer type the patron is inquiring about. Quite often people ask for information about a cancer in a specific organ such as "lung cancer" but do not provide a subtype, either because they were not given this information or because they just do not think it is important. Since subtypes may be completely different disease entities even in the same organ, it is important to try to find out the exact medical name of the cancer. If that is not possible, the librarian should provide general information on all possible subtypes in the organ. On the other hand, patrons may ask for information on a cancer cell type, such as adenocarcinoma, but not provide the tumor location in the body. Since adenocarcinomas may appear in many body parts, and are considered completely different disease entities in different organs, it would be impossible to give any information in response to this question. The patrons should be referred back to their health care provider to find out the exact cancer type and location. The key point here is that librarians do not want to give people information about a cancer they do not have.

Following are several questions a librarian can ask in order to determine the exact cancer type the patron is inquiring about:

1. What is the medical name of this disease?

    Oftentimes this would be the cancer subtype. If the patron does not know this information, the librarian may make suggestions using an authoritative reference source. Sometimes just hearing the name again may jog the patron's memory.

2. Where is the tumor located in the body (if not provided before)?

3. Do you know the stage?

    Since cancer treatment is determined by its stage, this information is useful for this type of question. If the stage is not known, the librarian should provide information on all stages.

4. Is the patient an adult or a child?

    The same cancers behave differently in adults and children. For example, information on acute lymphoblastic leukemia (ALL) in children is not relevant for adults with the same disease.

Keep in mind that many people may start looking for information before they have a confirmed diagnosis of cancer. They may start their search before they get results of a biopsy, which may turn out to be benign. In this case the librarian should provide very basic information and add a warning that it may not be relevant to the patron's situation. It is best if the patron can return after a diagnosis has been confirmed.

Another potential pitfall that may lead to a mistake is the confusion that patients have when cancer metastasizes. As explained above, many cancers metastasize to different organs. For example, breast cancer may metastasize to the bones, liver, bones, or brain. If a metastatic tumor is discovered in the bones, the disease is considered a metastatic form of breast cancer and not primary bone cancer. Librarians should pay attention especially when asked for information about brain, bone, liver, or lung cancer, since these are the organs to which most other cancers metastasize. In fact, the majority of bone, brain, lung, and liver tumors discovered in the United States are secondary and not primary tumors. It is a good idea to add the question "Did the cancer start in the liver/lung/brain/bones?" whenever a librarian is asked about one of these four diagnoses.

The Next Steps

Following is an annotated list of general cancer information sources arranged by format, from print to electronic materials. These quality resources offer authoritative information that covers the entire spectrum of cancer issues and topics, and may be consulted to answer any question about cancer.

Because these primary resources cover the topic in its entirety, they may not always be sufficient to answer all questions. In order to provide more comprehensive, detailed information, the reader should consult the index and look up a more specific topic. Parts II and III of the book list information sources that center around specific cancer types and topics. Each topic includes an introduction followed by a list of information sources. A discussion of key concepts in childhood cancer and an annotated list of primary information resources is presented in Chapter 2 beginning on page 23.

Chapter 3 of the book (page 41) suggests additional resources that provide advanced cancer information in patient-friendly language. Questions regarding rare cancer types, complex medical issues, and new research developments may be best answered utilizing the resources in this chapter.

Primary Print and Electronic Information Sources

Dictionaries

➤ Altman, Roberta, and Michael Sarg. 2006. *The Cancer Dictionary*. Rev. ed. New York: Facts on File.
This dictionary includes more than 2,500 definitions covering individual cancers, diagnostic tests, symptoms, surgeries, side effects, treatment methods, risk factors, carcinogens, acronyms, and abbreviations. The definitions are comprehensive, and some are cyclopedic in scope. Special features include photographs, illustrations, a pronunciation guide, a subject index, and directories of national organizations, comprehensive cancer centers, and clinical cancer centers arranged by state. Related terms are linked by cross- and see references.
➤ Laughlin, Edward H. 2002. *Coming to Terms with Cancer: A Glossary of Cancer-Related Terms*. Atlanta: American Cancer Society.
The ACS's comprehensive glossary consists of over a thousand technical-medical cancer terms listed in alphabetical order and explained in non-medical language. The terms include abbreviations, acronyms, drugs and medications as well as illustrations to explain anatomy. In addition to the glossary this book includes a highlights section with short overviews of selected cancers. The appendix provides cancer detection guidelines and a resource list.
➤ National Cancer Institute. *Dictionary of Cancer Terms*. Access at: www.cancer.gov

The NCI's dictionary contains more than 4,000 terms related to cancer and medicine. The simple search interface enables searching entries that start with a certain word or entries that contain a certain word. If unsure of spelling, it is possible to type in a few letters and the system will suggest all terms that start with the letters typed. It is also possible to browse by clicking on a letter in the alphabet. The definitions are very short, but the comprehensive coverage is extremely useful. This is the recommended dictionary to use with this book.

Encyclopedias

➤ Longe, Jacqueline L. 2005. *The Gale Encyclopedia of Cancer: A Guide to Cancer and Its Treatments*. 2nd ed. Jacqueline L. Longe, project ed. Detroit: Thomson/Gale.

This two-volume encyclopedia includes approximately 500 detailed entries that provide in-depth coverage of 120 cancer types, diagnostic procedures, cancer drugs, and traditional and alternative treatments. Entries range from 500 to 4,000 words, and many include short glossaries of key terms and questions to ask the doctor. Features comprise anatomical illustrations of major body systems affected by cancer, a glossary of medical terms, an extensive cross-referenced subject index, and 200 full-color illustrations, photos, and tables. In addition the set includes A–Z listings of cancer centers, national support groups, government agencies, and research groups.

➤ Turkington, Carol, and William LiPera. 2005. *The Encyclopedia of Cancer*. New York: Facts on File.

This A–Z reference tool includes more than 400 entries covering cancer types, treatments, and supportive care. The entries serve as thorough introductions to the topics explaining in detail national and global statistics, gender differences, and promising research. Appendixes provide an extensive list of associations arranged by topic, a list of comprehensive and clinical cancer centers, and a list of carcinogens. This text does not include photographs or illustrations. Some libraries may access this book free through NetLibrary.

Periodicals

➤ *Coping with Cancer* (ISSN 1043-8637).

An easy-to-read publication with many articles that focus on the psychosocial issues of cancer written by survivors and mental health specialists. Each issue features the story of a famous person who is a cancer survivor. Reputable cancer specialists write the articles that focus on medical and

symptom-management issues. This bimonthly publication is not indexed or included in any of the full-text databases. It is distributed to patients in doctors' offices and through subscriptions. Information on subscriptions may be found on the Web site at: www.copingmag.com
➤ *CURE: Cancer Updates, Research & Education* (ISSN 1534-7664).
This is a beautifully produced quarterly magazine that combines the science and humanity of cancer for those who have to deal with it on a daily basis. CURE provides scientific information in easy-to-understand language with equally understandable illustrations. The editor in chief, Vinay K. Jain, M.D., is an oncologist, and the magazine has a distinguished editorial board of physicians, nurses, and quality-of-life specialists. The complete content is archived, and the current issue is available free online at: www.curetoday.org. Free subscriptions are available through the Web site. CURE is indexed in CINHAL.
➤ *Women & Cancer* (ISSN 1557-5780).
Women & Cancer is a quarterly magazine developed specifically for women impacted by a cancer diagnosis. It aims to educate women about the effective management of cancer prevention and treatment and inform readers about wellness issues, news about medical advances, and legislative issues. Each issue presents inspiring stories of families and survivors, inside information about accessing the complicated medical system, and frequently updated resource listings for women affected by cancer. The editor-in-chief and medical editor are both physicians. Some full-text articles and subscriptions are available through the Web site: www.cancerconsultants.com

Reference Books

➤ Dollinger, Malin, et al. 2002. *Everyone's Guide to Cancer Therapy: How Cancer Is Diagnosed, Treated, and Managed Day to Day*. 4th ed. Kansas City, MO: Andrews & McMeel.
This is a thick volume of over 800 pages covering diagnosis, treatment, supportive care, quality-of-life issues, and cancer advances. Overviews of 51 specific cancer types also are included. The text provides explanations of the theories behind cancer research and treatment, as well as practical information written in easy-to-understand language with instructive illustrations. The authors address issues such as getting second opinions and cancer information seeking on the Internet. The editors are well-known cancer researchers and clinicians assisted by a 140-member board of medical advisers and contributing authors who are top specialists in all fields of cancer research and treatment.
➤ Eyre, Harmon J., et al. 2002. *Informed Decisions: The Complete Book of Cancer Diagnosis, Treatment, and Recovery*. 2nd ed. Atlanta: American Cancer Society.

The ACS offers this book with the goal of helping patients and families make informed decisions. The clear and organized text starts with a basic explanation of what cancer is, and then moves on to cover prevention and early detection, diagnosis, treatment, and living with cancer. The last part of the book, called "The Encyclopedia of Common and Uncommon Cancers," includes short overviews of specific cancers. This thick volume is made accessible and user friendly by the smart use of graphical elements such as icons and textboxes that contain case histories, checklists, dos and don'ts, tips and advice, and questions to ask the doctor.

➤ Morra, Marion E., and Eve Potts. 2003. *Choices.* 4th ed. New York: HarperCollins.

This book aims to be a complete sourcebook for cancer information, from diagnosis to recovery. The entire 1,000-page text is written in an easy-to-read question-and-answer format and has chapters focusing on topics such as choosing your doctor and hospital, searching the Web and cancer controversies. Other chapters concentrate on specific cancers and childhood cancers. The book includes many tables and illustrations and lists summarizing key points. The last chapter, titled "Where to Get Help," presents an extensive resource list.

➤ Sekeres, Mikkael, and Theodore A. Stern. 2004. *Facing Cancer: A Complete Guide for People with Cancer, Their Families, and Caregivers.* New York: McGraw-Hill.

This book was edited by a psychiatrist and an oncologist and has 33 chapters focusing on scientific and psychosocial aspects of cancer and written by specialists. The high reading level, small print, and scientific approach make this book suitable only for the sophisticated user looking for in-depth and comprehensive information on topics not covered by other, more accessible reference books. Chapters cover the meaning of cancer to children, stress reactions in caregivers, the use of medications to alter mood and behavior, the epidemiology of cancer, and more.

Guidebooks

➤ Bernay, Toni, and Saar Porrath. 2006. *When It's Cancer: The 10 Essential Steps to Follow After Your Diagnosis.* Emmaus, PA: Rodale; Distributed to the trade by Holtzbrinck Publishers.

This book was authored by a psychologist whose husband was an oncologist who died from leukemia. It summarizes the couple's strategy and vision of coping with cancer, which advocates patients being proactive about their treatment and care. The book includes self-assessments, worksheets, and checklists for tracing information to make sound, well-reasoned decisions.

➤ Coleman, C. Norman. 2006. *Understanding Cancer: A Patient's Guide to Diagnosis, Prognosis, and Treatment.* 2nd ed. Baltimore: Johns Hopkins University Press.

A professor of radiation oncology from Harvard Medical School guides patients through the decision-making process right after diagnosis and through the illness. Describing and explaining the various diagnostic tests and treatment options available, the book's purpose is to help patients evaluate risks and benefits and make decisions together with their doctors. Checklists and case studies help to illustrate how cancer patients can play an active role in determining their own treatment plan.

➤ Harpham, Wendy Schlessel. 2003. *Diagnosis, Cancer: Your Guide to the First Months of Healthy Survivorship.* Exp. and updated ed. New York: Norton.

The author, a physician and a cancer survivor, offers advice and guidance for newly diagnosed patients. The chapters focus on understanding the diagnosis, making the best treatment decisions, managing practical problems, and using the medical system, as well as information on the emotional adjustment and insights for healthy survivorship. Useful appendixes include tips for being an effective patient, resources for newly diagnosed patients, and explanations of commonly ordered tests.

➤ Silver, J. K. 2006. *After Cancer Treatment: Heal Faster, Better, Stronger.* Baltimore: Johns Hopkins Univ. Press.

This is a guidebook for people who completed cancer treatment. The author is a psychiatrist who directs a cancer support program and a breast cancer survivor herself. This book outlines her plan for a post-cancer life, addressing medical and mental issues of survivorship, including nutrition, exercise, fatigue, pain, spirituality, and emotional well-being. The author provides a detailed and specific health plan that helps redefine life after cancer treatment.

➤ Teeley, Peter, and Philip Bashe. 2005. *The Complete Cancer Survival Guide: The Most Comprehensive, Up-to-Date Guide for Patients and Their Families; With Advice from Dozens of Leading Cancer Specialists at More than 30 Major Cancer Centers.* Rev. and updated ed. New York: Broadway Books.

This comprehensive book offers detailed guidance based on interviews with cancer specialists from top cancer centers. The text covers the 25 most common forms of cancer, including diagnosis and staging, what to expect during treatment, and how to take control of symptoms, side effects, and complications. Suggestions on coping with the emotional impact of cancer; getting help from family, friends, and healthcare professionals; handling insurance; finances; and employment issues also are included. Graphical elements such as tables, lists, illustrations, and sidebars help readers navigate through the thousand-page volume.

Audiovisual Materials

➤ Johnson, Bill, et al. 2004. *Cancer Story*. Lebanon, NH; Sherborn, MA: Dartmouth-Hitchcock Medical Center; Aquarius Health Care Videos (dist.)

Cancer Story is a PBS television series of four one-hour programs presenting cancer in understandable layperson's terms. Each installment focuses on a different facet of the topic, such as an explanation of what cancer is, voices of people living with cancer, new directions in cancer research, and prevention and screening. Portions of the programs can be viewed online at www.cancerstory.org. Available in DVD and VHS.

Web Resources

Web Sites of Nonprofit National Organizations

➤ American Cancer Society. Access at: www.cancer.org

This comprehensive site offers information for patients undergoing treatment, survivors after treatment, caregivers, health-information seekers, the media, and people interested in getting involved with cancer advocacy. The overviews and detailed guides for specific cancer types are very useful for newly diagnosed patients and people during treatment. The detailed guides are written in a higher reading level than the overviews and can be printed as complete booklets or by section. In addition, the site offers detailed information about treatment, supportive care, prevention, and early detection. The ACS News Cancer includes stories about new developments in cancer research and lay-language summaries of articles published in the scientific medical literature. This site also provides an interactive section for patients, a drug database, and cancer statistics.

➤ National Cancer Institute. Access at: www.cancer.gov

At the core of this site is the Physician Data Query (PDQ®) database, which contains peer-reviewed summaries on cancer treatment, screening, prevention, genetics, complementary and alternative medicine, and supportive care. A registry of cancer clinical trials from around the world and directories of physicians, professionals, and organizations that provide cancer care also are part of the PDQ® database. Each PDQ® summary is presented in a health-professional version and a patient version and updated monthly. The site also includes the full-text of NCI publications and the *NCI Dictionary of Cancer Terms*, which contains more than 4,000 terms related to cancer and medicine explained in short, lay-language definitions. This dictionary is the recommended glossary to accompany this book.

➤ People Living with Cancer. Access at: www.plwc.org
The American Society of Clinical Oncology (ASCO) provides this patient information site that includes overviews on more than 85 types of cancer. Of special interest are the patient-friendly versions of ASCO's publications and recommendations for physicians, reports and summaries about research advances, and news from oncology conferences. Other features include a find-an-oncologist database, virtual lectures and presentations, and a medical illustrations gallery.

From Canada:

➤ Canadian Cancer Society. Access at: www.cancer.ca
The Canadian Cancer Society site contains a searchable database of local support services for cancer patients and families, as well as online versions of the Canadian Cancer Society publications. The *Canadian Cancer Encyclopedia (CCE)* is a comprehensive database of cancer information that covers a wide range of topics, including risk reduction, screening, diagnosis, treatment, and supportive care. This is a bilingual site in English and French. It includes a few publications in Chinese, Farsi, and Punjabi and links to other sites providing cancer information in languages other than English.

From the United Kingdom:

➤ Cancer BACKUP. Access at: www.cancerbackup.org.uk/Home
The British cancer information service offers news and data on specific cancer types and topics. Some of the terms, spelling, and treatment information may differ from what is used in the United States and other countries. The site is well organized, and the question-and-answer database is especially useful for librarians seeking answers to specific questions and situations. Each cancer topic has a Q&A section, and the database can be searched by keyword. The answers are written by cancer nurses and reviewed by specialists.

Commercial Sites

While it is possible to find quality, authoritative, and useful content on commercial sites, it is important to evaluate the information according to the guidelines in the "Evaluation Checklist..." section on page 20. Special attention should be given to sponsorship and advertising appearing onsite to ensure that the information is not biased.

The following commercial sites provide information written or reviewed by physicians or licensed health professionals:

➤ Cancersource.com
➤ Cancerconsultants.com
➤ Cancereducation.com

The unique content of this site are medclips, streaming video and audio educational programs addressing topics of interest to patients and their families and friends. Free registration is required.

➤ OncologyChannel.com

Cancer Listservs and E-mail Support Groups

Many cancer patients benefit from the easy accessibility and availability of online support groups. Information shared on these listservs varies from tips for coping with side effects and practical problems, to treatment and research news, alternative therapies, and more. Since the information is provided by individuals, mostly laypeople, the quality and reliability of information shared on listservs are questionable. Users should be made aware of the need to carefully evaluate the information and consult with their clinician before utilizing treatment suggestions obtained from listservs. That said, online support groups can be a valuable source of support for cancer patients and families who understand the reliability issues and are able to evaluate the information according to the guidelines on page 20.

➤ The Association of Cancer Online Resources (ACOR) hosts hundreds of disease-specific and topic-specific cancer listservs. The lists' content is archived, searchable, and browsable. To locate a specific list go to: www.acor.org and click on the link to "Mailing Lists."

Blogs

Thousands of blogs about cancer can be found on the Internet. Most of them are written by cancer survivors describing their experiences with the disease and treatment. Since nearly all of the blogs are written by laypeople and not by credentialed health professionals, facts may sometimes be erroneous, and the information biased. Blogs are not authoritative information sources about cancer.

Cancer Support and Advocacy Organizations

Cancer support and advocacy organizations publish patient education materials that may be very valuable for patients and families. It is always a good idea for patients to contact the relevant organization and ask for a new patient information packet. The packet may include brochures, list of physicians specializing in the particular cancer type, resource lists, patient support services, and information about educational and other events. In this book the sections that list information sources for particular cancer types include the contact information for relevant organizations.

Evaluation Checklist for Health Information on the Internet

This checklist is useful for quick evaluation of health Web sites. It includes three basic steps: check source, check accuracy, and check currency.

Step One: Check Source

➤ Check the site's URL (address): .gov sites are provided by government agencies and reflect the official opinion of the government. .edu sites are mostly from educational institutions. Information from reputable, well-known universities can be trusted. .edu sites from lesser-known institutions, as well as .org and .com sites, should be evaluated further by reading the "About us" or "Who are we?" section of the site. A reputable site should include this section; sites that do not should be avoided.

➤ Look for sites that offer information that was written or reviewed by credentialed health professionals. Sites of patient advocacy organizations should post a list of individuals serving on their medical advisory board (sometimes called "medical review board"). Check this listing to ensure that these are credentialed, reputable medical professionals. Avoid sites that offer information written by non-professionals or do not post a list of reputable experts reviewing the content.

➤ Identify the true motivation of the information provider and avoid biased sites. The information on sites that sell medical products, supplements, or drugs is likely to be biased, with the main purpose being promoting sales, not educating the public. Bias may also be present in Web sites that promote a political agenda.

➤ Be sure to check the original source of information. Many health and medical Web sites post information collected from other Web sites or sources.

If the source is determined to be reliable, continue to check the accuracy and currency as follows:

Step Two: Check Accuracy

➤ Look for sites that substantiate the information they provide with references to peer-reviewed, scientific literature. References to newspaper articles and the popular media are not authoritative.

➤ Avoid sites that offer testimonials and case studies. These are used when information cannot be validated by scientific research. Avoid sites that use emotional tone and include promises that sound too good to be true.

Step Three: Check Currency

➤ Check the date the information was last revised. Reliable Web sites are reviewed and updated frequently and regularly.

➤ In most cases, medical information that has been posted on the World Wide Web for longer than three years is outdated. Information on support, coping, and practical issues may be current for a longer period of time. Avoid sites that do not clearly display a revision or review date.

The National Cancer Institute's document "How to Evaluate Health Information on the Internet: Questions and Answers" (access at: www.cancer. gov/cancertopics/factsheet/Information/internet) is a useful handout for explaining the evaluation principles to library patrons. An audiovisual tutorial is available on the Medlineplus.gov site at: www.nlm.nih.gov/medlineplus/ webeval/webeval.html

Chapter 2

Cancer 101(b): Childhood Cancer Essentials

Key Concepts in Childhood Cancer

The National Cancer Institute estimates approximately 12,400 cancer diagnoses among children under the age of 20 in the United States per year. New developments in treatment and supportive care have greatly improved the five-year survival rates from 32% in the 1960s to 79% in 2001. Death rates have dramatically declined since the 1970s, but cancer still remains a major cause of death in children younger than 15, second only to accidents. It is estimated that more than 250,000 survivors of childhood cancer live in the United States.

Cancer behaves differently in children than in adults. The foremost difference is that cancer in children responds better to treatment and therefore cure rates are higher. Children can get cancer in the same parts of the body as adults do, but histologically many childhood cancer types differ from those of adults. Another difference between adult and childhood cancers is that anticancer treatment may have implications for the growth and development of children; sometimes the child's stage of growth is a determining factor in making treatment decisions. Experts observe that children are more resilient and can tolerate more aggressive therapy than adults who suffer from other health conditions that make treatment more difficult to endure.

Unlike many adult cancers, childhood cancers are not a result of lifestyle habits. A small number of childhood cancers are caused by inherited genetic mutations or as a result of exposure to carcinogenic materials in the environment. Causes of the great majority of childhood cancer are not known, and most cases cannot be linked to a specific risk factor.

The American Cancer Society recommends that children with cancer be treated in a specialized childhood cancer center that is a member of the Children's Oncology Group and affiliated with a university or a children's hospital. These centers have a multidisciplinary team of experts who are knowledgeable about the special needs of children and adolescents, committed to clinical care as well as research, and versed in the differences between adult and childhood cancers. The teams include pediatric oncologists, pediatric surgeons, radiation oncologists, and pediatric oncology nurses and nurse practitioners. In addition to these medical specialists the team also includes psychologists, social workers, nutritionists, and rehabilitation and physical therapists as well as educators who can support and educate the entire family. Child life specialists are essential members of the team and utilize a variety of therapeutic interventions to reduce the stress and anxiety associated with medical experiences. Child life specialists engage children in medical play, provide education opportunities for age-appropriate activities, enhance coping skills, and prepare and support children during medical tests and procedures. The goal is to foster understanding, comfort, and developmental progress while minimizing psychological trauma for the child and his or her siblings and parents.

The differences between adult and childhood cancer explain why information on the adult forms of cancer is not relevant to children. In addition to the differences in the diseases, outlook, and treatment, children with cancer and their families face unique psychosocial issues. Long periods of hospitalizations and vulnerability to infections cause kids and teens to miss many days of school as well as peer-activities and events. As a result, normal socialization and development may be negatively impacted. Educational and academic support during treatment is a major challenge. Parents need to become knowledgeable about children's educational rights so they can partner with school personnel in establishing plans for the child's unique needs and continued progress. Hair loss affects the child's perception of body image and self-esteem and may contribute to feelings of "being different," withdrawal, and depression. Relationships within the family may change along with relationships with extended family members and friends. Parents may need to alter work schedules, and as a result the family's income may suffer.

Major topics of interest to parents include how to explain the diagnosis and treatment to children with cancer and their siblings, advocating for the child within the medical environment and home community, and supporting the child's academic progress. Information is also available on parenting the ill child and meeting the needs of siblings. Children with cancer and their siblings also are information seekers who may benefit from learning about the illness, treatment methods, emotional coping, and socializing with peers during the illness. The key point in providing information to children with cancer and their siblings is to provide age-appropriate information in understandable language. The developmental level of children gives insight as to how they comprehend information and cope with illness. As children grow and mature, they require more detailed information and the topics that are of interest to them evolve and change. Some information sources on childhood cancer present similar content addressed separately to parents, children with cancer, and siblings in various age groups.

Listed below are the primary information sources on childhood cancer, appropriate for parents and caregivers of children with cancer. Information sources for children with cancer and their siblings are listed according to age starting on page 29.

Sections on specific types of childhood cancers are presented in Chapter 5 of this book, starting on page 159. Each type includes an introduction to the topic and an annotated list of information sources discussing the specific childhood cancer type. A section on childhood cancer survivors begins on page 36.

Primary Print and Electronic Information Sources

Dictionaries and Encyclopedias

The resources listed in the general cancer information sources on page 12 cover childhood cancer terms and topics.

Brochures, Booklets, and Other Short Print Publications

➤ Leukemia and Lymphoma Society. *Learning and Living with Cancer.*
  Written for parents of a child returning to school during or after cancer treatment, this booklet explains the challenges children with cancer may face at school and how to help them achieve their education potential. It explains the laws that protect children's educational needs and lists specific ways that schools can help. Access at: www.leukemia-lymphoma.org
➤ National Cancer Institute. *Young People with Cancer: A Handbook for Parents.*
  This publication discusses the most common types of childhood cancer, treatments, and side effects as well as issues that may arise when a child is diagnosed with cancer. It offers medical information and practical tips gathered from parents. Access at: https://cissecure.nci.nih.gov/ncipubs/
➤ National Childhood Cancer Foundation. *The Children's Oncology Group (COG) Family Handbook.*
  This 80-page handbook was written by nurses, doctors, and other childhood cancer professionals. The information is relevant to all types of childhood cancer and covers medical and psychosocial issues. The publication includes illustrations and has several areas that can be customized for a specific child. To download, access: www.curesearch.org.

➤ National Children's Cancer Society. *The Mountain You've Climbed: A Parent's Guide to Childhood Cancer Survivorship.*
This guide is designed to answer parent's questions regarding childhood cancer and offer suggestions on how to integrate the cancer experience into all areas of the family's life. It addresses issues beginning from the time of diagnosis through the completion of treatment and beyond. Order at: http://nationalchildrenscancersociety.com

Books

➤ Keene, Nancy. 2003. *Educating the Child with Cancer: A Guide for Parents and Teachers.* Kensington, MD: Candlelighters Childhood Cancer Foundation. This book was developed with the intent of promoting understanding and communication between parents, educators, and medical professionals so that together they can provide an appropriate education for children who have been treated for cancer. Learning issues that face children treated for cancer from infancy through adulthood are covered in depth, with some chapters written by experts and others by parents. Topics include gaining access to special education services, helping siblings in the classroom, physical activity in school, cognitive late effects, and grief in the classroom. Each chapter ends with a list of key points.

➤ Carroll, William L., and Jessica B. Reisman. 2005. *100 Questions and Answers about Your Child's Cancer.* Sudbury, MA: Jones and Bartlett. This book presents practical answers to questions about childhood cancer, treatment options, and post-treatment quality-of-life and coping strategies for both patients and parents. Two childhood cancer experts authored this book and incorporated comments from parents of children with cancer. The reviews of each cancer type are very short, but the book provides detailed information about diagnostic tests, supportive-care issues and side effects, and complications of treatment that are common to all children treated for cancer. The text is easy to read, and definitions for key terms are provided on the sidebar.

➤ Janes-Hodder, Honna, and Nancy Keene. 2002. *Childhood Cancer: A Parent's Guide to Solid Tumor Cancers.* 2nd ed. Sebastopol, CA: O'Reilly. This book provides detailed overviews of several childhood cancer types, but some of the chapters are relevant to all children with cancer. The authors offer practical advice on how to cope with procedures, hospitalization, family and friends, school, social and financial issues, communications, feelings, and, if treatment is not successful, grief and bereavement. The text includes stories from children and parents who have experienced childhood cancer. Appendixes include blood counts and what they mean and an extensive resource list.

➤ Woznick, Leigh A., and Carol D. Goodheart. 2002. *Living with Childhood Cancer: A Practical Guide to Help Parents Cope*. Washington, DC: American Psychological Assn.

The focus of this book is the psychological impact of childhood cancer. It provides guidance and advice to parents on managing the emotional and practical challenges of the disease and treatment. The book describes how adults, children, teenagers, and families may cope with illness and stress and offers strategies for successful coping. Topics include communication, stress, trauma, pain, side effects, encouraging child development, building self-esteem, dying and grieving, and long-term survivorship. Specific information is provided for different age groups and different types of families. The authors are a psychologist and her daughter, who is the mother of a child with cancer.

Web Resources

Sites Focusing on Childhood Cancer

➤ Candlelighters Childhood Cancer Foundation. Access at: www.candle lighters.org

The Candlelighters Childhood Cancer Foundation provides support, education, and advocacy for children and adolescents with cancer, survivors of childhood/adolescent cancer, their families, and the professionals who care for them. The site includes information about services to patients and families and a comprehensive annotated list of links to other sites, organizations, and resources arranged by topic.

➤ CureSearch. Access at: www.curesearch.org

The Children's Oncology Group and the National Childhood Cancer Foundation provide this comprehensive site about childhood cancer. It has separate sections for parents/families and for patients in different age groups: preschool, ages 5–10, 10–14, and 14–22. The site is divided into four major sections: newly diagnosed, in treatment, end of treatment, and after treatment. Topics covered include childhood cancer types, diagnostic tests, treatment methods, living with cancer, school and friends, the family, transition after treatment, long-term survivorship, and end of life. The site also includes a clinical-trials matching service, discussion boards, and a resource directory for national and local support groups and services.

➤ Penn State Hershey Medical Center. *Home Care Guide*. Access at: www. hmc.psu.edu/hematology/homeguide/

Nurses and physicians from the children's hematology/oncology team at Penn State Hershey Medical Center developed this guide for caregivers of children with childhood cancer. The guide provides treatment plans for a variety of supportive-care and psychosocial issues that may occur while a child is undergoing treatment. Each plan gives caregivers the information they need in order to solve problems, including understanding the problem, when to get professional help, what caregivers can do on their own, possible obstacles, and how to carry out and adjust the plan.

Detailed Sections in General Cancer Sites

➤ American Cancer Society. Access at: www.cancer.org

A section called Children and Cancer: Information and Resources (links from the Patients, Families and Friends page) has overviews and detailed guides for specific childhood cancer types that are very useful for parents of newly diagnosed children and those undergoing treatment. The detailed guides are written in a higher reading level than the overviews and may be printed as complete booklets, or by section. In addition this section includes detailed overviews discussing supportive care and coping issues such as: dealing with the diagnosis, insurance and financial issues, school re-entry and finding support sources.

➤ National Cancer Institute. Access at: www.cancer.gov

At the core of this site is the Physician Data Query (PDQ®) database, which contains peer-reviewed summaries of treatment for all cancer types, including childhood cancers. A registry of cancer clinical trials from around the world and directories of physicians, professionals, and organizations that provide cancer care also are part of the PDQ® database. Each PDQ® summary is presented in a health-professional version and a patient version and updated monthly. The site also includes the full-text of NCI publications and the *NCI Dictionary of Cancer Terms*, which contains more than 4,000 terms related to cancer and medicine explained in short lay-language definitions. This dictionary is the recommended glossary to accompany this book.

➤ National Coalition for Cancer Survivorship. Palliative Care and Symptom Management. Access at: www.canceradvocacy.org/resources/essential and click on "Care for Children"

This section has information about some of the most common side effects children experience when being treated for cancer. Each topic has information about symptoms, prevention, treatment, and questions to ask your health care team.

➤ People Living with Cancer. Access at: www.plwc.org
The American Society of Clinical Oncology (ASCO) hosts this patient information site that provides overviews of many cancer types, including childhood cancer. Other features of the site, such as news about research advances,
the find-an-oncologist database, the medical illustrations gallery, and drug
information resources, may be helpful to parents of children with cancer.

From Canada

➤ Canadian Cancer Society. Access at: www.cancer.ca
The Canadian Cancer Society site contains a searchable database of local
support services for cancer patients and families, as well as online versions of the Canadian Cancer Society publications in English, French, and
other languages. The section called "When Your Child Has Cancer" provides parents with practical advice on telling their children about their
cancer, nutrition for children with cancer, maintaining communication,
and supporting children through illness.

From the United Kingdom

➤ Cancer BACKUP. Access at: www.cancerbackup.org.uk/Home
The British cancer information service site has a section called "Children's
Cancers Information Centre" that links to overviews of specific childhood
cancers and information on treatment and living with cancer. The section
"Teen Info on Cancer" presents cancer information written for teenagers.
Some of the terms, spelling, and treatment data may differ from what is
used in the United States and other countries.

Patient-Support Organizations

➤ Candlelighters. Access at: www.candlelighters.org
Phone: 800-366-2223
➤ The National Children's Cancer Society. Access at http://nationalchildrens
cancersociety.com
Phone: 800-5-FAMILY

Resources for Children with Cancer

Brochures, Booklets, and Other Short Print Publications

➤ American Cancer Society. *What Happened to You, Happened to Me.*
Young people with cancer talk candidly about their feelings concerning
the hospital, treatment, side effects, school, and ways their illness has

changed their lives. For teenagers. To order, contact your local American Cancer Society or access at: www.cancer.org.

Books

For All Diagnoses (list arranged by age)

➤ Homer, Melodie, and Andy Lendway. 1999. *Chemo Crusader and the Cancer Fighting Crew*. Marlton, NJ: PEPCO.
This picture book for very young children describes chemotherapy as a team of superheroes fighting bad cancer cells. The text touches on chemotherapy side effects and includes colorful illustrations of chemotherapy infusion equipment, and a central line. For ages three to six.
➤ Klett, Amy, and David Klett. 2002. *The Amazing Hannah: Look at Everything I Can Do!* Kensington, MD: Candlelighters Childhood Cancer Foundation.
Appropriate for children ages one to five, the simple text is accompanied by photographs of a young girl with cancer as she goes though her day's routine. The photos show her at the doctor's office and the hospital room, getting her central line cleaned, playing with her baby sister, and taking medicine by mouth. Parents of children with cancer may obtain a free copy from the foundation at: www.candlelighters.org.
➤ Wilde, Daxton, and Sherry Wilde. 2006. *I'm a Superhero*. Salt Lake City, UT: Gibbs Smith.
The story chronicles the experiences of a four-year-old boy undergoing chemotherapy and radiation treatments for a brain tumor. The central character is a superhero fighting "a bad guy named Cancer" with the help of "Captain Chemo." For children ages two to five.
➤ Krisher, Trudy, and Nadine Bernard Westcott. 1992. *Kathy's Hats: A Story of Hope*. Morton Grove, IL: Albert Whitman.
Told in the first person by an elementary school–age girl, this story focuses on the girl's experiences with chemotherapy and especially with the ways she coped with losing her hair. For children ages four to eight.
➤ Gordon, Melanie Apel. 1999. *Let's Talk about When Kids Have Cancer*. New York: PowerKids Press.
The book discusses what cancer is, its treatment and side effects, and how it affects the lives of patients and their families. Includes color photographs. For children ages four to eight.
➤ Cranston, Lynda. 2001. *You and Your Cancer: A Child's Guide*. Lewiston, NY: BC Decker.
Written for children with cancer, the story follows the diagnosis and treatment of various cancers of three fictional children. The text covers

hospital stays, tests, treatment, feelings, school, getting help, why some kids die, and recovery. Includes color illustrations. For children ages 4 to 8.

➤ Romenesko, Ross. 2003. *I Had a Tumor, It Wasn't a Rumor*. Appleton, WI: The Ross Romensko Team.

This book started as a poem written as a class assignment by a seven-year-old boy undergoing treatment for lymphoma. The text discusses chemotherapy side effects and the importance of a positive attitude and includes 30 tips for making "life with cancer easier to swallow." The "Family Reflections" section is written by the boy's parents and sibling, who candidly share how cancer has affected their lives. To download the book as an Adobe Acrobat (.pdf) file or order the print copy, access at: www.rossromenesko.org. For children ages 5 to 12.

➤ Keene, Nancy. 2002. *Chemo, Craziness and Comfort: My Book about Child-hood Cancer*. Washington, D.C.: Candlelighters Childhood Cancer Fnd.

This comprehensive, 200-page resource provides practical advice for children diagnosed with cancer between 6 and 12 years of age. Warm and funny illustrations and easy-to-read text help the child (and parents) understand cancer and its treatment. The book offers detailed explanations of the body, cancer, hospital routines, diagnostic tests, and ways to cope with treatment side effects. Parents of children with cancer may obtain a free copy from the foundation at: www.candlelighters.org

➤ Trillin, Alice Stewart, and Edward Koren. 1996. *Dear Bruno*. New York: New Press; Norton (dist.).

The text is a letter written by an adult cancer survivor to a friend's 12-year-old son, who had just been diagnosed with cancer. The author shares the feeling she experienced during her treatment and attempts to cheer the boy up with humor and a matter-of-fact attitude toward the illness. For children ages 12 to 16.

➤ Gill, Kathleen A. 1999. *Teenage Cancer Journey*. Pittsburgh: Oncology Nursing Press.

The author is a cancer survivor who was diagnosed and treated during her teenage years. The book provides insight into the special issues cancer presents to teenagers and addresses philosophical questions as well as practical dilemmas. Topics include coping with hair loss, relating to friends and family, and balancing school responsibilities during treatment.

For Children Undergoing a Bone Marrow or Stem-Cell Transplantation (list arranged by age)

➤ Leukemia & Lymphoma Society. *The Stem Cell Transplant Coloring Book*. This book is intended for preschool and elementary school–age children with blood cancer who are coping with having a stem cell transplant. Siblings, friends, and classmates can learn from the experiences of Sam and Serena, two young stem cell transplant patients who are the main characters in the story. The book can be printed as an Adobe Acrobat (.pdf) file. Access at: www.leukemia-lymphoma.org.

➤ Lilleby, Kathryn Ulberg, and Chad Chronick. 2002. *Stevie's New Blood*. Pittsburgh: Oncology Nursing Press.

The story described bone marrow transplantation (BMT) from a child's point of view with cartoon characters and colorful illustrations. The goal is to help children know what to expect before, during, and after transplantation. Each page features two text levels: a large-print version for kids ages 6 to 10 and a small-print version for ages 10 to 17. Younger children can follow the illustrations.

➤ Crowe, Karen. 1999. *Me and My Marrow: A Kid's Guide to Bone Marrow Transplants*. Deerfield, IL: Fugisawa Healthcare.

Humorous illustrations accompany the text in this comprehensive nonfiction overview of bone marrow transplantation. The three main parts—before, during, and after transplantation—provide detailed explanations of medical and emotional issues. Appropriate for children between the ages of 10 and 18. Access at: www.meandmymarrow.com. It is possible to view the book as a series of Web pages, or download a PDF file for printing.

For Children with Leukemia (list arranged by age)

➤ Schulz, Charles M. 2002. *Why, Charlie Brown, Why?: A Story about What Happens When a Friend Is Very Ill*. New York: Ballantine Books.

Linus and Snoopy, the Peanuts characters, explore what happens when a friend is diagnosed with leukemia. The friends have varying reactions as they follow her treatment and ultimate recovery. For children ages 4 to 8.

➤ Baker, Lynn S., Charles G. Roland, and Gerald S. Gilchrist. 2002. *You and Leukemia: A Day at a Time*. 2d ed. Philadelphia: Saunders.

This book was written by a pediatric oncologist to answer many questions that children with leukemia and their parents may have at the time of diagnosis or initial treatment. It provides a basic explanation of leukemia, including the biology of the disease, its causes, and its effects. The author also provided advice on living with leukemia and explanations of therapies, side effects, central lines, and blood transfusions. For children ages 6 to 12.

➤ Westcott, Patsy. 2000. *Living with Leukemia*. Austin, TX: Raintree Steck-Vaughn.

This book follows two children who have been treated for leukemia and one who was recently diagnosed. Color illustrations and photographs help describe leukemia and its treatments and how to cope in the hospital and school. For children ages 4 to 12.

➤ Apel, Melanie Ann. 2001. *Coping with Leukemia*. New York: Rosen Pub. Group.

This book for teenagers describes leukemia and explains its symptoms and diagnosis. It includes a discussion of chemotherapy and bone marrow transplants and tips from teenage patients. The emotional side of living with leukemia also is covered and the book has a special chapter for teenage siblings.

Audiovisual Materials (list arranged by age)

➤ 2000. *Kidz with Leukemia: A Space Adventure*. Arlington, VA: Degge Group. An interactive educational CD-ROM program with three separate sections: one for children ages 4 to 6, one for children ages 7 and up, and one for adults. The CD-ROM combines games, videos, and text to teach children about acute leukemia. Friendly cartoon characters present information about tests, treatments, communicating with peers, food issues, and pain control. To order, access: www.kidzwithleukemia.com

➤ National Marrow Donor Program. *Discovery to Recovery: A Child's Guide to Bone Marrow Transplant*. Minneapolis, MN: National Marrow Donor Program, 2005.

This is an educational, interactive DVD and booklet for children ages 5 to 9, who will be undergoing a marrow or cord blood transplant. The DVD tells the transplant story through two engaging puppets and provides interviews from children and their families who have been through the transplant process. The accompanying booklet is designed as a supportive tool to promote transplant discussion within the family. To order a free copy, access: www.marrow.org.

➤ *Emily's Story: Back to School After Cancer*. Los Angeles, CA: Cancervive, 1999. This 15-minute documentary follows Emily, a nine-year-old girl with leukemia, from her hospitalization to her successful return to classmates and school life. The partnership between the patient, school, and hospital is stressed, as well as raising awareness about the challenges of school re-entry. For elementary school–age children. Available in DVD and VHS. To order, access: www.cancervive.org

➤ *Alex's Journey: The Story of a Child with a Brain Tumor*. 2000. American Brain Tumor Assn. 1 videocassette (30 min.).

This is a story of a nine-year-old boy with a brain tumor. It describes several symptoms, diagnostic procedures, and treatments for brain tumors. The boy eventually gets better with the help of many people who care for him. Suitable for children ages 9 to 13. Available in VHS and DVD formats from the American Brain Tumor Association at: www.abta.org.

➤ *Making the Grade: Back to School after Cancer for Teens.* Los Angeles, CA: Cancervive, 1999.

This 18-minute documentary profiles the lives of three teens as they return to school. It is a useful tool for educating classmates, school staff, and family members about what teenagers experience when they re-enter school after treatment for cancer. Available in DVD and VHS. To order, access: www.cancervive.org

➤ Degge Group. 2005. *Conquering Cancer Network: Empowering Teens with Tools, Info and Inspiring Stories.* Arlington, VA: Degge Group.

This interactive educational CD-ROM aims to teach 12–18-year-olds with cancer about their illness, its treatment, its side effects, and potential late effects, as well as to provide coping skills to help support them through this challenge. Produced with funding from the National Cancer Institute. To order, access: www.conqueringcancer.net

Web Resources (list arranged by age)

➤ Cancer Characters. Access at: www.nursing.uiowa.edu/sites/PedsPain/BancerCh/index.htm

Developed by a pediatric-oncology nurse and an art teacher. These characters help children ages 3 to 6 understand cancer and its treatment.

➤ Blood Count Information for Kids with Cancer. Access at: www.nursing.uiowa.edu/sites/PedsPain/Bcounts/index.htm

Pediatric-oncology nurses developed special characters to explain blood counts to children ages five to nine. Color illustrations help children to understand medical terminology such as different blood cell types, clotting, and hemoglobin.

➤ ABTA Kids. Access at: www.abta.org/kids/home.htm

The kids' section ("ABTA KIDS") of the American Brain Tumor Association provides child-friendly information about brain tumors. The site has interactive features and enables children to share their thoughts and engage in activities.

➤ CureSearch. Access at: www.curesearch.org

This site has information for children with cancer written in kid-friendly language. Users can learn about different childhood cancer types, diagnostic tests, and treatment methods. Other topics include living with cancer, school and friends, the family, transition after treatment, long-term survivorship, and end of life.

➤ Teens Living with Cancer. Access at: www.teenslivingwithcancer.com
This Web site is suitable for children ages 12 to 17 who are undergoing
cancer treatment. It provides detailed information about specific cancer
types, medications, tests, central lines, and other medical issues. Quality-
of-life concerns such as body issues, school, and friends also are discussed.
The site has a medical dictionary and interactive features. A medical
review board and a teen advisory board are responsible for the content.

Resources for Siblings of Children with Cancer

Brochures, Booklets, and Other Short Print Publications

➤ American Cancer Society. *When Your Brother or Sister Has Cancer.*
This publication for children ages 6–12 addresses the feelings siblings
may experience, such as sadness, guilt, jealousy, anger, being worried
about their sibling and parents, and missing their parents.
➤ CancerCare. *Helping the Sibling of the Child with Cancer.*
A short, two-page handout for parents with suggestions on communicating with children who have a sibling with cancer. Access at: www.cancer
care.org
➤ National Cancer Institute. *When Your Brother or Sister Has Cancer: A
Guide for Teens.*
This 100-page booklet describes how teens deal with the challenges facing
the family when a sibling is diagnosed with cancer. It suggests ways for
teens to help themselves and their families and provides information
about cancer treatments and where to go for more support. Access at
www.cancer.gov and click on "NCI Publications"
➤ SuperSibs. *Parent Guide.*
A two-page handout for parents with practical tips for helping siblings redefine the cancer experience. Access at: www.supersibs.org

Books for Siblings

➤ Dodd, Michael, and Candlelighters Childhood Cancer Fnd. 2004. *Oliver's
Story for "Sibs" of Kids with Cancer.* Kensington, MD: CCCF.
This 40-page illustrated book is written through the eyes of a six-year-
old boy whose sister has cancer. The text addresses many of the questions
that siblings may have when their brother or sister is diagnosed with
cancer, and it offers constructive ways on how they can provide support.
Children between the ages of 3 and 8 are the primary audience for this

book. Families of children with cancer may request a free copy online at www.candlelighters.org or by calling 800-366-2223.

➤ Sonnenblick, Jordan. 2004. *Drums, Girls, and Dangerous Pie*. New York: Scholastic.

When his younger brother is diagnosed with leukemia, 13-year-old Steven tries to deal with his complicated emotions, his school life, and his desire to support his family. This novel is suitable for children ages 11–16.

Audiovisual Materials

➤ *Kids Tell Kids What It's Like When Their Brother or Sister Has Cancer.* 1998. Los Angeles, CA: Cancervive.

Kids do all the talking in this 17-minute video for and about children who have a brother or sister with cancer. They share the ways they cope with changes in their family life, fears about their siblings, and lack of attention. Available in DVD and VHS. To order access: www.cancervive.org

Web Resources

➤ CureSearch. Access at: www.curesearch.org

The section "Impact on the Family" includes tips and suggestions for parents, as well as essays written by siblings.

➤ SuperSibs. Access at: www.supersibs.org

SuperSibs is an organization that reaches out to the brothers and sisters of children in the United States and Canada who are diagnosed with cancer. The organization's site has information on events, activities, and services provided by SuperSibs, a guide for parents, and age-appropriate newsletters for siblings of children with cancer.

Support Organizations

➤ SuperSibs. Access at www.supersibs.org
Phone: 866-444-7427

Childhood Cancer Survivors

Cure rates for childhood cancer have improved dramatically in the second half of the 20th century. Up until the 1950s, very few children survived cancer; now almost 80% of children and adolescents diagnosed with cancer are alive at least five years after diagnosis. Most children ultimately will be considered cured. Out of the ten million cancer survivors living in the United States in 2005, at least 270,000 were diagnosed and treated before age 20.

In many cases, cure has health and emotional consequences. Adults who survived childhood cancer have unique medical and psychosocial needs. Chemotherapy, radiation therapy, and surgery typically cause side effects: various symptoms and problems that occur when treatment affects healthy tissues or organs. Most side effects are reversible and resolve once treatment is completed. Side effects that persist after treatment are called "long-term effects" or "late effects." Late effects can surface months, years, and even decades after treatment has ended.

While some survivors do not develop any late effects from treatment, others experience mild, moderate, or severe ones. The type and intensity of the effects vary from child to child and depend on the specific type and dose of therapy received. The age of the child during treatment is another factor in the severity and type of problems that may arise as a result of anticancer treatment. Younger children are at higher risk.

One of the most devastating late effects is loss of fertility. This topic is discussed on page 274, and the information sources provided in this section are relevant to childhood cancer survivors. Neurological difficulties are more common in children who had brain surgery, received radiation therapy aimed at the head, or received chemotherapy delivered directly to the fluid around the spinal cord. These children may suffer cognitive difficulties, learning disabilities, and even retardation. Heart damage may occur after chemotherapy with a class of drugs called anthracyclines. These drugs can weaken the heart muscle and cause congestive heart failure. Radiation to the chest increases the risk for heart disease and may cause injury to the lungs. Late effects may cause damage to the child's growth, hearing, kidneys, liver, thyroid gland, and other body systems and organs.

Chemotherapy and radiation therapy increase the risk for developing a secondary cancer years after treatment. The level of risk depends on the types and dosages of therapy given, and the age of the child during treatment. Overall, the chance of getting a second cancer is very small for most survivors.

The mental health of childhood cancer survivors may also be affected. Survivors of childhood cancer may experience anxiety and depression related to physical changes, appearance, or the fear of cancer coming back. These difficulties may cause problems with personal relationships, education, and employment.

Regular follow-up of childhood cancer survivors is essential in order to identify and address problems as early as possible. Many childhood cancer treatment centers have specialized clinics that screen survivors for late effects and inform them about ways to promote health and lower health-related risks. Another important goal of the long-term follow-up clinics is to educate survivors on becoming educated healthcare consumers, and enable them to locate quality providers in their communities who are capable of treating the complex ongoing medical and emotional needs of childhood cancer survivors.

In addition to the medical and mental issues childhood cancer survivors face, they also confront educational and occupational challenges. Knowledge of children's rights with regards to education is also important, as many children who were treated for cancer require special education services to maximize their educational potential. Understanding the law as it is specified in the Individuals with Disabilities in Education Act (IDEA) and the process of obtaining special education services from school systems is the first step in ensuring that children receive the appropriate special education services they need and to which they are entitled. Many of the information sources listed below provide information for parents on advocating for their children within the education system and working effectively with school systems and teachers. Adult survivors of childhood cancer may encounter job discrimination and difficulties in obtaining health insurance due to their health history. Information about employment and insurance issues is covered in the practical matters section on page 296.

Information Sources

Brochures, Booklets, and Other Short Print Publications

➤ Leukemia and Lymphoma Society. *Learning and Living With Cancer*. Written for parents of a child returning to school during or after cancer treatment, this booklet explains the challenges children with cancer may face at school and how to help them achieve their education potential. The booklet discusses the laws that protect the child's educational needs and lists specific ways that schools can help. Access at: www.leukemia-lymphoma.org

➤ National Children's Cancer Society. *The Mountain You've Climbed: A Young Adult's Guide to Childhood Cancer Survivorship*. This guide is designed to answer questions and address issues related to cancer survivorship for people ages 15–24. Topics include: employments, health insurance, fertility, healthy living, medical issues, spirituality, grief, psychological issues, relationships, and educational challenges. Includes an extensive list of resources and a bibliography. Access at: http://national childrenscancersociety.com

➤ National Cancer Institute. *Facing Forward Series: Life After Cancer Treatment*. This booklet covers post-treatment issues such as follow-up medical care, physical and emotional changes, changes in social relationships, and workplace issues. It also shows ways to educate and empower cancer survivors as they face the challenges associated with life after cancer treatment. Access at: https://cissecure.nci.nih.gov/ncipubs/

Book

➤ Keene, Nancy, Wendy Hobbie, and Kathy Ruccione. 2006. *Childhood Cancer Survivors: A Practical Guide to Your Future*, 2nd ed. Cambridge, MA: O'Reilly.
This book provides a comprehensive overview of all topics of interest to children, adolescents, and adults after treatment for childhood cancer. The text combines information and personal stories on topics such as medical late effects of treatment, emotional aspects of surviving cancer, schedules for follow-up care, challenges in the healthcare system, and lifestyle choices to maximize health and discrimination in employment or insurance.

Web Resources

➤ Beyond the Cure. Access at: www.beyondthecure.org
Provided by the National Children's Cancer Society, this site offers extensive information pertaining to all areas of a survivor's life. Detailed articles offer practical information on medical, educational, and financial long-term effects. Users can find in-depth information on many topics such as fertility, psychological conditions, grief, insurance, and employment challenges.
➤ Lance Armstrong Foundation. LIVESTRONG SurvivorCare. Access at: www. laf.org
The Cancer Support section of this site contains information on many topics of interest to cancer survivors including physical, emotional, and practical issues. Each topic has detailed information, suggestions of what to do, and a list of resources. The site also offers downloadable survivorship tools that can help manage the information and documents needed to maintain a healthy survivorship.
➤ Long-Term Follow-Up Study. Access at: www.cancer.umn.edu/ltfu
The Long-Term Follow-Up Study is a collaborative, multi-institutional study of individuals who survived five or more years after treatment for childhood cancer. Some study results are published in the newsletters accessible from the left side bar. The newsletters feature articles about specific subgroups of survivors and psychosocial issues.
➤ Long-Term Follow-Up Guidelines for Survivors of Childhood, Adolescent, and Young Adult Cancers. Access at: www.survivorshipguidelines.org
Developed by the Children's Oncology Group, these guidelines provide recommendations for screening and management of late effects that may

potentially arise as a result of therapeutic exposures used during treatment for childhood cancer.

➤ Outlook—Life Beyond Childhood Cancer. Access at: www.outlook-life. org/
A Web portal for survivors of childhood cancer and their families with information on insurance and financial issues, health issues and concerns, job and school challenges, and features an interactive section. This site is provided by the University of Wisconsin Comprehensive Cancer Center.

Patient Support Organizations

➤ Lance Armstrong Foundation. LIVESTRONG SurvivorCare. Access at: www.laf.org
Phone: 866-235-7205

➤ National Coalition for Cancer Survivorship. Access at: www.canceradvocacy. org
Phone: 877-622-7937

Chapter 3

Beyond Cancer 101

ancer is a complex disease that may have an unpredictable path with many twists and turns. Along this winding road the information needs of patients and their caregivers vary. The amount of information sought, the degree of detail, and the topics of interest shift during the course of the illness. Newly diagnosed patients require basic, introductory-level information that describes the disease, the common treatments for cancer, and some of the support/coping issues relating to persons affected by cancer. This type of "Cancer 101" information is easily accessible in brochures, books, and the Web sites listed in this book. On the other hand, information sought by patients with rare cancer types or by patients whose disease has progressed is not so easily found. These patients have very specific questions on complex medical issues and new therapies still under investigation. For example, at the Patient Education Resource Center (PERC) at the University of Michigan Comprehensive Cancer Center, patients have requested information on topics such as

➤ Latest results of clinical trials evaluating targeted therapies for treatment of head and neck cancer
➤ The significance of minimal residual disease in childhood leukemia
➤ Open versus closed MRI: the pros and cons of each option

While it is possible to answer such queries by searching MEDLINE to find articles in the peer-reviewed medical literature, the average person would find it difficult to understand and analyze articles written for professionals in technical language. The challenge for librarians working with cancer patients and families is to provide current, reliable, and comprehensive information on complex issues and cutting-edge therapies, and presented in lay language.

If searching the resources listed under specific cancer types and topics does not produce a satisfactory result, the librarian should move on to plan B and search the sources listed in this chapter. Although it is possible to type the term in a general search engine such as Google or Yahoo!, the list of hits would have to be carefully screened for quality, currency, and educational level. The first part of this chapter offers a number of authoritative sources where one may find answers to questions beyond the introductory level. The second part offers strategies for locating information on rare cancers, unique treatments, illustrations, and information in languages other than English.

Advanced Information Sources

Cancer News

The Web sites below offer news databases on cancer. Most are short articles explaining medical articles published in peer-reviewed scientific medical journals. In a way, these articles provide "translations" of medical articles from technical to lay language and explore topics currently being explored in cancer research. These are excellent starting points for information on new therapies or to answer questions such as "What's new in non-Hodgkin's lymphoma?"

Following is a list of a few general cancer sites offering searchable news item databases.

➤ www.cancer.org
   Under the heading "ACS News Today" and select the topic from a pull-down menu
➤ www.cancer.gov
   Click on the "NEWS Center" button
➤ medlineplus.gov
   At the top of every health topic page
➤ www.oncolink.com
   Under the heading "Cancer News" or click on the advanced search interface and limit your search to "Cancer News"
➤ www.peoplelivingwithcancer.org
   Click on "News and Events"
➤ www.cancerpage.com/news/
➤ www.patient.cancerconsultants.com
   Click on "Cancer News"

Question-and-Answer Archives

"Question-and-Answer" (Q&A) databases contain expert answers to questions asked by cancer patients and caregivers. The questions on these databases tend to relate to specific topics and personal situations; however, the same situations may apply to other patients. For example: a PERC user was considering stopping tamoxifen treatment because of bothersome side effects. The "Cancer Q and As" section of CancerBACKUP provided an answer to a similar question, explaining, in lay terms, that clinical trials have demonstrated that taking Tamoxifen for five years is more effective in breast cancer prevention than taking the drug for two years. Moreover, taking Tamoxifen for ten years offers little or no more protection than taking it for five years. By stopping Tamoxifen after fewer than five years, a patient would potentially lose a great deal of the protective benefit of the drug. This answer provided the information seeker with concrete and understandable information that helped her to make an informed decision.

Listed here are two sites with a large and searchable archive of answers provided by reputable specialists. It is of outmost importance to check the credentials of people who provide answers in other sites.

➤ www.oncolink.com
  Click on "Ask the Experts" or click on the advanced search interface and limit your search to "Ask the Experts"
➤ www.cancerbacup.org.uk
  Click on "Cancer Q&As"

Webcasts, Lectures and Articles

Webcasts

Healthology.com contains transcripts of Webcasts and lectures given by cancer specialists for patients. This content may be very useful for patients seeking more comprehensive, current, and in-depth information. Webcasts are virtual conferences that offer patients the opportunity to interact with cancer specialists through the Internet in real time, utilizing RealAudio or RealVideo software. During the Webcasts oncologists provide detailed, lay-language explanations of the diseases and new developments in research that have not yet been incorporated into books or brochures. After the live broadcasts, transcripts and video files of the event are posted on the site. Several sites that offer access to Webcasts and transcripts are listed below.

➤ www.healthology.com
  Click on " Consumer Health Library" and then on "View All Health Topics"
➤ www.cancereducation.com
  Click on "Patient & Family Center" (audio and video clips available)
➤ www.plwc.org
  Click on "News and Events" and then on "Ask the ASCO Expert Series"

In-depth Articles

Medical articles in peer-reviewed scientific journals are not appropriate for patients and families who lack the education and professional knowledge to fully understand and interpret the information correctly. Using articles from popular magazines and newspapers is not recommended because they are not written or reviewed by medical professionals and may contain inaccuracies and misrepresentations. Librarians should look for articles that are either written by credentialed professionals or published in a publication that has a medical advisory board with reputable advisors.

Articles written or reviewed by health professionals can be found in cancer advocacy organizations' newsletters and in the four magazines listed below. Access to these publications is difficult, since most are not indexed in any bibliographic indexes or databases. The following magazines are the primary serial publications aimed at cancer patients and families; they offer articles written or reviewed by credentialed professionals.

➤ *Coping with Cancer* (ISSN 1043-8637).
   This is an easy-to-read publication with many articles that focus on the psychosocial issues of cancer written by survivors and mental health specialists. Information on subscriptions may be found on the Web site at: www.copingmag.com/

➤ *MAMM* (ISSN 1099-563X).
   This publication is geared to women with breast and gynecological cancers. Information on subscription can be found on the Web site at: www.mamm.com. Access to content is available online for a fee.

➤ *CURE: Cancer Updates, Research & Education* (ISSN 1534-7664).
   This beautifully produced quarterly offers articles on the science and the human side of cancer. *CURE* is indexed in CINHAL and the Web site (access available at: www.curetoday.com) contains the full-text of all articles ever published.

➤ *Women & Cancer* (ISSN 1557-5780).
   Women & Cancer is a quarterly magazine developed specifically for women impacted by a cancer diagnosis. Some full-text articles and subscriptions information are available at: www.cancerconsultants.com

Professional Medical Information Sources

There are occasions when it is appropriate to provide professional-level information to nonprofessional patrons in a public or hospital library. Sometimes lay-language information just does not exist to answer questions about rare cancers and complex issues. It is also appropriate to provide professional-level information to patrons who have the education and ability to understand scientific literature. Since the scope of this book is lay-language information sources, only one professional resource is listed.

➤ Kufe, Donald W., and James F. Holland. 2005. *Holland-Frei Manual of Cancer Medicine.* Lewiston, NY: BC Decker.

The intended audience of this cancer reference book is medical oncologists, radiation oncologists, internists, and surgical oncologists. The chapters are written by specialists from the relevant disciplines and present a comprehensive overview of cancer from basic science to clinical practice, including clinical trials, prevention, screening and early detection, pathology, imaging, and therapies. The full-text of this medical textbook is available free online through PubMed, the National Library of Medicine gateway to MEDLINE, and other scientific databases. To access, go to: www.pubmed.gov and click on "books" on the top selection bar.

Strategies for Locating Advanced Cancer Information

Rare Cancers

Patient-friendly information about rare cancers may be difficult to find. For information about cancers others than the ones listed separately in this book, several steps can be taken.

1. Search the term in one of the primary cancer information sources listing on page 12. If the topic concerns childhood cancer, information seeking can start by consulting the information sources listed in the childhood cancer primary information sources listing on page 25. The information sources listed in the cancer supportive care section on page 258 can be used to start a search on quality-of-life issues.
2. Search the National Organization for Rare Disorders (NORD) database at: www.rarediseases.org. The NORD reports are overviews of specific rare diseases and may be downloaded free by subscribers. Users who do not have a subscription to the database may purchase the reports for a nominal fee.
3. Enter the term in on one of the Q & A databases listed above.
4. If the steps above did not produce sufficient results it may be necessary to search the medical literature and provide professional-level information.

Information from a medical textbook such as the *Holland-Frei Manual of Cancer Medicine* listed above tends to be more understandable than a journal article. If a MEDLINE search is still needed, it is better to provide a recent review article on the topic rather than articles about a specific clinical trial or a case study.

Procedures and Therapies

Chapter Seven includes treatment methods that are utilized in many cancers, such as radiation therapy, drug therapies, and complementary therapies. There are, however, many treatments and surgical procedures that are used in a more limited way, for specific cancer diseases. These include surgical procedures that are specific to the anatomy of the cancer, and other treatments such as laser surgeries, photodynamic therapy, radiofrequency ablation, and more. For information on treatment modalities that do not have a section in Chapter Seven, please search the information sources listed for the specific cancer type for which they are used.

Illustrations

Illustrations are key to enabling lay people to understand medical conditions. Good information products are those that include good color graphics in addition to text. Each cancer type description in this book includes a reference to an illustration accessible on the Web. In addition, the following sites offer collections of cancer images:

➤ People Living with Cancer Medical Illustrations Gallery offers a collection of full-color illustrations of common sites where cancer occurs, organized by cancer type. Each illustration is offered in a Web version and a print version that may be downloaded and printed on an 8.5" x 11" page. The gallery includes both anatomical illustrations and illustrations of the cancers by stage. To access go to: www.plwc.org and click on Library on the left sidebar.

➤ NCI Visuals Online—this database contains images from the National Cancer Institute including general biomedical and science-related images, cancer-specific scientific and patient care-related images. To access, go to: http://visualsonline.cancer.gov/

➤ The A.D.A.M. Medical Encyclopedia available at Medlineplus.gov includes color medical photographs and illustrations. Enter a term in the search box and click on the "Medical Encyclopedia" folder in the search results to find the images.

Information in Other Languages

Several cancer Web sites such as the American Cancer Society, the National Cancer Institute and a few other cancer organizations' sites offer Spanish-language Web sites. The American Cancer Society is developing a collection of Asian-language cancer materials, which may be accessed through a link on the home page at: www.cancer.org

The Canadian Cancer Society site at www.cancer.ca offers a mirror site in French and a large number of publications translated to other languages, such as Punjabi, Farsi, and Chinese. The page "Cancer information in other languages" links to cancer Web sites from other countries.

Cancerbackup, the cancer information service from the United Kingdom, has a collection of fact sheets in several Asian languages. To access, go to: www.cancerbackup.org.uk/Home.

The Cancer Council of South Australia offers cancer information in a number of languages. To access go to: http://old.cancersa.org.au/ and click on "Other Languages" on the left sidebar.

Librarians can also look for cancer information in other languages in a few multilingual health information sites, such as:

➤ www.ethnomed.org
➤ http://spiral.tufts.edu

Not Recommended

It is not recommended to use information from listservs, Wikis, and blogs to answer reference questions. One must remember that the medical information in listservs and blogs is anecdotal and not scientifically proven. It may even be biased, misleading, and erroneous. Since it may be difficult to find the credentials and motives of information providers in listservs, Wikis, and blogs, it is best to use the other sources listed in this book to answer patrons' questions.

Part II

Key Resources for Finding Information on Specific Types of Cancer

Chapter 4

Main Types of Adult Cancer

Biliary Tract Cancer:
Bile Duct and Gallbladder Cancers

Anatomical facts: Bile is a fluid that contains enzymes needed to digest fat. It is secreted by the liver and stored in the gallbladder, a small organ located underneath the liver. Bile is released and delivered from the gallbladder to the small intestine when a person eats. A complex system of hollow tubes, called ducts, delivers bile from the liver to the gallbladder and from the gallbladder to the duodenum, which is the first section of the small intestine. This system is referred to as the biliary tract. The part of the system located inside the liver is called the intrahepatic bile duct, and the part located outside the liver is called the extrahepatic bile duct.

Illustrations available at: Johns Hopkins Pathology. *Gallbladder and Bile Duct Cancer.*

Access at: http://pathology2.jhu.edu/gbbd/index.htm

About 9,000 people in the United States are diagnosed with extrahepatic bile duct cancer or gallbladder cancer each year. Most biliary tract cancers are discovered in late stages, when cure is very difficult to achieve. The five-year survival rate for both gallbladder cancer and extrahepatic bile duct cancer is about 15%.

Bile duct cancer is more common in men, and most patients are diagnosed between the ages of 50 and 70. Gallbladder cancer, on the other hand, is more common in women because one of the risk factors for this disease are gallstones, which are more frequent in women. Gallbladder cancer has a higher incidence among the Native American population in New Mexico and Alaska. Most patients are diagnosed after age 70. Bile duct cancer has a higher incidence in the Middle East and Asia because a parasite infection common in those parts of the world is one of the causes of this disease.

The majority of tumors that develop in the biliary tract are adenocarcinomas. Cholangiocarcinoma is a synonym for an adenocarcinoma that grows in the biliary tract. Cholangiocarcinomas also grow in the intrahepatic bile duct, and although these tumors are counted as liver cancer, their treatment and behavior are similar to those for cholangiocarcinomas that grow in the extrahepatic biliary tract. Some information sources present separate sections for gallbladder and bile duct cancer, but others present the information together.

A rare subtype of cholangiocarcinomas, papillary cholangiocarcinoma, is less invasive and carries a better prognosis. Other tumors that may appear in the biliary tract are neuroendocrine carcinoma, adenosquamous carcinoma, melanoma, and lymphoma. These tumors are treated differently than cholangiocarcinomas.

Surgery is the only treatment that has the potential for cure of biliary tract cancer. The type and extent of the surgery depends on the location of the tumor. A number of surgical procedures may be used with the goal of removing the diseased section of the biliary tract and reconnecting the tubes to the small intestine. If the disease has spread, parts of other organs, such as the pancreas, the small intestine, and the liver, also are removed. Cancers that are confined to the intrahepatic bile duct are treated with removing part of the liver (partial hepatectomy). Surgery in the biliary tract area is very complicated, requires a long recovery period, and has significant side effects, some of which may be long term. Radiation therapy and chemotherapy are used to alleviate symptoms and improve the quality of life of patients whose disease is inoperable or has metastasized to distant organs.

Information Sources

Web Resources

Sites focusing on biliary tract cancers

➤ Johns Hopkins Pathology. *Gallbladder* and *Bile Duct Cancer*. Access at: http://pathology2.jhu.edu/gbbd/index.htm
A detailed overview of biliary tract cancers includes color illustrations that explain the anatomy of this complex system. The site also includes a news section and a coping section with information on supportive-care issues such as nutrition and physical activity.

Detailed sections in general cancer sites

➤ American Cancer Society. *Learn about Bile Duct Cancer* and *Learn about Gallbladder Cancer*. Access at: www.cancer.org and select from the menu under "Choose a Cancer Type or Topic." Disease-specific detailed guides can be printed by section or as Adobe Acrobat (.pdf) files.

➤ National Cancer Institute. *Extrahepatic Bile Duct Cancer* and *Gallbladder Cancer*. Access at: www.cancer.gov and click on "Types of cancer." The top page of the sections links to patient versions of PDQ® (Physician Data Query) statements, clinical trial information, and other NCI publications on this topic.

➤ People Living with Cancer. *Bile Duct Cancer* and *Gallbladder Cancer*. Access at: www.plwc.org and click on "Cancer Type." The PLWC oncologist-approved guides can be printed in their entirety or by subtopic.

Sections about bile duct cancer and gallbladder cancer are also available at the following sites:

➤ Cancerbackup. Access at: www.cancerbackup.org.uk/Home and click on "Cancer Types."

➤ CancerSource.com. Access at: www.cancersource.com/Patient.pg and make a selection from the "Diagnosis & Treatment" pull-down menu.

Patient-Support Organizations

➤ American Cancer Society. Access at: www.cancer.org
Phone: 800-ACS-2345

Bladder Cancer

Anatomical facts: The bladder is a hollow balloon-shaped organ in the lower abdomen. It stores urine, the liquid waste produced by the kidneys. Urine passes from each kidney into the bladder through a tube called a ureter. Urine empties from the bladder through another tube called the urethra.

Illustrations available at the Medical Illustrations Gallery of the People Living with Cancer Web site .
Access at: www.plwc.org and click on Library on the left sidebar.

Approximately 67,000 Americans are diagnosed with bladder cancer each year. It is more prevalent in men than in women and more common in whites than in African Americans. The average age of diagnosis is 68. If caught in its early stages, bladder cancer can be successfully treated with minimal side effects.

The greatest risk factor for bladder cancer is smoking. Smokers are two to three times more likely to develop bladder cancer than are nonsmokers. Carcinogenic chemicals in the tobacco smoke get absorbed into the blood, are filtered by the kidneys, and collect in the urine. This urine damages the bladder cells. Exposure to other chemicals and frequent bladder inflammation also may damage the bladder cells and their ability to control their growth.

The most common tumor type in the bladder is urothelial carcinoma, which is also known as transitional cell carcinoma or TCC. Less than 10% of bladder cancers are squamous cell carcinomas, or adenocarcinomas. For treatment purposes, bladder cancers are divided into two groups: superficial and invasive. Superficial cancer is confined to the inner lining of the bladder, while invasive cancers spread deeper into the muscle wall of the bladder and possibly to other tissues and organs.

The surgical procedure for treating superficial bladder cancer is called transurethral resection (TUR). TUR is performed by inserting a tube called a cystoscope through the urethra. This procedure enables the preservation of bladder function. Cancers that invade the muscle wall are removed with open surgery. The extent of the surgery depends on the spread of the tumors. Sometimes it is possible to preserve part of the bladder and normal bladder function, but in advanced disease the entire bladder and even other organs, such as the prostate in men and uterus in women, will be removed. The extent of surgery also determines if it will be possible to reconstruct a bladder internally ("neobladder") or if the urine will have be removed manually through a bag ("urostomy"). Another option is an internal diversion of the urine to the small bowel.

In addition to surgery, bladder cancer can be treated with chemotherapy and/or radiation therapy. In the early stages, chemotherapy can be delivered directly to the bladder ("intravesical") to help minimize the systemic side effects of chemotherapy. Another treatment option for superficial bladder cancer is immunotherapy. With this method, a bacteria called BCG (Bacillus Calmette-Guérin) is injected directly into the bladder through a catheter in order to stimulate the immune system to attack the cancer.

Sex and intimacy may be a concern to some bladder cancer survivors who might have to adapt to having sexual activity with a urostomy bag. In men, sexual function may be impaired if their surgery included the removal of the prostate and adjacent nerves.

Information Sources

Brochures, Booklets, and Other Short Print Publications

➤ National Cancer Institute. *What You Need to Know about Bladder Cancer.*
A concise introduction to bladder cancer describing the diagnostic tests, staging treatment options, getting a second opinion, and coping with side effects. Access at: https://cissecure.nci.nih.gov/ncipubs/

➤ National Comprehensive Cancer Network (NCCN). *Bladder Cancer: Treatment Guidelines for Patients.*
Overview of bladder cancer as well as treatment decision "trees" explaining the treatment choices for different stages and conditions in breast cancer. This resource is developed from the NCCN Clinical Practice Guidelines in Oncology—the standard for clinical policy in cancer care. A Spanish-language version is also available. Access at: www.nccn.org/patients/

Books

➤ Ellsworth, Pamela, and Brett Carswell. 2006. *100 Questions and Answers about Bladder Cancer.* Sudbury, MA: Jones and Bartlett.
Detailed information about bladder cancer is presented in an easy-to-read question-and-answer format. Terms are explained on the sidebar, and the book includes lists of Web sites, organizations, literature, and resources on general and specific topics related to bladder cancer. This book was co-authored by two urologists from the University of Massachusetts Memorial Medical Center.

➤ Schoenberg, Mark P., Johns Hopkins University, and Genitourinary Oncology Group. 2000. *The Guide to Living with Bladder Cancer.* Baltimore: Johns Hopkins University.
Dr. Schoenberg and the faculty and staff of the Johns Hopkins Genitourinary Oncology Group discuss the symptoms, diagnosis, and treatment of bladder cancer. The contents include anatomy of the bladder, diagnostic tests, and descriptions of different surgical procedures, including laparoscopic surgery, bladder removal, urinary tract reconstruction, and bladder preservation strategies. Other chapters cover life after surgery and chemotherapy principles. The insights and personal stories of patients who were treated by Dr. Schoenberg are presented in the last chapter.

Web Resources

Sites focusing on bladder cancer

➤ The Bladder Cancer Advocacy Network (BCAN). Access at: www.bcan.org
The Web site of the Bladder Cancer Advocacy Network provides education and information for people affected by bladder cancer. The site includes bladder cancer facts, news about new developments in bladder cancer, and information about support services for patients and families.

➤ Bladder Cancer WebCafé. Access at: www.blcwebcafe.org
Detailed and comprehensive information about bladder cancer, diagnostic procedures, staging, and treatment options. This site has an extensive

interactive section including a message board and survival guides written by patients about how they coped with different aspects of the disease, such as hospitalization, recovering from surgery, chemotherapy, and sexual side effects.

Detailed sections in general cancer sites

➤ American Cancer Society. *Learn about Bladder Cancer.* Access at: www. cancer.org and select from the menu under "Choose a Cancer Topic." A detailed guide about bladder cancer can be printed by section or as an Adobe Acrobat (.pdf) file.

➤ National Cancer Institute. *Bladder Cancer.* Access at: www.cancer.gov and click on "Types of Cancer." The top page of the section links to patient versions of PDQ® statements, clinical trial information, and other NCI publications on this topic.

➤ People Living with Cancer. *Bladder Cancer.* Access at: www.plwc.org and click on "Cancer Types." The PLWC oncologist-approved bladder cancer guide can be printed in its entirety or by subtopic.

Sections about bladder cancer are also available at the following sites:

➤ Canadian Cancer Society. Access at: www.cancer.ca and click on "About Cancer."

➤ Cancerbackup. Access at: www.cancerbackup.org.uk/Home and click on "Cancer Types."

➤ Cancerconsultants.com. Access at: www.cancerconsultants.com and make a selection under "Links to Specific Cancer type Information."

➤ CancerSource.com. Access at: www.cancersource.com/Patient.pg and make a selection from the "Diagnosis & Treatment" pull-down menu.

➤ OncologyChannel.com. Access at: www.oncologychannel.com and select a condition from the left sidebar.

Patient Support Organizations

➤ The Bladder Cancer Advocacy Network (BCAN). Access at: www.bcan.org Phone: 301-469-6865

Brain and Central Nervous System Tumors

Anatomical facts: The brain is the center of thought, memory, emotion, and speech, as well as the coordinator of the body's voluntary and involuntary actions and processes. A network of nerves located in the brain itself and in the spinal cord exchanges messages between the brain and the rest of the body. These messages tell our muscles how to move, transmit information gathered by our senses, and help coordinate our internal organs. The soft, spongy mass of brain tissue is located in the head and protected by the bones of the skull and three thin membranes called meninges. Watery fluid called cerebrospinal fluid cushions the brain. This fluid flows through spaces between the meninges and through spaces within the brain called ventricles. The brain and spinal cord compose the central nervous system.

Illustrations available in the American Brain Tumor Association publication *A Primer of Brain Tumors: A Patient's Reference Manual.*
Access at: www.abta.org and click on Tumor Information.

The brain and spinal cord have a complex structure that includes many cell types and tissues; consequently, there are over 50 types of tumors that start in the central nervous system (CNS). Brain and spinal cord tumors vary greatly in clinical behavior, outlook, and treatment. The American Cancer Society estimates about 20,000 new diagnoses of CNS tumors per year in the United States. (These statistics includes tumors in children. For information about childhood Brain tumors, please refer to Chapter 5, p. 159).

The majority of brain tumors are secondary tumors of cancers that started in a different organ and metastasized to the brain. Secondary tumors are treated differently than primary brain tumors, and the information about them should be found under the primary site. Information sources about CNS tumors focus only on tumors that started in the brain or spinal cord.

Most primary brain tumors are not associated with any specific risk factor. A very small number of tumors are the result of radiation to the head that was given as treatment for a previous cancer. Other environmental factors such as exposure to certain chemicals or to cellular phones have been suggested as risk factors, but studies have not shown a clear connection. Immune system disorders, including AIDS (acquired immune deficiency syndrome), increase the risk for lymphoma of the brain or spinal cord. Information about CNS lymphoma can be found in either the CNS tumors or lymphoma information sources.

There are approximately 50 types of primary CNS tumors. About 35% of them are astrocytomas that start in brain cells called astrocytes. Most astrocytomas cannot be cured because they spread widely throughout the surrounding normal brain tissue. About two-thirds of astrocytomas are glioblastoma multiform tumors that grow and spread very quickly. Intermediate-grade astrocytomas, or anaplastic astrocytomas, grow at a moderate rate, and low-grade astrocytomas are the slowest growing. A few rare types of astrocytoma have a better prognosis than the ones mentioned above.

Other types of primary CNS tumors are oligodendrogliomas, ependymomas, gangliogliomas, schwannomas, and medulloblastomas. The term *glioma* is a general category that includes astrocytomas, oligodendrogliomas, and ependymomas.

Meningiomas, which originate in the meninges tissue surrounding the outer part of the brain and spinal cord, make up about 25% of all brain tumors and the majority of spinal cord tumors. Most meningiomas (about 85%) are benign and can be cured by surgery. Some meningiomas, however, are located dangerously close to vital structures within the brain and cannot be completely removed by surgery. Meningiomas do not metastasize beyond the CNS.

The first step in treating CNS tumors is usually surgery. Surgeons who operate in this delicate area require additional training in the subspecialty of neurosurgery. Cure is possible if the tumor is completely removed by surgery, but oftentimes a complete removal is not possible because of the tumor's proximity to structures that control essential functions. In some cases it is even impossible to perform a biopsy because the potential for damage is greater than the benefit of knowing the exact histology of the tumor. The surgery to open the skull and enable access to the brain is called craniotomy. Another procedure sometimes required is the placement of a shunt to bypass blockage in the flow of cerebrospinal fluid. Some tumors may cause an obstruction to the flow of cerebrospinal fluid, and the excess fluid may increase the pressure in the brain and cause severe symptoms or even death.

Most brain tumor patients are also treated by radiation either as adjuvant therapy or as the main therapy if surgery is not feasible. Radiation to the brain is delivered in several methods, including stereotactic radiosurgery. With this method narrow, high-dose beams of radiation are directed at the tumor while minimizing radiation delivered to normal brain tissue.

Chemotherapy is less effective against CNS cancers because of its difficulty in penetrating through the blood-brain barrier. The blood-brain barrier is a system of thin membranes that filter chemical molecules from the blood, including many drugs, in order to protect the sensitive brain tissue. There is controversy regarding which anticancer drugs are able to penetrate the blood-brain barrier; however, some chemotherapy drugs have been shown to have activity against brain tumors. Researchers are working on developing methods to bypass the blood-brain barrier. One such method is implantation of dissolvable wafers that are saturated with chemotherapy at the tumor site during surgery.

A large number of brain tumor patients are treated with steroids to reduce swelling and inflammation in the brain. Some patients are also treated with drugs that prevent seizures.

Tumors in the brain and spinal cord and their treatment may cause difficulties in speech, movement, memory, and cognitive ability. Rehabilitative services such as speech, physical, and occupational therapy can greatly improve or even restore function. Survivors and their families may need to adjust to life with certain limitations and changes in their employment and social environments. For information on support and services, it is best to contact the brain tumor patient organizations listed below.

Information Sources

Brochures, Booklets, and Other Short Print Publications

➤ American Brain Tumor Association. *Living with a Brain Tumor: A Guide for Brain Tumor Patients.*
A step-by-step, reassuring guide for newly diagnosed patients and their families. Includes finding information, getting second opinions, reacting to the diagnosis, telling family and friends, and nurturing the caregiver. Access at: www.abta.org

➤ Brain Tumor Society. *Our Diagnosis: Brain Tumor.*
A brief overview for newly diagnosed patients. Includes questions to ask the doctor, tips on managing the illness, definitions of important terms, and Brain Tumor Society resources. Access at: ww.tbts.org

➤ CancerCare. *Brain Tumors: Current Treatment and Hope for the Future.*
This short booklet with color photographs and illustrations focuses on new treatments and medications for brain tumors. Includes frequently asked questions, a short glossary, and a list of resources. Access at: www.cancercare.org

➤ National Cancer Institute. *What You Need to Know about Brain Tumors.*
This booklet on brain tumors discusses possible causes, symptoms, diagnosis, treatment, emotional issues, and questions to ask the doctor. Includes a glossary of terms and other resources. Access at: https://cissecure.nci.nih.gov/ncipubs/

Books

➤ Segal, Gail, and American Brain Tumor Association. 2002. *Dictionary for Brain Tumor Patients.* Des Plaines, IL: American Brain Tumor Association. This dictionary contains short definitions of terms the patient with a brain tumor is likely to hear or read. In addition to medical terms the dictionary includes lists of medical abbreviations, prefixes, roots, and suffixes that can help a layperson understand medical lingo, as well as useful measurement tables. Available at the ABTA site www.abta.org.

➤ Stark-Vance, Virginia, and M. L. Dubay. 2004. *100 Questions and Answers about Brain Tumors*. Sudbury, MA: Jones and Bartlett.
Detailed information about brain tumors presented in an easy-to-read question-and-answer format. Terms are explained on the sidebar, and the book includes lists of Web sites, organizations, literature, and resources on general and specific topics related to brain tumors. This book was co–authored by a neurooncologist and a brain tumor survivor.

➤ Zeltzer, Paul M. 2004. *Brain Tumors: Leaving the Garden of Eden: A Survival Guide to Diagnosis, Learning the Basics, Getting Organized and Finding Your Medical Team*. Encino, CA: Shilysca Press.
This 400-page comprehensive reference guide for people living with a brain tumor was authored by a renowned neuro-oncologist. The book starts with the basics about brain tumors and advises readers on finding a good medical team, getting a second opinion, and using the Internet to search for information. The text includes chapters on all major types of brain tumors as well as brain metastases of other cancers. The chapter about medications explains how to deal with side effects and avoid drug interactions of drugs used for pain control, seizures, fatigue, and brain swelling.

Audiovisual Resources

➤ Patient Education Institute. *Brain Cancer Interactive Tutorial*. Access at: www.medlineplus.gov and click on: "Interactive Tutorials," then select from a list.
This slide show utilizes illustrations, sound, and animations to provide basic, easy-to-understand explanations of brain anatomy, primary and metastatic tumors, and the most common therapies. It is possible to turn on a voice-over or print a text version.

Web Resources

Sites focusing on brain and spinal cord tumors

➤ American Brain Tumor Association. Access at: www.abta.org
This organization offers information and support services for people diagnosed with brain tumors. The "Tumor Information" section offers tumor-specific information as well as Adobe Acrobat (.pdf) files of two premier publications: *A Primer of Brain Tumors: A Patient's Reference Manual* and *Dictionary for Brain Tumor Patients*. Both publications are updated periodically and sent to patients and families free of charge. The "Care and Support" section provides information about living with a brain tumor and coping with emotional and physical challenges.

➤ The Brain Tumor Society Online. Access at: www.tbts.org
This site is provided for the entire brain tumor community, from newly diagnosed patients to survivors, families, and health care professionals. The "Patients Resources" section provides detailed medical information including pathology, nutrition, and lay-language summaries of published professional articles. This site also includes information about support services for patients and families and downloadable files of brochures and fact sheets published by the Brain Tumor Society. The book *Color Me Hope: A Resource Guide for People Affected by Brain Tumors* is the premier publication covering medical as well as employment and financial matters.

➤ Musella Foundation For Brain Tumor Research Information. *Clinical Trials & Noteworthy Treatments for Brain Tumors.* Access at: www.virtualtrials.com
At the heart of this site is a comprehensive database of clinical trials for brain tumors. The site also includes a 48-page brain tumor guide for the newly diagnosed, which is downloadable as an Adobe Acrobat (.pdf) file; lay-term summaries of published studies, medical news, an online dictionary, and many interactive features. The extensive video library featuring brain tumor experts discussing various treatments is especially interesting.

➤ National Brain Tumor Foundation (NBTF). Access at: www.braintumor.org
This site presents information regarding treatment options and community resources for brain tumor patients and families. Features include a database of questions answered by health professionals, a link library arranged by topic, and a treatment center database. Adobe Acrobat (.pdf) files of publications such as fact sheets and brochures are available, including *The Essential Guide to Brain Tumors*, a comprehensive 80-page booklet that covers symptoms, treatments, brain anatomy, and survivorship.

Detailed sections in general cancer sites

➤ American Cancer Society. *Learn about Brain/CNS Tumors in Adults.* Access at: www.cancer.org and select from the menu under "Choose a Cancer Type or Topic." A detailed guide about the topic can be printed as an Adobe Acrobat (.pdf) file.

➤ National Cancer Institute. *Brain Tumors.* Access at: www.cancer.gov and click on "Types of Cancer." The top page of the section links to patient versions of PDQ® statements on specific tumor types, clinical-trials information, and other NCI publications on this topic.

➤ People Living with Cancer. *Brain Tumor.* Access at: www.plwc.org and click on "Cancer Type." The PLWC oncologist-approved guides may be printed in their entirety or by subtopic.

Sections about brain tumors are also available at the following sites:

➤ Cancerbackup. Access at: www.cancerbackup.org.uk/Home and click on "Cancer Types."

➤ Canadian Cancer Society. Access at: www.cancer.ca and click on "About Cancer."

➤ CancerSource.com. Access at: www.cancersource.com/Patient.pg and make a selection from the "Diagnosis & Treatment" pull-down menu.

➤ Cancerconsultants.com. Access at: www.cancerconsultants.com and make a selection under "Links to Specific Cancer type Information."

➤ OncologyChannel.com. Access at: www.oncologychannel.com and select a condition from the left sidebar.

Patient Support Organization

➤ American Brain Tumor Association. Access at: www.abta.org
Patient Line: 800-886-2282

➤ The Brain Tumor Society. Access at: www.tbts.org
Phone: 800-770-8287

➤ National Brain Tumor Foundation (NBTF). Access at: www.braintumor.org
Phone: 800-934-CURE

Breast Cancer

Anatomical facts: The breasts are a pair of glands capable of producing milk for nursing babies. These organs have a complex structure made of lobules, ducts, and fatty connective tissue. The lobules are small glands that produce milk; the ducts are thin, hollow tubes that deliver the milk from the lobules to the nipple, which is located in the center of a dark area of skin called the areola. Fat and ligament tissue fill the spaces between the lobules and ducts. The breasts also contain blood vessels and lymphatic vessels that drain lymphatic fluid to lymph nodes.

Illustrations available at the Medical Illustrations Gallery of the People Living with Cancer Web site.
Access at: www.plwc.org and click on Library on the left sidebar.

Breast cancer is the most common cancer among women in the United States. Approximately 180,000 new cases of invasive breast cancer and 60,000 cases of noninvasive breast cancer are diagnosed every year. Men also can develop breast cancer, but the great majority of people with breast cancer are women (for more on male breast cancer, see below on page 64). Breast cancer is the second leading cause of cancer death among American women after lung cancer. Death rates have been declining in the past few decades, probably because of earlier detection and improved treatment. Wide use of regular mammograms, which can detect breast lumps before they can be felt in a physical exam, has contributed greatly to the improvement in cure rates.

Breast cancer is one of the few cancers for which specific inherited genetic mutations have been identified as causes. The most common mutations occur on the BRCA1 and BRCA2 genes, but other genetic mutations have been identified as well. For information on breast cancer genetics, please refer to the cancer genetics section in Chapter 6 of this book (p. 223). Only 5% to 10% of breast cancers occur among women who inherited an abnormal gene. Another risk factor for breast cancer is exposure to estrogen; women with a long menstrual history (women who started to menstruate at an early age and/or stopped menstruating at a late age), women who have never had children, and women taking hormone replacement therapy (HRT) after menopause have an increased risk. Obese women have a higher risk because their bodies produce more estrogen than normal-weight women. Women who have had previous breast biopsies, previous breast cancer, and previous radiation therapy to the chest area also have a higher risk.

Most breast tumors develop in the ducts, and some develop in the lobules. Ductal and lobular carcinomas are the most common cell types. Breast cancer is divided into two major groups: noninvasive and invasive (infiltrating). The noninvasive types are ductal carcinoma in situ (DCIS) and lobular carcinoma in situ (LCIS). In both these conditions, the malignant cells are confined to the lobules or ducts and have not spread into the connective tissue of the breast or lymph nodes. DCIS tumors may become invasive if left untreated. Surgery in combination with radiation therapy is the standard care for DCIS and has very high cure rates. LCIS is not considered a true cancer because it does not turn into invasive cancer, but women with a history of LCIS have a higher risk of developing an invasive breast cancer in both breasts and need to be monitored closely.

More than 80% of invasive breast cancers are invasive ductal carcinomas (IDC). About 10% are invasive lobular carcinomas (ILC). The rest are rare types such as medullary carcinoma, colloid carcinoma, mucinous carcinoma, and tubular carcinoma. These rare types have a slightly better prognosis than IDC or ILC, but all invasive breast cancers are treated in a similar manner according to stage. Inflammatory breast cancer (IBC) is a rare subtype of invasive breast cancer that has a high likelihood of spreading and a worse prognosis than invasive ductal or lobular cancers. Paget's disease of the nipple is another rare type of breast cancer that starts in the ducts and spreads to the skin of the nipple and areola. In many cases, patients with

Paget's disease also have a carcinoma in situ or an invasive tumor inside the breast. Phyllodes tumor is a rare type of sarcoma that develops in the connective tissue of the breast. It is treated differently than invasive breast cancer. Overall, breast cancers that are diagnosed in an early stage are highly curable.

Men's breast tissue is less developed than women's and contains a much smaller number of ducts, and only a few, if any, lobules. Cancer may develop in the male breast, but it is very rare; only 1,700 men are diagnosed each year in the United States. Eighty to ninety percent of male breast cancers are invasive ductal carcinomas, and the rest are DCIS. Very few rare cancers such as inflammatory breast cancer and Paget's disease of the nipple have been seen in men, but lobular breast cancer has never been diagnosed in males. Treatment approaches for male and female breast cancer are similar.

There are many treatment approaches in breast cancer. All invasive breast cancer patients are treated with surgery in order to remove the cancerous tumor. Most patients also receive radiation and/or chemotherapy. About two-thirds of breast cancers are dependent on estrogen and respond well to hormonal therapy that reduces the level of estrogen in the body or blocks its effect. The drug Herceptin slows the progression of tumors that express a high level of the HER2/neu protein. About one-third of breast tumors have too much of this protein that promotes the growth and spread of the malignant cells.

The variety of treatment approaches means that many patients are presented with treatment options and will seek information to help them make informed decisions. Following are a few topics that require patients to make decisions:

Surgery: Some women can choose between a lumpectomy, which is the removal of the lump with a surrounding margin of normal tissue, or a mastectomy, which is the removal of the entire breast. A lumpectomy, also called breast-conserving surgery, is typically followed by radiation, which may not be needed after mastectomy. Women treated with a mastectomy need to decide if and when to reconstruct the breast and what method of reconstruction to use.

Hormonal Therapy: Hormonal therapy is recommended for women with hormone-sensitive breast cancer. The drug most commonly used is Tamoxifen, which is taken in pill form for a period of five years. This drug does have side effects, and many women seek information to help them assess its benefit for their particular situation. A new class of drugs called aromatase inhibitors has been proven to be as effective as Tamoxifen for postmenopausal women, hence librarians may be asked for information to help women decide between taking Tamoxifen or taking one of the aromatase inhibitors.

The American Cancer Society estimates that approximately 2 million women in the United States have a history of breast cancer. This population has many and diverse information needs that include medical, emotional, and practical issues. Some survivors struggle with long-term side effects of treatment. One troublesome side effect that may occur after removal of lymph nodes and radiation therapy is lymphedema, which is excessive swelling of the arms. This topic is discussed in detail in Chapter 8 (p. 277). A subset of breast cancer survivors, women who were diagnosed before age 40, struggle with early onset of menopause and fertility issues. Another group that has specific information needs are healthy women who have a high risk for breast cancer. These women may seek information on genetic counseling, lifestyle changes, and hormonal therapy for breast cancer prevention.

Information Sources

Brochures, Booklets and Other Short Print Publications

➤ BreastCancer.org. *Your Guide to Breast Cancer Treatment.*
This booklet focuses on treatment options including surgery, radiation therapy, chemotherapy hormone therapy, immune therapy, and experimental therapies. Access at: www.breastcancer.org/booklet_intro.html
Other publications available on this site are: *Your Guide to the Breast Cancer Pathology Report* (available also in Spanish) and *Overcoming Your Fears of Breast Cancer Treatment.*
➤ National Cancer Institute. *Surgery Choices for Women with Early-Stage Breast Cancer.*
This publication has useful information for women faced with a decision between having a breast-spring surgery (lumpectomy) and surgery that removes the whole breast (mastectomy). It includes a comparison table and a list of questions for the doctor. Access at: https://cissecure.nci.nih.gov/ncipubs/
➤ National Cancer Institute. *What You Need to Know about Breast Cancer.*
A concise introduction to breast cancer covering staging and treatment options, emotional support, and a list of questions for the doctor. Access at: https://cissecure.nci.nih.gov/ncipubs/
➤ National Comprehensive Cancer Network (NCCN). *Breast Cancer: Treatment Guidelines for Patients.*
Overview of breast cancer as well as treatment decision "trees" explaining the treatment choices for different stages and conditions in breast cancer. This resource is developed from the NCCN Clinical Practice Guidelines in Oncology™—the standard for clinical policy in cancer care. A Spanish-language version also is available. Access at: www.nccn.org/patients/
➤ Singletary, S. Eva, and Alice F. Judkins. 2005. *Breast Cancer: Myths and Facts: What You Need to Know.* 4th ed. Manhasset, NY: Oncology Pub. Group of CMP Healthcare Media.

This 64-page handbook with a detailed overview of breast cancer includes many color illustrations and photographs. The sidebar features facts that dispel common myths about breast cancer and repeat key points. Includes a list of resources, a glossary, and a step-by-step guide for breast self-exam with photographs. The authors are a breast surgeon and an advanced-practice nurse from M. D. Anderson Cancer Center. To view online, download an Adobe Acrobat (.pdf) file, or order access at: www.cancernetwork.com.

➤ Y-ME. *Every Woman's Guide to Breast Cancer.*
This booklet was designed for newly diagnosed women and covers the treatment options as well as coping, intimacy, reconstruction and prosthesis decisions, lifestyle, and practical matters. Other Y-ME publications address issues such as living with advanced breast cancer, reading the pathology report, tumor markers, fatigue, and more. Access at: www.y-me. org and click on "Y-ME Publications." Some publications available in Spanish.

Periodicals

➤ *MAMM* (ISSN 1099-563)
This publication is geared to women with breast and gynecological cancers. It offers news and in-depth articles about medical and survivorship issues. Professional writers who interview reputable cancer physicians write the articles. *MAMM* is indexed in CINHAL, and information on subscription can be found on the Web site at: www.mamm.com. Access to content is available online for a fee.

Books

➤ American Cancer Society. 2004. *Breast Cancer Journey: Your Personal Guidebook.* 2d ed. Atlanta: American Cancer Society.
A step-by-step guide through the emotional and physical aspects of the breast cancer experience, from the moment of diagnosis to thinking about the future. The text includes quotes from women living with breast cancer, tips on managing the emotions, reactions and side effects, and a special section aimed at family, friends, and caregivers. Many of the topics include questions to ask the medical team. An extensive resource section at the end of the book includes national and local organizations.

➤ Breast Cancer Support Group of the Penn State Milton S. Hershey Medical Center. 2004. *Show Me: A Photo Collection of Breast Cancer Survivors' Lumpectomies, Mastectomies, Breast Reconstruction and Thoughts on Body Image.* 3d ed. Hershey, PA: Milton S. Hershey Medical Center.
A visual resource book presenting color photographs of thirty breast

cancer survivors showing the choices they made about breast reconstruction. The goal was to enable newly diagnosed women to see in color the lumpectomy, mastectomy, and reconstruction scars of women of different sizes, shapes, ages, and skin colors. Comments provided by the women and some of the significant others provide an intimate look at their decision-making process, their relationships, and their feelings about what is most important in their lives. To order and see a few of the testimonials, access: www.hmc.psu.edu/womens/showme/testimonials.htm

➤ Brown, Zora. 2007. *100 Questions and Answers about Breast Cancer*. 2d ed. Sudbury, MA: Jones and Bartlett Publishers, 2007.

Detailed information about breast cancer is presented in an easy-to-read question-and-answer format. Terms are explained in the sidebar, and the book includes lists of Web sites, organizations, literature, and resources on topics that may be of interest to women with breast cancer. This book was co–authored by Zora Brown, a breast cancer advocate; Harold P. Freeman, M.D., a breast cancer surgeon; and Elizabeth Platt, a medical and scientific writer.

➤ Chan, David. 2006. *Breast Cancer: Real Questions, Real Answers*. New York: Marlowe & Company.

A comprehensive overview of breast cancer is presented in a question-and-answer format accompanied by many black-and-white illustrations and tables. The sections on chemotherapy and hormonal therapy are very detailed. Lifestyle and supportive-care issues include many practical suggestions. The author is an experienced breast cancer specialist who also presents real-life situations faced by his patients.

➤ Elk, Ronit. 2003. *Breast Cancer for Dummies*. New York: Wiley.

This comprehensive and detailed book is rich in graphical elements, such as bold headings, bullet points, icons, illustrations, and tables, that may help comprehension. The first chapter discusses adjusting and coming to grips with a breast cancer diagnosis. Additional chapters cover diagnostic procedures, prognosis and treatment options, undergoing treatment, and life after treatment. The last chapter provides a list of the ten best hospitals for breast cancer treatment and a list of the best resources. This book was co–authored by Ronit Elk, a psychologist and scientific program director at the American Cancer Society, and Monica Morrow M.D., director of the Lynn Sage Breast Center at Northwestern Memorial Hospital in Chicago.

➤ Kaelin, Carolyn M. 2005. *Living through Breast Cancer: What a Harvard Doctor and Survivor Wants You to Know about Getting the Best Care While Preserving Your Self-Image*. New York: McGraw-Hill.

This book was written from the unique perspective of a breast cancer surgeon who was diagnosed with the disease. It is divided into three parts: the first explains the medical management of breast cancer; the second focuses on body image, appearance, reconstruction options, and hair and mouth care; and the third covers nutrition, exercise, menopause, fertility, and sexuality. Includes a list of resources, photographs, and illustrations.

➤ Lange, Vladimir. 2005. *Be a Survivor: Your Guide to Breast Cancer Treatment*. 3d ed. Los Angeles: Lange Productions.

This book is rich with color illustrations and photographs as well as comments from patients and partners that bring the breast cancer experience to life. Written by a physician whose wife was treated for breast cancer, the book includes a separate section addressed to partners of women with breast cancer. Includes a glossary, a resource section, and a list of questions to ask health care professionals. The book is accompanied by a free DVD.

➤ Love, Susan. 2005. *Dr. Susan Love's Breast Book*. 4th ed. rev. Cambridge, MA: Da Capo Press.

This fourth edition of the book by this highly respected breast cancer surgeon offers a comprehensive overview of breast health, including common benign conditions. The majority of the book focuses on breast cancer, and every aspect of the disease is covered in great detail suitable for sophisticated readers. Includes a list of drugs used in breast cancer treatment, a list of NCI-designated cancer centers by state, and a pathology checklist.

Audiovisual Resources

➤ Bosom Buddies. 2001. *Partners in Hope: A Man's Guide to Women's Breast Cancer*. Chicago: Bosom Buddies.

This program looks at breast cancer from a man's point of view. Couples who have faced the illness and its related issues discuss how they experienced this serious challenge. Additionally, experts in the field of family and couples counseling bring perspective and offer advice to men and couples about methods for coping with breast cancer. Available in VHS and DVD.

➤ Bosom Buddies. 1998. *Woman to Woman: Breast Cancer and Reconstruction Options*. Chicago: Bosom Buddies.

Breast cancer survivors share their insights about reconstruction choices they made after mastectomy. Includes medical animation of a number of procedures, including lumpectomy, tissue expanders, saline and silicone implants, and tissue flap procedures. Available in VHS and DVD formats.

➤ Bosom Buddies. 2003. *Will Mom Be OK? Families Talk About Breast Cancer.* Chicago: Bosom Buddies.

Child/family counseling experts discuss family communications during and after the treatment, managing the daily routine, and recognizing a child's distress signals. Children and parents share their stories and insights. Available in VHS and DVD formats.

➤ Information Television Network. 2005. *Breast Cancer: Early Detection.* Boca Raton, FL: Information Television Network (30 min.). Available in DVD and VHS formats. Access at: www.itvisus.com or Amazon.com

Part of the public television series *Healthy Body/Healthy Mind,* this episode features cancer specialists explaining how digital mammograms help detect breast cancer in its earliest form. Also highlighted are new treatments and targeted therapies that improve survival rates and quality of life. The program also features breast cancer patients and color graphics and animations that illustrate the scientific content.

➤ Patient Education Institute. *Breast Cancer Interactive Tutorial.* Access at: www.medlineplus.gov and click on "Interactive Tutorials," then select from a list.

This slideshow utilizes illustrations, sound, and animations to provide basic, easy-to-understand explanations of breast anatomy, breast cancer staging, surgery, and adjuvant treatment. It is possible to turn on a voice-over or print a text version.

➤ WomenStories. 2001. *Psychosocial Video Series.* Buffalo, NY: WomenStories.

Each 15–20-minute program addresses a specific issue from the perspective of breast cancer survivors, who share their experiences and what they have learned from them. Topics include initial discovery and diagnosis, intimacy, young women and breast cancer, surgical choices, chemotherapy, family support, recurrence and metastasis, hormone treatment, radiation, and life after breast cancer. Available in VHS and DVD formats. May be purchases together or separately and viewed free online at: www.womenstories.org

Web Resources

Sites focusing on breast cancer

➤ Breastcancer.org. Access at: www.breastcancer.org

This site offers a wealth of information about every aspect of breast cancer. Topics are explained in a very thorough and detailed manner. Special features include an extensive talking dictionary with terms read by celebrities, ask-the-expert online conferences and transcripts, and monthly reports summarizing research news. The site also has a large community section where users can interact with other users or with breast cancer experts.

Breastcancer.org is headed by Dr. Marisa Weiss, a Philadelphia oncologist, and has an impressive list of breast cancer specialists on the medical advisory board.

➤ Living Beyond Breast Cancer. Access at: www.lbbc.org
Living Beyond Breast Cancer is an organization that provides education and support for breast cancer survivors. The site focuses on news concerning breast cancer treatment and clinical trials. News stories and articles along with recordings and transcripts of educational events are presented, as well as information about LBBC support services and events.

➤ Michigan Breast Reconstruction Outcome Study (MBROS). *Consumer Guide to Breast Reconstruction*. Access at: www.lifehealth.net/breastrecon.htm
The purpose of this site is to help women facing breast surgery decide if they want to have breast reconstruction, when to have the reconstruction, and what kind of reconstruction would be the best for them. Detailed explanations of the different options are provided along with photos, illustrations, and a comparison chart. It is possible to download the entire content of the site as an Adobe Acrobat (.pdf) file. Dr. Edwin Wilkins, a plastic surgeon from the University of Michigan, developed the content.

➤ Susan G. Komen Foundation. Access at: www.komen.org
The site of this important breast cancer advocacy organization contains an enormous amount of information about the foundation and about breast cancer. Linking to "About Breast Cancer" takes the user to the main page, which further links to information about diagnosis and treatment, risk factors and screening, and a host of other topics such as complementary therapies, life after treatment, and quality medical care. The site contains many interactive tools and downloadable educational materials. A multimedia library features innovative audiovisual programs covering a variety of topics, such as early detection and screening, reducing your risk, diagnosis, and new treatment advances. Also in Spanish.

➤ Susanlovemd.com. Access at: www.susanlovemd.com
The author of *Dr. Susan Love's Breast Book* (described above) is also one of the "founding mothers" of the breast cancer advocacy movement and founder of this Web site. The information is designed to assist women in making treatment decisions, dealing with the changes and challenges brought on by breast cancer, and improving their general health. An extensive section of frequently asked questions (FAQs) is organized by topics and presents expert answers to hundreds of questions.

➤ Y-ME National Breast Cancer Organization. Access at: www.y-me.org
Y-ME is a national organization supporting and empowering women who have breast cancer. The extensive site enables users to locate programs,

support services, and events. It also includes broad information about breast cancer diagnosis, treatment, coping, and quality-of-life issues. A Spanish-language version is available.

Detailed sections in general cancer sites

➤ American Cancer Society. *Learn about Breast Cancer* and *Learn about Male Breast Cancer.* Access at: www.cancer.org and select from the menu under "Choose a Cancer Type or Topic." Disease-specific detailed guides can be printed as a Adobe Acrobat (.pdf) files.

➤ Healthology. *Breast Cancer.* Access at: www.healthology.com and click on "Consumer Health Library." This site offers detailed articles, Webcasts, and transcripts featuring cancer professionals.

➤ National Cancer Institute. *Breast Cancer.* Access at: www.cancer.gov and click on "Types of Cancer." The top page of the section links to patient versions of PDQ® statements, clinical trial information, and other NCI publications on this topic.

➤ People Living with Cancer. *Breast Cancer* and *Breast, Male.* Access at: www.plwc.org and click on "Cancer Type." The PLWC oncologist-approved breast cancer guide may be printed in its entirety or by subtopic.

Sections about breast cancer are also available at the following sites

➤ Canadian Cancer Society. Access at: www.cancer.ca and click on "About Cancer."

➤ Cancerbackup. Access at: www.cancerbackup.org.uk/Home and click on "Cancer Types."

➤ Cancerconsultants.com. Access at: www.cancerconsultants.com and make a selection under "Links to Specific Cancer Type Information."

➤ CancerSource.com. Access at: www.cancersource.com/Patient.pg and make a selection from the "Diagnosis & Treatment" pull-down menu.

➤ OncologyChannel.com. Access at: www.oncologychannel.com and select a condition from the left sidebar.

Patient-Support Organizations

➤ Living Beyond Breast Cancer
Survivors' helpline: 888-753-5222

➤ The Susan G. Komen Breast Cancer Foundation
National toll-free breast care helpline: 800-462-9273

➤ Y-ME National Breast Cancer Organization
Phone: 800-221-2141 (English); 800-986-9505 (Spanish)
Staffed 24 hours, 7 days a week

Cervical Cancer

Anatomical facts: The cervix is part of a woman's reproductive system. It is the lower, narrow part of the uterus that connects the uterus to the vagina. The cervix produces mucus that helps sperm move from the vagina into the uterus. During childbirth, the cervix dilates to allow the baby to pass through the vagina.

Illustrations available at the Medical Illustrations Gallery of the People Living with Cancer Web site.

Access at: www.plwc.org and click on Library on the left sidebar.

Cervical cancer may be the first cancer to be prevented with a vaccine. In 2006, the FDA approved the use of a new vaccine that prevents infection from two types of the human papillomavirus (HPV) that are responsible for about 70% of the cases of cervical cancer worldwide. Clinical trials demonstrated that it was nearly 100% effective in preventing precancerous cervical changes caused by HPV.

Up until the 1950s, cervical cancer killed more women than any other cancer in the United States. Death rates have dropped dramatically, by more than 70%, since the widespread implementation of Pap smear exams. The Pap smear test consists of removing cells from a woman's cervix with a swab and examining the cells under a microscope. This simple test, which can be performed by a clinician during a woman's annual physical exam, can detect precancerous changes in the cervix called cervical intraepithelial neoplasia (CIN). Left untreated, precancerous changes may bring about the formation of a cancerous tumor in the cervix. The American Cancer Society estimates 11,000 new cases of cervical cancers per year in the United States and 3,700 deaths (before implementation of the new vaccine). Fifty percent of cervical cancer cases are discovered in women between the ages of 35 and 55, but this cancer occurs in older women as well; about 20% of cases are diagnosed in women over 65.

The vast majority of cervical cancers are caused by HPVs. HPVs are a class of over 100 common viruses transmitted through sexual contact. Most adults have been infected with HPV at some time in their life. Only a few specific strains of HPV are associated with cervical cancer, and most women infected with HPVs will never develop cervical cancer. Women who had many sexual partners or had sex with a partner that had multiple partners may be at higher risk for cervical cancer. Other factors that increase risk are smoking and having many full-term pregnancies. Lack of regular pap tests is a huge risk factor. Most new diagnoses occur among women who have not been screened, many of whom are of low socioeconomic status and lack access to medical care.

There are two main types of cervical cancer: approximately 85% are squamous cell carcinomas, and the remaining 15% are adenocarcinomas. Both types have similar prognosis and are treated similarly.

Some preinvasive and early-stage tumors can be treated with minor surgical procedures that destroy only the cancerous tissue while preserving the cervix. Most early-stage cancers are treated with a simple hysterectomy, which includes the removal of the uterus and cervix. Sometimes it is possible to treat early-stage tumors without surgery, utilizing radiation therapy alone. Treatment options for advanced-stage tumors include surgery, radiation therapy, and chemotherapy. The surgical procedure to treat advanced cervical cancer is a radical hysterectomy, which is the removal of the cervix, uterus, and the upper part of the vagina. In some cases, the removal of the ovaries, fallopian tubes, or pelvic lymph nodes may be necessary as well. Cancers that have spread to distant organs are treated with chemotherapy and/or radiation therapy, with the goal of alleviating symptoms and improving quality of life.

Premenopausal women who are treated with a radical hysterectomy that includes the removal of the ovaries experience early onset of menopause and lose the ability to become pregnant. These women may ask for information on treating menopausal symptoms and side effects, on sexuality, and on fertility.

Information Sources

Brochures, Booklets, and Other Short Print Publications

➤ Gynecologic Cancer Foundation. *Understanding Cervical Cancer: A Woman's Guide.*
   This overview of cervical cancer covering mainly treatment options and quality-of-life issues, including fatigue, work life, relationships, and intimacy, offers tips for talking with the treatment team and a resource list. Access at: www.thegcf.org.

➤ National Cancer Institute. *What You Need to Know about Cancer of the Cervix.*
   A concise introduction to cervical cancer covering staging, treatment options, and emotional issues. Includes a glossary and a list of questions for the doctor. Access at: https://cissecure.nci.nih.gov/ncipubs/

Book Chapters

➤ Hartmann, Lynn C., and Charles L. Loprinzi. 2005. *Mayo Clinic Guide to Women's Cancers.* Rochester, MN: Mayo Clinic.
   This book was edited by two physicians from the Mayo Clinic, and book chapters have been written and reviewed by Mayo Clinic experts. Part two of the book focuses on gynecologic cancer, with a few chapters on cervical

cancer. The third part of the book, "Living with Cancer," provides supportive care information that is relevant to all women with cancer. A unique feature of this book is the visual guide that includes color illustrations explaining the cancer process, anatomical facts, surgery, and radiation. Other photos and illustrations, tables, and text boxes throughout the text help in understanding and comprehension.

➤ McGinn, Kerry Anne, and Pamela J. Haylock. 2003. *Women's Cancers: How to Prevent Them, How to Treat Them, How to Beat Them.* 3d ed., fully updated ed. Alameda, CA: Hunter House.
This book provides practical information for women with cancer and includes a chapter about cervical cancer. Other chapters discuss working with the medical team, sources of support, complementary and alternative treatments, and feelings. The part called "Life after Cancer" focuses on the physical, emotional, and social challenges women may experience after treatment ends. The authors are oncology nurses.

Web Resources

Sites focusing on cervical cancer

➤ National Cervical Cancer Coalition. Access at: http://www.nccc-online. org/
This site has information relevant to women with, or at risk for, cervical cancer and HPV disease. It contains many articles written by health professionals about screening for, treatment for, and living with cervical cancer. The site includes information about outreach events, conferences, and support services for patients and caregivers. Links to other sites of interest and information in Spanish also are available.

➤ Women's Cancer Network. Access at: www.wcn.org
This site is provided by the Gynecologic Cancer Foundation, which is affiliated with the Society of Gynecologic Oncologists. Detailed information about cancer in women, including reproductive cancer is included. Special features provide an extensive news section; a "Find a Doctor" database, which helps locate oncologists specializing in gynecologic cancers; and links to clinical trial databases.

Detailed sections in general cancer sites

➤ American Cancer Society. *Learn about Cervical Cancer.* Access at: www. cancer.org and select from the menu under "Choose a Cancer Topic." A detailed guide about cervical cancer can be printed by section or as an Adobe Acrobat (.pdf) file.

➤ National Cancer Institute. *Cervical Cancer.* Access at: www.cancer.gov and click on "Types of Cancer." The top page of the section links to patient versions of PDQ® statements, clinical trial information, and other NCI publications on this topic.

➤ People Living with Cancer. *Cervical Cancer.* Access at: www.plwc.org and click on "Cancer Type." The PLWC oncologist-approved cervical cancer guide can be printed in its entirety or by subtopic.

Sections about cervical cancer are also available at the following sites:

➤ Canadian Cancer Society. Access at: www.cancer.ca and click on "About Cancer."

➤ Cancerbackup. Access at: www.cancerbackup.org.uk/Home and click on "Cancer Types."

➤ Cancerconsultants.com. Access at: www.cancerconsultants.com and make a selection under "Links to Specific Cancer Type Information."

➤ CancerSource.com. Access at: www.cancersource.com/Patient.pg and make a selection from the "Diagnosis & Treatment" pull-down menu.

➤ OncologyChannel.com. Access at: www.oncologychannel.com and select a condition from the left sidebar.

Patient-Support Organizations

➤ EyesOnThePrize.org
An online support group for gynecologic cancer survivors. Access at: www.eyesontheprize.org

Colon and Rectal Cancer

Anatomical facts: The colon and rectum are parts of the digestive system. They form a long, muscular tube called the large intestine (also called the large bowel). The colon is the first four-to-five feet of the large intestine, and the rectum is the last four-to-five inches. Partly digested food enters the colon from the small intestine. The colon removes water and nutrients from the food and stores the rest as waste. The waste passes from the colon into the rectum and then out of the body through the anus.

Illustrations available at the Medical Illustrations Gallery of the People Living with Cancer Web site.

Access at: www.plwc.org and click on Library on the left sidebar.

Even though the colon and rectum are two separate organs, most of the cancers found in these structures are of the adenocarcinoma type, thus they are sometimes called "colorectal cancer," and information on both types is usually presented together. Most colorectal cancer information sources focus on adenocarcinomas and may not include information about carcinoid tumors, stromal tumors, or lymphomas which rarely affect the colon or rectum.

Colorectal cancer is the fourth most common cancer in men and women in the United States. The American Cancer Society estimates approximately 110,000 new diagnoses of colon cancer and 41,000 new diagnoses of rectal cancer per year. The average age at diagnosis is mid-60s. The exact cause for this cancer has not been found; however, a few risk factors have been identified. Studies have shown that a diet high in fat and low in vegetable consumption may increase the risk for colorectal cancer. Three percent of colorectal cancer patients have one of the two known genetic mutations that greatly increase a person's chance to develop colorectal cancer. People with a history of benign polyps called adenomas and people with a history of inflammatory bowel diseases such as colitis or Crohn's disease have a higher risk of developing colorectal cancer. People with a family history of the disease have a higher risk even if they do not have one of the known genetic mutations.

Colorectal cancer is one of the few cancers to have an effective screening method, called colonoscopy. Most colon cancers develop from benign polyps called adenomas. Examining the colon through a long lighted tube called a colonoscope enables finding and removing these polyps before they turn into cancerous tumors. The American Cancer Society recommends colon cancer screening for every person over 50 years old, or younger if they have one of the known risk factors listed above.

Treatment decisions on colorectal cancer depend on staging, which is determined by the size of the tumor, its location, and how far it has spread. Tumors that affect only the inner layer of the colon or rectum are treated only with surgery and have a very high cure rate. As the tumors spread deeper into the colon or rectal wall and to lymph nodes and neighboring organs, the survival rate decreases and more extensive treatment is needed.

Surgery is the main treatment method for colorectal cancer. The goal of surgery is to remove the sick part of the colon or rectum and maintain normal digestive flow and function. In some cases, however, the surgeon will have to create an opening in the abdomen, called a colostomy, in order to remove waste from the body. In most cases, the colostomy is temporary and would be closed when the colon heals, but for some people, especially those with a tumor in the lower rectum, the colonoscopy would be permanent.

Radiation therapy and/or chemotherapy are added after surgery for tumors that involve more than just the inner lining of the colon or rectal wall or when lymph nodes are affected. Chemotherapy is the treatment of choice in all cases of metastatic disease. The organ most affected when colorectal cancer spreads is the liver. To treat liver metastases, chemotherapy may be delivered directly to the liver through a catheter. This method of drug delivery is called hepatic artery infusion. Metastases can also be removed with open surgery or with minor surgical procedures depending on the extent and size of the tumors.

New therapies for treatment of colorectal cancer include targeted therapies that attempt to kill only the cancerous cells while avoiding healthy cells. Targeted therapies can be taken in pill form and seem to cause less side effects than does chemotherapy. Targeted therapies are usually given in combination with chemotherapy.

Nutrition is a major issue for colorectal cancer patients because treatment may cause many digestive side effects such as poor appetite, nausea, vomiting, diarrhea, or mouth sores. Colorectal cancer survivors that have a colostomy deal with issues related to body image, intimacy, and sexuality. In men, a certain type of surgery may cause nerve damage and impair sexual function.

Information Sources

Brochures, Booklets, and Other Short Print Publications

➤ CancerCare. *Advances in the Treatment of Colorectal Cancer.*
A review of new drug combinations and targeted treatments for colorectal cancer includes color illustrations, frequently asked questions, a glossary, and resources. Access at: www.cancercare.org/reading.html

➤ National Cancer Institute. *What You Need to Know about Cancer of the Colon and Rectum.*
A concise introduction to colorectal cancer that covers staging, treatment options, rehabilitation, nutrition, and emotional support. Includes a glossary. Access at: https://cissecure.nci.nih.gov/ncipubs/

➤ National Comprehensive Cancer Network (NCCN). *Colon and Rectal Cancer: Treatment Guidelines for Patients.*
This publication includes an overview of colon and rectal cancer as well as treatment decision "trees" explaining the treatment choices for different disease stages and conditions. Developed from the NCCN Clinical Practice Guidelines in Oncology, the standard for clinical policy in cancer care. A Spanish-language version also is available. Access at: www.nccn.org/patients/

➤ Pazdur, Richard, and Melanie E. Royce. 2004. *Myths and Facts about Colorectal Cancer: What You Need to Know.* 3d ed. New York: Oncology Group. Division of SCP Communications.

This 52-page handbook with a detailed overview of colorectal cancer includes many color illustrations and photographs. The sidebar features facts that dispel common myths about colorectal cancer and repeat key points. Includes a list of resources and a glossary. The authors are colorectal cancer specialists. To view online, download an Adobe Acrobat (.pdf) file or order access at: www.cancernetwork.com.

➤ The Wellness Community. *Frankly Speaking About New Discoveries in Cancer: Special Focus on Colorectal Cancer.*
This 36-page publication explains the newest advances in colorectal cancer treatment, how to manage side effects, how to be active in managing the disease, and communicating with the healthcare team. Access at: www.thewellnesscommunity.org

Books

➤ Bub, David S., Susannah Rose, and W. Douglas Wong. 2003. *100 Questions and Answers about Colorectal Cancer.* Boston: Jones and Bartlett.
Detailed information about colon and rectal cancer is presented in an accessible question-and-answer format. Terms are explained in the sidebar, and the book includes a list of Web sites, organizations, literature, and resources on general and specific topics related to colorectal cancer. This book was co–authored by two colorectal cancer specialists and an oncology social worker.

➤ Larson, Carol Ann. 2005. *Positive Options for Colorectal Cancer: Self-Help and Treatment.* Alameda, CA: Hunter House.
Presented from the perspective of a colon cancer survivor, this book follows the path of a person who received a colorectal cancer diagnosis, starting with a chapter called "Facing the Unknown" and moving to gathering information, working with medical professionals, dealing with feelings, making treatment decisions, possible complications after treatment, and survivorship. Positive stories of 12 colon cancer survivors help illustrate key points. Each chapter ends with a list of practical suggestions and tips.

➤ Levin, Bernard, et al. eds., 2006. *American Cancer Society's Complete Guide to Colorectal Cancer.* Rev. ed. Atlanta: American Cancer Society.
The American Cancer Society's all-inclusive guide to colorectal cancer takes a helpful, matter-of-fact approach to explaining risk factors and prevention, screening, diagnosis, symptom management, and treatment options. The book also explores such psychosocial issues as coping with emotions, relationships, and practical issues. Tips and stories from real people with colorectal cancer help personalize the topic.

➤ Metz, James M., and Margaret K. Hampshire. 2005. *OncoLink Patient Guide: Colorectal Cancer.* 2d ed. Philadelphia: Elsevier/Saunders.

This pocket book is the compilation of answers to questions submitted by cancer information seekers through the oncolink site to cancer experts at the University of Pennsylvania. The book covers prevention, screening, genetics, diagnostic tests, treatment methods including alternative therapies, and nutrition. Each answer is accompanied by a one-sentence highlight summarizing the key point.

➤ Pochapin, Mark Bennett. 2004. *What Your Doctor May Not Tell You about Colorectal Cancer: New Tests, New Treatments, New Hope.* New York: Warner Books.

The author, a colon cancer specialist and an early-screening advocate, devotes a large portion of this book to colorectal cancer prevention and screening—including nutrition, supplements, and chemoprevention of this disease. Other parts of the book are aimed at people who have already gotten a cancer diagnosis. It discusses different surgical procedures, chemotherapy drugs, and radiation treatment, as well as complementary therapies that may be beneficial.

➤ Ruggieri, Paul. 2001. *Colon and Rectal Cancer: A Patient's Guide to Treatment.* Omaha, NE: Addicus Books.

This easy-to-read overview of colon cancer covers the topic systematically, starting with anatomy and symptoms to emotional coping, basic treatments, and follow-up care. The author is a surgeon who provides clear explanations with black-and-white illustrations. Each chapter ends with a list of questions to ask the doctor, and the book includes a glossary and a list of resources.

Audiovisual Resources

➤ Patient Education Institute. *Colon Cancer Interactive Tutorial.* Access at: www.medlineplus.gov and click on: "Interactive Tutorials," then select from a list.

This slideshow utilizes illustrations, sound, and animations to provide basic, easy-to-understand explanations of the anatomy, diagnosis, and treatment options of colon cancer. It is possible to turn on a voice-over or print a text version.

➤ Patient Education Institute. *Colon Cancer Surgery Interactive Tutorial.* Access at: www.medlineplus.gov and click on "Interactive Tutorials," then select from a list.

This slideshow informs users on preparing and recovering from colon cancer surgery and includes color illustrations describing the surgical procedure.

➤ Information Television Network. 2005. *Advanced Colon Cancer*. Boca Raton, FL: Information Television Network. (30 min.). Available in DVD and VHS formats. Access at: www.itvisus.com or Amazon.com.
Part of the public television series *Healthy Body/Healthy Mind*, this program features cancer specialists discussing the ways to manage and control advanced colon cancer. The program also features patients and families coping with advanced colon cancer, as well as color graphics and animations that illustrate the scientific content.

➤ Information Television Network. 2005. *Colon Cancer*. Boca Raton, FL: Information Television Network (30 min.). Available in DVD and VHS formats. Access at: www.itvisus.com or Amazon.com.
Part of the public televisions series *Healthy Body/Healthy Mind*, this program features cancer specialists explaining how colon cancer is graded and detailing the new treatment advances for this disease. The program also introduces patients and families living with colon cancer and features color graphics and animations that illustrate the scientific content.

➤ Information Television Network. 2005. *Colon Cancer: Early Detection*. Boca Raton, FL: Information Television Network. (30 min.). Available in DVD and VHS formats. Access at: www.itvisus.com or Amazon.com
Part of the public televisions series *Healthy Body/Healthy Mind*, this program features cancer specialists explaining how colon cancer develops, who is at risk, and the importance of early detection that, in many cases, can actually prevent colon cancer or improve survival if cancer is already present. The program also introduces patients and families living with colon cancer and features color graphics and animations that illustrate the scientific content.

Web Resources

Sites focusing on colon and rectal cancer

➤ Colon Cancer Alliance. Access at: www.ccalliance.org
The Colon Cancer Alliance (CCA) is a national patient advocacy organization dedicated to ending the suffering caused by colorectal cancer. The site offers extensive information relevant to people affected by this disease, including disease information, symptoms, screening, and genetics. The news section follows new developments in treatment, genetics, clinical trials, prevention, and screening. The site also includes information about support services for patients and families

➤ Colorectal Cancer Coalition. Access at: www.fightcolorectalcancer.org
Detailed information accompanied by color illustrations is accessible by

clicking on the link "For Patients." Easy-to-read summaries discuss prevention, screening, diagnosis, treatment, and drugs. Users may also access a clinical trials matching service and links to other organizations offering support to people with colorectal cancer.

➤ Colorectal Cancer Network. Access at: www.colorectal-cancer.net/
The purpose of this site is to assist people with colorectal cancer by helping them find the information needed to make decisions regarding treatment and management of their disease. In addition to original content about the disease and treatment, the site offers many links to other Web resources, as well as information about local support groups, listservs, chat rooms, and a peer-matching service that connects the newly diagnosed with long-term survivors.

➤ The National Colorectal Cancer Research Alliance. Access at: www. eifoundation.org/national/nccra/splash/
The site of the National Colorectal Cancer Research Alliance (NCCRA), a program co–founded by Katie Couric, provides detailed information about colon cancer screening and prevention. Simple explanations accompanied by photos discuss how colon cancer starts, what the risk factors are, and how to reduce risk. The testing section describes in detail the different diagnostic and screening tests for colon and rectal cancer.

Detailed sections in general cancer sites

➤ American Cancer Society. *Learn about Colon and Rectum Cancer.* Access at: www.cancer.org and select from the menu under "Choose a Cancer Topic." A detailed guide about colorectal cancer can be printed as an Adobe Acrobat (.pdf) file.

➤ Healthology. *Colon Cancer.* Access at: www.healthology.com and click on "Consumer Health Library." This site offers detailed articles, Webcasts, and transcripts featuring cancer professionals.

➤ National Cancer Institute. *Colon Cancer* and *Rectal Cancer.* Access at: www. cancer.gov and click on "Types of Cancer." The top page of the section links to patient versions of PDQ® statements, clinical trial information, and other NCI publications on this topic.

➤ People Living with Cancer. *Colorectal Cancer.* Access at: www.plwc.org and click on "Cancer Type." The PLWC oncologist-approved colorectal cancer guide may be printed in its entirety or by subtopic.

Sections about colorectal cancer are also available at the following sites

➤ Canadian Cancer Society. Access at: www.cancer.ca and click on "About Cancer."

➤ Cancerbackup. Access at: www.cancerbackup.org.uk/Home and click on "Cancer Types."

➤ Cancerconsultants.com. Access at: www.cancerconsultants.com and make a selection under "Links to Specific Cancer Type Information."

➤ CancerSource.com. Access at: www.cancersource.com/Patient.pg and make a selection from the "Diagnosis & Treatment" pull-down menu.

➤ OncologyChannel.com. Access at: www.oncologychannel.com and select a condition from the left sidebar.

Patient-Support Organizations

➤ Colon Cancer Alliance. Access at: www.ccalliance.org
Toll-free Help Line: 877.422.2030

➤ Colorectal Cancer Network. Access at: www.colorectal-cancer.net
Phone: 301-879-1500

Esophageal Cancer

Anatomical facts: The esophagus is a hollow muscular tube that carries food and liquids from the mouth to the stomach. The esophagus is about 10–13 inches long, and in its smallest point it is a little less than 1 inch wide. The esophagus connects to the mouth at the top and to the stomach at the bottom through special round-shaped muscles calls sphincters. The sphincters have the ability to open and close in order to enable food to go in and out while preventing stomach acids from entering the esophagus.

Illustrations available at the Medical Illustrations Gallery of the People Living with Cancer Web site.

Access at: www.plwc.org and click on Library on the left sidebar.

The American Cancer Society estimates that every year, about 15,000 new cases of this cancer are diagnosed in the United States. This disease affects three-to-four times more men than women and is about 50% more common in African Americans than in white Americans. Even though survival rates are still poor, they have been improving steadily since the 1960s.

Esophageal cancer is associated with gastroesophageal reflux disease (GERD) and especially with Barrett's esophagus. This condition develops if GERD has caused a change in the cells of the esophagus. The abnormal cells are still not cancer, but they may become malignant over time. It is estimated that people with Barrett's esophagus are about 50 times more likely to develop esophageal cancer than the general population. Alcohol and tobacco are major risks for esophageal cancer, and the combination of smoking and drinking alcohol raises a person's risk much more than using either alone.

There are two main types of cancer of the esophagus. Squamous cell carcinoma may occur anywhere along the length of the esophagus and accounts for slightly less than half of esophageal cancers. The majority of esophageal cancers are adenocarcinomas that grow near the intersection of the esophagus and the stomach. Adenocarcinomas develop in cells that were damaged as a result of GERD.

Early-stage esophageal cancer is treated with surgery, chemotherapy, and radiation therapy. One of two surgical procedures may be used. An esophagectomy is the removal of the part of the esophagus containing the cancer and the connection of the upper part of the esophagus to the stomach. An esophagogastrectomy is the removal of part of the lower esophagus containing the cancer as well as the upper part of the stomach next to the esophagus. The remaining part of the stomach is then connected to the upper part of the esophagus to allow food to pass into the stomach.

Unfortunately, most esophageal cancer cases are discovered at the advanced stage, when cure is not possible. In these cases, the goal of surgery is to improve swallowing and nutritional status. Photodynamic therapy and mechanical stents also may relieve this problem. Advanced esophageal cancer patients may also benefit from radiation therapy and chemotherapy, which may help reduce the severity of symptoms and improve quality of life.

Esophageal cancer survivors may suffer from swallowing problems that cause severe weight loss. A soft diet of calorie-rich food may be helpful, but sometimes patients need additional nutritional support through artificial feeding. Food in liquid form is delivered directly to the stomach through a tube inserted into the stomach through an opening in the skin of the abdomen. Pain control is another concern and can be managed effectively by the patient's medical team.

Information Sources

Brochures, Booklets, and Other Short Print Publications

➤ National Cancer Institute. *What You Need to Know about Cancer of the Esophagus.*
This booklet on esophageal cancer discusses possible causes, symptoms, diagnosis, treatment, emotional issues, and questions to ask the doctor. Includes resources for additional information. Access at: https://cissecure. nci.nih.gov/ncipubs/

Books

➤ Ginex, Pamela, Jacqueline Hanson, and Bart L. Frazzitta. 2005. *100 Questions and Answers about Esophageal Cancer.* Sudbury, MA: Jones and Bartlett. Detailed information about esophageal cancer is presented in an easy-to-read question-and-answer format. Terms are explained in the sidebar, and the book includes lists of Web sites, organizations, literature, and resources on general and specific topics related to esophageal cancer. This book was co–authored by a lymphoma specialist, an oncology nurse, and a lymphoma survivor.

Web Resources

Detailed sections in general cancer sites

➤ American Cancer Society. *Learn about Esophagus Cancer.* Access at: www.cancer.org and select from the menu under "Choose a Cancer Topic." A detailed guide about esophageal cancer can be printed by section or as an Adobe Acrobat (.pdf) file.

➤ National Cancer Institute. *Esophgeal Cancer.* Access at: www.cancer.gov and click on "Types of cancer." The top page of the section links to patient versions of PDQ® statements, clinical trial information, and other NCI publications on this topic.

➤ People Living with Cancer. *Esophageal Cancer.* Access at: www.plwc.org and click on "Cancer Type." The PLWC oncologist-approved esophageal cancer guide can be printed in its entirety or by subtopic.

Sections about esophageal cancer are also available at the following sites

➤ Canadian Cancer Society. Access at: www.cancer.ca and click on "About Cancer."

➤ Cancerbackup. Access at: www.cancerbackup.org.uk/Home and click on "Cancer Types."

➤ Cancerconsultants.com. Access at: www.cancerconsultants.com and make a selection under "Links to Specific Cancer type Information."

➤ CancerSource.com. Access at: www.cancersource.com/Patient.pg and make a selection from the "Diagnosis & Treatment" pull-down menu.

➤ OncologyChannel.com. Access at: www.oncologychannel.com and select a condition from the left sidebar.

Patient-Support Organizations

➤ Esophageal Cancer Awareness Association. Access at: www.ecaware.org
Phone: 866-370-3222

Head and Neck Cancer

Anatomical facts: The head and neck region includes many complex anatomical structures. These organs are responsible for functions necessary for breathing, eating, and speaking. A more detailed description of the head and neck structures is presented later on in this section.

Illustrations available at the Medical Illustrations Gallery of the People Living with Cancer Web site.

Access at: www.plwc.org and click on Library on the left sidebar. Select either Laryngeal and Hypopharyngeal Cancer or Oral and Oropharyngeal Cancer.

Head and neck cancer is an umbrella term used to describe a complex group of cancers affecting different structures in the head and neck. Most of these tumors originate in the thin cell layer that lines the majority of the head and neck organs, called squamous cells; but other types of cancer can be found there as well.

Approximately 50,000 people are diagnosed with head and neck cancer each year in the United States. Consuming tobacco in all forms including pipes, cigars, cigarettes, and chewing tobacco and prolonged use of alcohol are the main causes for head and neck tumors.

Most information sources divide head and neck cancers into five groups according to the anatomic structure in which the cancer originated; hence the librarian must find out which subtype of head and neck cancer the client is inquiring about.

➤ Oral cancer includes tumors on the lips, gums, tongue, and tonsils. More than half of all head and neck cancers occur in the oral cavity.
➤ Larynx cancer is cancer of the voice box and vocal cords.
➤ Nasopharyngeal cancer affects the nasopharynx, the air passageway in the upper part of the throat, behind the nose.
➤ Nasal cavity cancer affects the nose and sinuses.
➤ Salivary glands cancer affects the glands that produce saliva.

Non-Hodgkin's lymphomas and melanomas may also appear in the head and neck region, but the information on these types of tumors will be found in information sources specific to these cancer types. Brain tumors are not considered part of the head and neck cancers.

Determining the treatment for head and neck cancers is a complex process and requires the input, cooperation, and coordination of many specialists in the field: surgeons, medical oncologists, radiation oncologists, pathologists, radiologists, dentists, maxillofacial surgeons, plastic surgeons, prosthodontic specialists, speech pathologists, and dieticians are consulted in order to decide on a treatment plan. In general, patients with early-stage disease that has not spread to the lymph nodes are treated with surgery or radiation therapy and have the best chance of a cure. Patients whose disease has spread to nearby lymph nodes but not to organs outside of the head and neck are treated with simultaneous administration of radiation and chemotherapy in addition to surgery. People with disease that has spread to organs outside of the head and neck are treated with chemotherapy. The goal of treatment at this stage is to decrease symptoms and improve quality of life.

New ways to treat head and neck cancers include new methods of delivering drugs directly into the blood vessels feeding the tumors, thus decreasing the chemotherapy side effects. Biological therapies such as vaccines, viruses and targeted therapies that block specific substances in cancer cells that cause uncontrolled growth are explored in clinical trials.

Tumors in the head and neck region may have devastating consequences on the patient's quality of life. Side effects of these cancers and their treatment may include difficulties in eating and drinking, severe weight loss, dry mouth, dental problems, speech impairments, and facial deformities. Some patients may need to use assistive devices such as feeding tubes and communication tools. The physical changes and difficulties may put a strain on the patient's emotional well-being and social relationships. In addition, many patients struggle with guilt because lifestyle choices cause so many of these cancers. Patients who smoke need information on smoking cessation. It has been demonstrated that people with head and neck cancers who quit smoking during treatment have a better chance of a cure.

Information Sources

Brochures, Booklets, and Other Short Print Publications

➤ CancerCare. *A Team Approach to Treating Head and Neck Cancer.*
This booklet, with color photographs and illustrations, explains the importance of a team approach to treating head and neck cancer. It discusses the roles of various professions and how they help maintain quality of life and manage such side effects as difficulties in swallowing and speech. Includes frequently asked questions, a short glossary, and a list of resources. Access at: www.cancercare.org

➤ National Cancer Institute. *What You Need to Know about Cancer of the Larynx and What You Need to Know about Oral Cancer.*
These booklets discuss possible causes, symptoms, diagnosis, treatment,

emotional issues, and questions to ask the doctor. Includes a glossary of terms and other resources. Access at: https://cissecure.nci.nih.gov/ncipubs/
➤ National Institute of Dental and Craniofacial Research. *Head and Neck Radiation Treatment and Your Mouth.*
This booklet discusses how radiation affects the mouth and the importance of seeing a dentist before, during, and after cancer treatment. Also included are self-care tips for patients to keep their mouth healthy during treatment. Access at: www.nidcr.nih.gov/

Books

➤ Carper, Elise, Hu Kenneth, and Kuzin, Elena. 2007. *100 Questions and Answers about Head and Neck Cancer.* Sudbury, MA: Jones and Bartlett.
Detailed information about head and neck cancer is presented in an easy-to-read question-and-answer format. Terms are explained in the sidebar, and the book includes lists of Web sites, organizations, literature, and resources on general and specific topics related to head and neck cancer. This book was co–authored by two nurses and a physician.
➤ Lydiatt, William M., and Perry J. Johnson. 2001. *Cancers of the Mouth and Throat: A Patient's Guide to Treatment.* Omaha NE: Addicus Books.
This easy-to-read, comprehensive overview explores the diagnosis and treatment of mouth and throat cancer. Part three focuses on post-treatment considerations, including quality-of-life and end-of-life issues. The appendix provides short descriptions of different surgical procedures to treat mouth and throat cancers.
➤ Leupold, Nancy E. 2005. *Eat Well—Stay Nourished: A Recipe and Resource Guide for Coping with Eating Challenges.* Lenexa, KS: Cookbook Publisher.
A recipe and resource guide that addresses the unique eating challenges of oral and head and neck cancer patients. This book contains 270 recipes as well as information about swallowing problems and nutrition, tips, suggestions, and survivors' cancer journeys. The recipes include full nutritional information. Order at: www.spohnc.org or by phone: 800-377-0928
➤ Thomas, Jack E., and Robert L. Keith. 2005. *Looking Forward: The Speech and Swallowing Guidebook for People with Cancer of the Larynx or Tongue.* 4th ed. New York: Thieme Medical.
The first part of this guidebook explains the anatomy of the head and neck region and the various therapies used to treat cancers of the larynx or tongue, including surgery, radiation therapy, and chemotherapy. The second part provides techniques and exercises for improving speech and swallowing, tips on tube feeding and speaking with assistive devices, and sources of support. Numerous illustrations help understand the anatomy,

equipment, and processes involved in swallowing and communication. This book was authored by two speech pathologists who provide many tips and advice to help people live a full and complete life after treatment.

Web Resources

Detailed sections in general cancer sites

➤ American Cancer Society
  ➤ *Learn about Laryngeal and Hypopharyngeal Cancer*
  ➤ *Learn about Nasal Cavity and Paranasal Cancer*
  ➤ *Learn about Nasopharyngeal Cancer*
  ➤ *Learn about Oral Cavity and Oropharyngeal Cancer*
  ➤ *Learn about Salivary Gland Cancer*
  Access at: www.cancer.org and select from the menu under "Choose a Cancer Topic." Disease-specific detailed guides may be printed as Adobe Acrobat (.pdf) files.
➤ National Cancer Institute. *Head and Neck Cancer.* Access at: www.cancer. gov and click on "Types of Cancer." The top page of the section links to patient versions of PDQ® statements for specific head and neck cancer types.
➤ People Living with Cancer. *Head and Neck Cancer.* Access at: www.plwc. org and click on "Cancer Type." PLWC oncologist-approved guides about different types of head and neck cancer can be printed in their entirety or by subtopic.

Sections about head and neck cancer are also available at the following sites

➤ Canadian Cancer Society. Access at: www.cancer.ca and click on "About Cancer."
➤ Cancerbackup. Access at: www.cancerbackup.org.uk/Home and click on "Cancer Types."
➤ Cancerconsultants.com. Access at: www.cancerconsultants.com and make a selection under "Links to Specific Cancer type Information."
➤ CancerSource.com. Access at: www.cancersource.com/Patient.pg and make a selection from the "Diagnosis & Treatment" pull-down menu.
➤ OncologyChannel.com. Access at: www.oncologychannel.com and select a condition from the left sidebar.

Patient-Support Organizations

➤ *Support for People with Oral and Head and Neck Cancer—S.P.O.H.N.C.*
  Access at: www.spohnc.org
  Phone: 800-377-0928
  Fax: 516-671-8794

Hodgkin's Disease

Anatomical facts: *The lymphatic system is a network of vessels, similar to blood vessels, that carry the lymph fluid to different parts of the body. Lymph is a colorless fluid that contains infection-fighting white blood cells called lymphocytes. Lymphocytes are made and stored in lymph nodes, small bean-shaped organs that cluster along the lymphatic system. There are two types of lymphocytes: B lymphocytes (B cells) and T lymphocytes (T cells). Other parts of the lymphatic system include the spleen, thymus, tonsils, and bone marrow. Lymphatic tissue is also found in other parts of the body, including the stomach, intestines, and skin. The lymphatic system is part of the body's immune system.*

Illustrations available at the Medical Illustrations Gallery of the People Living with Cancer Web site.

Access at: www.plwc.org and click on Library on the left sidebar.

Hodgkin's disease is one of the most curable cancers. Improvements in treatment contributed to a 60% drop in death rates since the 1970s. The overall five-year survival rate is 85%. The American Cancer Society estimates approximately 8,000 new cases of Hodgkin's lymphoma per year. The disease has a peak incidence in two age groups: early adulthood (ages 15 to 40) and late adulthood (after age 55). About 10% to 15% of cases are found in children aged 16 years old and younger. Information on Hodgkin's disease in children is discussed in the childhood lymphomas section in Chapter 5.

People who have a history of infectious mononucleosis (sometimes called "mono" for short) are four times more likely to develop Hodgkin's than are people who have not had the disease. People with a weakened immune system, such as those infected with AIDS; people who received an organ transplant; or people with other immunodeficiency disorders have a slightly increased risk. There does not appear to be a connection between lifestyle factors or occupational exposures and Hodgkin's disease.

Hodgkin's disease is one of two cancers that start in the lymphatic system. Non-Hodgkin's lymphoma is a different disease, discussed later in this chapter on p. 116. Hodgkin's disease is characterized by the development of unique abnormal B lymphocytes called Reed-Sternberg cells. Reed-Sternberg cells are much larger than normal lymphocytes and also look different from the cells of non-Hodgkin's lymphoma and other cancers. The disease may affect one or more lymph nodes in any part of the body, but it usually starts in the upper part of the body, most typically in the chest, or neck or under the arms. Hodgkin's disease spreads through the lymphatic vessels in an orderly manner, from one lymph node cluster to the other, from nearby clusters to distant ones. A spread through the bloodstream to organs beyond the lymphatic system is rare. The enlargement of the lymphatic tissue may pressure healthy structures and cause pain. The two main types of Hodgkin's disease are classical Hodgkin's disease (which has several subtypes) and nodular lymphocyte-predominant Hodgkin's disease.

The majority of newly diagnosed Hodgkin's disease patients can be cured with a combination of chemotherapy and radiation therapy. Chemotherapy for Hodgkin's disease is a regimen of several drugs given in combination. These regimens are named with an acronym derived from the first letters of the individual drugs. For example, ABVD is a combination of doxorubicin, bleomycin, vinblastine and dacarbazine; BEACOPP is a combination of bleomycin, etoposide, adriamycin, cyclophosphamide, vincristine, procarbazine, and prednisone.

The exact type and combination of anticancer drugs depends on the stage and grade of the disease. Bone marrow or stem cell transplantations are used in patients who relapsed after first-line treatment with chemotherapy and radiation. Most patients do not undergo surgery, except for biopsy and staging purposes.

Chemotherapy regimens for Hodgkin's disease have a high likelihood of causing fertility problems in men and women. Since many patients are diagnosed before and during their reproductive years, it is important to provide information about fertility options to all newly diagnosed patients.

It is estimated that 123,000 long-term survivors of Hodgkin's disease live in the United States. Long-term effects of treatment are weighty concerns for people treated for Hodgkin's disease. Young women and girls who have been treated with radiation therapy to the chest area have a high risk for breast cancer. Treatment also increases the risk for developing other secondary cancers and may cause thyroid disease or heart damage. Long-term survivors need to be watched very closely for the development of any of those conditions.

Information Sources

Brochures, Booklets, and Other Short Print Publications

➤ The Leukemia & Lymphoma Society. *The Lymphomas: A Guide for Patients and Families: Hodgkin and Non-Hodgkin Lymphoma Information.* This basic introduction to lymphoma starts with the anatomy of the lymphatic system and continues with a text description of diagnostic tests, subtypes, and treatments for Hodgkin's and non-Hodgkin's lymphoma. An easy-to-read version of this publication is *The Lymphomas: A Guide for Patients and Their Families.* Larger print and bullet points summarize the topic in a concise manner. Access at: www.leukemia-lymphoma.org

➤ Lymphoma Research Foundation. *Lymphoma Resource Guide.*
A listing of organizations, online resources, audio and videotapes, publications, and therapies that are of interest to lymphoma patients and families. Access at: www.lymphoma.org

➤ Lymphoma Research Foundation. *Understanding Hodgkin's Lymphoma: A Guide for Patients.*
This 84-page booklet provides a comprehensive review of Hodgkin's lymphoma, including diagnosis, treatment, coping with side effects, clinical trials experimental treatments, and living with cancer. Includes a glossary. Individual copies are free and can be obtained by calling the Lymphoma Research Foundation at 800-500-9976.

➤ National Cancer Institute. *What You Need to Know about Hodgkin's Disease.*
A concise introduction to Hodgkin's disease covering staging, treatment options, and emotional support. Includes a glossary and a list of questions for the doctor. Access at: https://cissecure.nci.nih.gov/ncipubs/

Books

➤ Adler, Elizabeth M. 2005. *Living with Lymphoma: A Patient's Guide.* Baltimore, MD: Johns Hopkins Univ. Press.
Written by a neurobiologist and a lymphoma survivor, this book offers a detailed explanation of cell biology that helps understand the disease and its treatment. While this book provides an in-depth look at the medical side of lymphoma and provides detailed descriptions of specific drugs, drug combinations, and treatment approaches, psychosocial issues are not as meticulously covered. Sophisticated readers who are interested in learning the scientific aspects of lymphoma will appreciate this book.

➤ Holman, Peter, Jodi Garrett, and William D. Jansen. 2004. *100 Questions and Answers about Lymphoma.* Sudbury, MA: Jones and Bartlett.
Detailed information about lymphoma is presented in an easy-to-read question-and-answer format. Terms are explained on the sidebar, and the book includes lists of Web sites, organizations, literature, and resources on general and specific topic related to Hodgkin's lymphoma. This book was co–authored by a lymphoma specialist, an oncology nurse, and a lymphoma survivor.

Web Resources

Sites focusing on Hodgkin's lymphoma

➤ The Leukemia & Lymphoma Society. Access at: www.leukemia-lymphoma.org

The site of the world's largest organization dedicated to blood cancers includes many sections and features for people with lymphoma. Live and archived versions of educational teleconferences and Webcasts enable users to study complicated topics explained by top experts. The site also includes medical news about lymphoma, short and longer overviews of the disease, and information about the organization's support services for patients.

➤ Leukaemia Research. Access at: www.lrf.org.uk/
Leukaemia Research is a British research charity focusing on blood cancers and disorders. The "Information and Education" section offers printable booklets on adult and childhood blood cancers, including some on rare subtypes and conditions. The "News" section includes stories about research developments and other related articles.

➤ Lymphoma Information Network. Access at: www.lymphomainfo.net
This well-organized directory of lymphoma information sources presents short, concise introductions to information about many types of lymphoma. Each section has a list of references with links to other sites, PubMed abstracts, or books on Amazon. This site has been maintained for over ten years by an Non-Hodgkin's lymphoma survivor and is useful as a starting point for a search on specific or complex issues in lymphoma.

➤ Lymphoma Research Foundation. Access at: www.lymphoma.org
The Lymphoma Research Foundation is a patient-support and advocacy organization providing support and education to lymphoma patients and families. Information about the disease, its treatment, and research news is presented in fact sheets, Webcasts, newsletters, and other formats. This site also includes information about support programs and services for patients and families.

Detailed sections in general cancer sites

➤ American Cancer Society. *Learn about Hodgkin's Disease*. Access at: www. cancer.org and select from the menu under "Choose a Cancer Topic." A detailed guide about Hodgkin's disease can be printed by section or as an Adobe Acrobat (.pdf) file.

➤ Healthology. *Lymphoma*. Access at: www.healthology.com and click on "Consumer Health Library." This site offers detailed articles, Webcasts, and transcripts featuring cancer professionals.

➤ National Cancer Institute. *Hodgkin's Lymphoma, Adult*. Access at: www. cancer.gov and click on "Types of Cancer." The top page of the section links to patient versions of PDQ® statements, clinical trial information, and other NCI publications on this topic.

➤ People Living with Cancer. *Lymphoma, Hodgkin.* Access at: www.plwc.org and click on "Cancer Type." The PLWC oncologist-approved Hodgkin's lymphoma guide can be printed in its entirety or by subtopic.

➤ The Wellness Community. *Frankly Speaking about Lymphoma.* Access at: www.thewellnesscommunity.org and click on "Cancer Information" on the left sidebar. This section explains lymphoma and its treatment, integrating mind-body practices into lymphoma treatment, and managing the personal impact of the illness.

Sections about Hodgkin's lymphoma are also available at the following sites

➤ Canadian Cancer Society. Access at: www.cancer.ca and click on "About Cancer."

➤ Cancerbackup. Access at: www.cancerbackup.org.uk/Home and click on "Cancer Types."

➤ Cancerconsultants.com. Access at: www.cancerconsultants.com and make a selection under "Links to Specific Cancer Type Information."

➤ CancerSource.com. Access at: www.cancersource.com/Patient.pg and make a selection from the "Diagnosis & Treatment" pull-down menu.

➤ OncologyChannel.com. Access at: www.oncologychannel.com and select a condition from the left sidebar.

Patient Support Organizations

➤ The Leukemia & Lymphoma Society. www.leukemia.org
Phone: 800-955-4572

➤ Lymphoma Research Foundation. www.lymphoma.org
Phone: LA office 800-500-9976; New York office 800-235-6848

Kidney Cancer

Anatomical facts: The kidneys are two fist-size organs located on either side of the spine in the lower abdomen. The adrenal glands are attached to the top of each kidney. The kidneys are part of the urinary tract, and their main function is to produce urine by collecting wastes and extra water from the blood. Urine passes from the kidneys to the bladder through a tube called a ureter. It is stored in the bladder until it leaves the body through another tube called a urethra. It is possible to live with only one kidney.

Illustrations available at the Medical Illustrations Gallery of the People Living with Cancer Web site.

Access at: www.plwc.org and click on Library on the left sidebar.

The American Cancer Society estimates more than 52,000 new kidney cancer cases in the United States per year and 13,000 deaths. The disease is more common in men than in women, and most cases are diagnosed in people between 50 and 70. In early stages, tumors growing in the kidney produce vague symptoms that may be attributed to other conditions; as a result, the majority of new diagnoses occur after the cancer has already spread. (Childhood kidney cancer, Wilms' tumor, is a different disease and is discussed in Chapter 5, p. 206.)

Risk factors for kidney cancer include exposure to cancer-causing substances in cigarettes and other chemicals. People who are obese, people on dialysis, and people taking medication for high blood pressure have an increased risk. Kidney cancer has a genetic factor: 25% to 45% of people with von Hippel–Lindau (VHL) syndrome develop kidney cancer. There are other forms of hereditary kidney cancer, and people with a strong family history of the disease have a higher risk.

Of tumors in the kidney, 90% are renal cell carcinomas, with 5% to 10% being transitional cell carcinomas, which have similar symptoms to renal cell but their treatment is slightly different. Renal sarcomas are very rare and account for less than 1% of all kidney tumors. Relevant information on renal sarcomas should be looked for in the soft tissue sarcoma information sources. It is important to find out the exact cancer type since many information sources provide data relevant only to renal cell carcinomas and some have separate sections for renal cell and transitional cell carcinomas.

Nephrectomy—surgical removal of the kidney—is the primary treatment for kidney cancer that is discovered before spreading to distant regions of the body. Early-stage kidney cancer is treated only with nephrectomy and has a 95% survival rate after ten years. Nephrectomies can be performed as minimally invasive laparoscopic procedures instead of open surgery. In some early-stage cases, it may be possible to perform a partial nephrectomy and remove only a portion of the kidney.

Cancers that have spread beyond the kidney are typically treated with a combination of radiation therapy and chemotherapy. In recent years, the biologic therapy interleukin (IL-2) has produced longer remission periods in about 10% to 20% of patients. Doctors are also testing and evaluating the drug thalidomide and other targeted and biological therapies. Encouraging results have been observed in an early trial utilizing stem cell transplants to treat advanced-stage renal cell carcinomas that failed to respond to other therapies.

Information Sources

Brochures, Booklets, and Other Short Print Publications

➤ CancerCare. *Progress in the Treatment of Kidney Cancer.*
This short booklet with color photographs and illustrations focuses on targeted treatments for kidney cancer. Includes frequently asked questions, a short glossary, and a list of resources. Access at: www.cancercare.org

➤ Kidney Cancer Association.
   ➤ *A Closer Look at Renal Cell Carcinoma*
   ➤ *We Have Kidney Cancer*
   ➤ *Kidney Cancer: Emotional vs. Rational*
   Access at: www.curekidneycancer.org. Free registration is needed to obtain the printable versions of these and other brochures concerning kidney cancer.

➤ National Cancer Institute. *What You Need to Know about Kidney Cancer.*
This booklet on kidney cancer discusses possible causes, symptoms, diagnosis, treatment, emotional issues, and questions to ask the doctor. Includes glossary of terms and other resources. Access at: https://cissecure.nci.nih.gov/ncipubs/

Audiovisual Resource

➤ Information Television Network. 2005. *Kidney Cancer: The Silent Destroyer.*
Boca Raton, FL: Information Television Network. (30 min.). Available in DVD and VHS formats. Access at: www.itvisus.com or Amazon.com
Part of the public television series *Healthy Body/Healthy Mind*, this episode features cancer specialists explaining kidney cancer and the latest treatment approaches. The program also features kidney cancer patients discussing their experience with the disease. Color graphics and animations illustrate the scientific content.

Web Resources

Sites focusing on kidney cancer

➤ Kidney Cancer Association. Access at: www.curekidneycancer.org/
A free registration enables access to a wealth of information about kidney cancer, including full text of brochures and publications, detailed information about dealing with kidney cancer, video presentations by medical experts and leading researchers, and access to a clinical trial dababase, news, and support services offered by this organization.

Detailed sections in general cancer sites

➤ American Cancer Society. *Learn about Kidney Cancer.* Access at: www.cancer.org and select from the menu under "Choose a Cancer Topic." A detailed guide about kidney cancer can be printed by section or as an Adobe Acrobat (.pdf) file.

➤ National Cancer Institute. *Kidney Cancer.* Access at: www.cancer.gov and click on "Types of Cancer." The top page of the section links to patient versions of PDQ® statements, clinical trial information, and other NCI publications on this topic.

➤ People Living with Cancer. *Kidney Cancer.* Access at: www.plwc.org and click on "Cancer Type." The PLWC oncologist-approved kidney cancer guide can be printed in its entirety or by subtopic.

Sections about kidney cancer are also available at the following sites:

➤ Canadian Cancer Society. Access at: www.cancer.ca and click on "About Cancer."

➤ Cancerbackup. Access at: www.cancerbackup.org.uk/Home and click on "Cancer Types."

➤ Cancerconsultants.com. Access at: www.cancerconsultants.com and make a selection under "Links to Specific Cancer type Information."

➤ CancerSource.com. Access at: www.cancersource.com/Patient.pg and make a selection from the "Diagnosis & Treatment" pull-down menu.

➤ OncologyChannel.com. Access at: www.oncologychannel.com and select a condition from the left sidebar.

Patient-Support Organizations

Kidney Cancer Organization. Access at: www.curekidneycancer.org
Phone: 800-850-9132

Leukemia

Anatomical facts: Bone marrow is the soft material in the center of most bones. It contains blood-forming cells called stem cells that mature in the marrow and then move into the blood vessels. Stem cells mature into different types of blood cells. Each type has a special function. Red blood cells carry oxygen from the lungs to all other tissues of the body and carry away carbon dioxide, a waste product of cell activity. Platelets help form blood clots that control bleeding. White blood cells help fight infection. The two main types of white blood cells are granulocytes and monocytes. Lymphocytes are the main cell of the lymphoid tissue, a major part of the immune system. Lymphocytes also originate in the bone marrow.

Illustration available at the National Cancer Institute publication *What You Need to Know about Leukemia.*

Access at: https://cissecure.nci.nih.gov/ncipubs

Leukemia is a group of distinct blood cancers diagnosed in about 44,000 adults and children per year. Of new cases, 11%, or approximately 3,800, are diagnosed in children. Childhood leukemia behaves differently then adult leukemia. Additional information sources specific to childhood leukemia can be found in Chapter 5 on page 173.

Two main subgroups of leukemias affect adults: acute leukemias and chronic leukemias. Acute leukemias are a group of diseases that progress very rapidly; abnormal blood cells prevent the normal functioning of the blood and bone marrow, and symptoms worsen very quickly if left untreated. In contrast, chronic leukemias are diseases that progress slowly. Some of the normal blood cells are still able to function properly; hence many patients do not have symptoms when diagnosed. Chronic leukemias get worse over time and at some point become acute. This process may take years. At the time of diagnosis, approximately 45% of leukemia cases in adults are chronic and 55% are acute. The overall five-year survival rate for all types of leukemia is 48%, but survival rates differ greatly by age at diagnosis, gender, race, and type of leukemia.

Risk factors for adult leukemia include exposure to chemicals such as benzene, excessive amounts of radiation, and certain chemotherapy drugs.

Different leukemia diseases originate from different types of blood cells. Acute lymphocytic leukemia (ALL) and chronic lymphocytic leukemia (CLL) start in the lymphocytes. Acute myelogenous leukemia (AML) starts in the granulocytes, and chronic myelogenous leukemia (CML) starts in blood-forming cells in the bone marrow. Hairy cell leukemia (HCL) is a rare type of chronic leukemia in which abnormal lymphocytes appear to be covered with tiny hairlike projections. AML is the most common type of acute leukemia in adults and accounts for over 83% of cases. CLL accounts for 63% of chronic leukemias.

When responding to questions about leukemia, librarians should provide disease-specific information because the different types of leukemias are completely distinct diseases, each with its own characteristics, treatment, and outlook. The Leukemia & Lymphoma Society, the American Cancer Society, and other Web sites and organizations offer separate overviews for the different leukemia diseases.

People diagnosed with one of the acute leukemias need to start treatment immediately with an aggressive regimen of chemotherapy. The goal of the first phase of treatment, called induction, is to bring about a remission. After symptoms disappear, more chemotherapy is given to prevent a relapse. This phase of treatment is called maintenance therapy.

People with chronic leukemia may not require immediate treatment; however, if symptoms worsen, treatment will be initiated, with the goal of controlling the disease and symptoms. Chronic leukemia can seldom be cured, but therapy may keep the disease in remission for prolonged periods. People with CML usually receive the targeted therapy imatinib mesylate (brand name: Gleevec), which blocks the production of leukemia cells but does not harm normal cells. People with CLL usually start treatment with chemotherapy. Other treatment options to treat all types of leukemia are biological therapies and bone marrow transplants. Patients are not typically treated with surgery. Radiation therapy is used sometimes to treat leukemia cells that collect in certain parts of the body or before a bone marrow transplantation.

Leukemia survivors need a lot of support and information with regard to short- and long-term effects of chemotherapy and/or bone marrow transplantation. Topics of interest may include nutrition, fertility, sexuality, financial, employment, and insurance issues.

Information Sources
Brochures, Booklets, and Other Short Print Publications

➤ The Leukemia & Lymphoma Society.
  ➢ *Acute Lymphocytic Leukemia (ALL).*
  ➢ *Acute Myelogenous Leukemia (AML)*
  ➢ *Chronic Lymphocytic Leukemia (CLL)*
  ➢ *Chronic Myelogenous Leukemia (CML)*
  ➢ *Hairy Cell Leukemia*
  This is a series of detailed overviews of specific leukemia types. Each booklet covers anatomy, subtypes, diagnosis, side effects of treatment, and social and emotional aspects. Easy-to-read versions of these publications are titled:
  ➢ *Acute Lymphocytic Leukemia: A Guide for Patients and Their Families*
  ➢ *Acute Myelogenous Leukemia: A Guide for Patients and Their Families*
  ➢ *Chronic Lymphocytic Leukemia: A Guide for Patients and Their Families*
  ➢ *Chronic Myelogenous Leukemia: A Guide for Patients and Their Families*
  Larger print and bullet points summarize the topic in a concise manner. Access at: www.leukemia-lymphoma.org
➤ National Cancer Institute. *What You Need to Know about Leukemia.*
  This booklet on leukemia discusses possible causes, symptoms, diagnosis, treatment, emotional issues, and questions to ask the doctor. Includes glossary of terms and other resources. Access at: https://cissecure.nci.nih.gov/ncipubs/

Book

➤ Ball, Edward D., and Gregory A. Lelek. 2003. *100 Questions and Answers about Leukemia.* Sudbury, MA: Jones and Bartlett.

Detailed information about leukemia is presented in an easy-to-read question-and-answer format and covers treatment options, post–treatment quality of life, and sources of support. Terms are explained in the sidebar, and the book includes lists of Web sites, organizations, literature, and resources on general and specific topics related to leukemia. This book was co–authored by a physician specializing in leukemia and a survivor.

Audiovisual Resources

➤ Patient Education Institute. *Leukemia Interactive Tutorial.* Access at: www. medlineplus.gov and click on: "Interactive Tutorials," then select from a list. This slideshow utilizes illustrations, sound, and animations to provide basic, easy-to-understand explanations of blood cells and the diagnosis and treatment options of leukemia. It is possible to turn on a voice-over or print a text version.

Web Resources

Sites focusing on Leukemia

➤ The Leukemia & Lymphoma Society. Access at: www.leukemia-lymphoma. org
The site of the world's largest organization dedicated to blood cancers includes many sections and features for people with all types of leukemia. Live and archival versions of educational teleconferences and Webcasts enable users to study complicated topics explained by top experts. The site also includes medical news about leukemia, short and longer overviews of the diseases, and information about the organization's support services for patients.

➤ Leukaemia Research. Access at: www.lrf.org.uk
Leukaemia Research is a British research charity focusing on blood cancers and disorders. The "Information and Education" section offers printable booklets on adult and childhood blood cancers, including some on rare subtypes and conditions. The "News" section includes stories about research developments and other related articles.

Detailed sections in general cancer sites

➤ American Cancer Society.
  ➢ *Learn about Leukemia—Acute Lymphocytic (ALL)*
  ➢ *Learn about Leukemia—Acute Myeloid (AML)*
  ➢ *Learn about Leukemia—Chronic Lymphocytic (CLL)*
  ➢ *Learn about Leukemia—Chronic Myeloid (CML)*

Access at: www.cancer.org and select from the menu under "Choose a Cancer Topic." Detailed guides about specific types of leukemia can be printed by section or as Adobe Acrobat (.pdf) files.

➤ Healthology. *Leukemia.* Access at: www.healthology.com and click on "Consumer Health Library." This site offers detailed articles, Webcasts, and transcripts featuring cancer professionals.

➤ National Cancer Institute. *Leukemia.* Access at: www.cancer.gov and click on "Types of Cancer." The top page of the section links to patient versions of PDQ® statements on specific leukemia types, clinical trial information, and other NCI publications on this topic.

➤ People Living with Cancer.
  ➤ *Leukemia, Acute Lymphocytic (ALL)*
  ➤ *Leukemia, Acute Myeloid (AML)*
  ➤ *Leukemia, B-Cell*
  ➤ *Leukemia, Chronic Lymphocytic (CLL)*
  ➤ *Leukemia, Chronic Myeloid (CML)*
  ➤ *Leukemia, Eosinophilic*
  ➤ *Leukemia, T-Cell*
  Access at: www.plwc.org and click on "Cancer Type." The PLWC oncologist-approved guides for leukemia diseases can be printed in their entirety or by subtopic.

Sections about leukemia are also available at the following sites:

➤ Canadian Cancer Society. Access at: www.cancer.ca and click on "About Cancer."

➤ Cancerbackup. Access at: www.cancerbackup.org.uk/Home and click on "Cancer Types."

➤ Cancerconsultants.com. Access at: www.cancerconsultants.com and make a selection under "Links to Specific Cancer Type Information."

➤ CancerSource.com. Access at: www.cancersource.com/Patient.pg and make a selection from the "Diagnosis & Treatment" pull-down menu.

➤ OncologyChannel.com. Access at: www.oncologychannel.com and select a condition from the left sidebar.

Patient Support Organizations

➤ *The Leukemia & Lymphoma Society.* Access at: www.leukemia.org
  Phone: 800-955-4572

➤ *Leukemia Research Foundation (LRF).* Access at: www.leukemia-research. org
  Phone: 888-558-5385

Liver Cancer

Anatomical facts: *The liver is the largest internal organ in the body and is located behind the ribs on the right side of the abdomen. It is a pyramid-shaped organ divided into right and left lobes. This is the only organ in the body that receives blood from two sources: the hepatic artery delivers oxygen-rich blood from the heart, and the portal vein carries nutrient-rich blood from the intestines. The liver is responsible for a number of essential functions in the body. It processes and stores nutrients, removes toxic materials from the blood, secretes enzymes and bile that help in digestion, and produces clotting factors necessary to stop bleeding.*

Illustrations available at the Medical Illustrations Gallery of the People Living with Cancer Web site.

Access at: www.plwc.org and click on Library on the left sidebar.

Approximately 19,000 people are diagnosed with primary liver cancer every year in the United States. Symptoms do not usually appear until the disease is already advanced; as a result, only about 30% of liver tumors are found at a stage that enables the removal of the tumor with surgery. The overall five-year relative survival rate from liver cancer is poor. In the United States, the majority of cancerous tumors found in the liver are metastasized from a different site in the body, such as the colon, pancreas, breast, and so forth. These secondary tumors are considered a metastatic form of the primary site cancer and are completely different disease entities from cancer that started in liver cells, called primary liver cancer. Before starting to look for information about liver cancer, it is important to find out if the cancer started in the liver or metastasized from a different organ.

People who have long-term viral liver infection (hepatitis B or C) and people who have cirrhosis of the liver have a higher risk of developing cancer in the liver. Cirrhosis is a condition where scar tissue forms in the liver. In most cases cirrhosis is caused by alcohol abuse, but exposure to other drugs and chemicals and some inherited metabolic disorders also may cause cirrhosis and increase the risk for liver cancer. Obesity and smoking also have been linked to liver cancer. This disease is more common in men than in women and has a higher incidence in developing countries in Asia and Africa than in Europe and the United States.

The most common subtype of liver cancer is hepatocellular carcinoma (HCC), which accounts for about 75% of all primary liver cancers. It is sometimes called hepatoma because it originates in the hepatocytes (the main type of liver cells). About 10% to 20% of primary liver tumors are cholangiocarcinomas that start in the bile ducts located inside the liver (intrahepatic bile ducts). Cholangiocarcinomas can also start in bile ducts located outside the liver (extrahepatic) and the gallbladder. Although intrahepatic cholangio-carcinomas are counted as liver cancer, they are similar to extrahepatic cholangiocarcinomas, and the information about treatment and prognosis of these tumors should be found under bile duct and/or gallbladder cancer. Angiosarcomas and hemangiosarcomas are very rare and start in the liver's blood vessels. Most information sources on liver cancer focus on hepatocellular carcinomas.

The only possibility for curing liver cancer is with surgery. If the disease has not spread to nearby lymph nodes and other organs, it is possible to remove only the diseased portion of the liver with a procedure called partial hepatectomy. Because the body cannot function without a liver, total removal of the entire organ is not possible, unless a new liver can be transplanted. To alleviate symptoms of patients who have a few small tumors but for whom surgery is not possible, doctors use ablation techniques to destroy tumors without surgery. Chemotherapy and radiation therapy help improve symptoms, but unfortunately none of these treatments is capable of curing this type of cancer.

Information Sources

Brochures, Booklets, and Other Short Print Publications

➤ National Cancer Institute. *What You Need to Know about Liver Cancer.* This booklet on liver cancer discusses possible causes, symptoms, diagnosis, treatment, emotional issues, and questions to ask the doctor. Includes a glossary of terms and other resources. Access at: https://cissecure.nci. nih.gov/ncipubs/

Books

➤ Abou-Alfa, Ghassan K., and Ronald DeMatteo. 2006. *100 Questions and Answers about Liver Cancer.* Sudbury, MA: Jones and Bartlett.
Detailed information about liver cancer is presented in an easy-to-read question-and-answer format and covers treatment options, quality-of-life isssues, and sources of support. Terms are explained in the sidebar, and the book includes lists of Web sites, organizations, literature, and resources on general and specific topics related to leukemia. This book was co–authored by two physicians from Memorial Sloan-Kettering Cancer Center.

Web Resources

Detailed sections in general cancer sites

➤ American Cancer Society. *Learn about Liver Cancer.* Access at: www. cancer.org and select from the menu under "Choose a Cancer Type or

Topic." A detailed guide about liver cancer can be printed by section or an Adobe Acrobat (.pdf) file.

➤ National Cancer Institute. *Liver Cancer*. Access at: www.cancer.gov and click on "Types of cancer." The top page of the section links to patient versions of PDQ® statements, clinical trial information, and other NCI publications on this topic.

➤ People Living with Cancer. *Liver Cancer*. Access at: www.plwc.org and click on "Cancer Type." The PLWC oncologist-approved liver cancer guide can be printed in its entirety or by subtopic.

Sections about liver cancer are also available at the following sites:

➤ Canadian Cancer Society. Access at: www.cancer.ca and click on "About Cancer."

➤ Cancerbackup. Access at: www.cancerbackup.org.uk/Home and click on "Cancer Types."

➤ Cancerconsultants.com. Access at: www.cancerconsultants.com and make a selection under "Links to Specific Cancer Type Information."

➤ CancerSource.com. Access at: www.cancersource.com/Patient.pg and make a selection from the "Diagnosis & Treatment" pull-down menu.

➤ OncologyChannel.com. Access at: www.oncologychannel.com and select a condition from the left sidebar.

Patient Support Organization

➤ American Liver Foundation. Access at: www.liverfoundation.org
Phone: 800-465-4837

Lung Cancer

Anatomical facts: The lungs are a pair of spongy, cone-shaped organs and are part of the respiratory system. The right lung is a bit larger and has three sections, called lobes; the left lung has two lobes. With each breath, the lungs take in oxygen, which our cells need to live and carry out their normal functions. When we breathe out, the lungs get rid of carbon dioxide, which is a waste product of the body's cells.

Illustrations available at the Medical Illustrations Gallery of the People Living with Cancer Web site.
Access at: www.plwc.org and click on Library on the left sidebar.

Approximately 213,000 Americans are diagnosed with lung cancer each year. It represents 13% of all cancer diagnoses in the United States and 28%

of all cancer deaths. This disease is very rare under age 40. The average age of diagnosis is 70. Cigarette smoking is the cause for the vast majority (87%) of lung cancers, although it is possible for a nonsmoker to develop this disease.

Lung cancer is the leading cause of cancer death for both men and women. More Americans die each year of lung cancer than of colon, breast, melanoma, and prostate cancers combined. It kills more women than breast cancer and more men than prostate cancer. The reason lung cancer is such a deadly disease is because its early signs such as coughing, shortness of breath, and chest pain tend to be disregarded in smokers or attributed to other conditions. Consequently, most cases are diagnosed after the disease has already spread beyond the lung to other organs and cure is no longer possible.

Lung cancers are divided into two major types: small-cell lung cancer (SCLC) and non-small-cell lung cancer (NSCLC). These two cancer types originate from different lung cells and look and behave differently from each other. Accordingly, each type requires different treatment. Most information sources have separate sections describing treatment for NSCLC and SCLC, but the information on symptoms, diagnostic procedures, and supportive care is the same for both types. Other rare tumor types that appear in the lungs are carcinoid tumors and mesotheliomas. These diseases are very different from NSCLC or SCLC, and information on them should be obtained from disease-specific resources and not from lung cancer information sources.

The three major treatment methods for lung cancer are surgery, chemotherapy, and radiation therapy. Surgery may include the removal of part of a lobe, known as a segmentectomy or wedge resection; removal of a lobe, called lobectomy; or removal of an entire lung, called a pneumonectomy. Surgery can potentially cure early-stage lung cancer that has not metastasized to distant organs or lymph nodes, but since most lung cancer cases are discovered after they have already spread, the majority of patients are treated with radiation and/or chemotherapy without surgery.

In recent years, new treatment options for lung cancer have been developed. Targeted therapies that attempt to kill only the cancerous cells while avoiding healthy ones are taken in pill form and cause fewer side effects than chemotherapy. Researchers are still trying to determine if these drugs enable patients to have a longer survival and better quality of life than other treatments.

Lung cancer patients have unique information needs. Breathing difficulties may occur in later stages of the illness and require special treatments. Pain is another concern and can be controlled by medications or radiation therapy to bone metastases. Patients may ask for information on smoking cessation because their doctors advise them that stopping smoking will increase their ability to tolerate treatment and greatly improve their quality of life. Emotionally, lung cancer patients often experience strong feelings of guilt and shame because lung cancer is perceived as a disease that they have brought on themselves.

Information Sources

Brochures, Booklets, and Other Short Print Publications

➤ CancerCare. *Coping with Lung Cancer.*
   A concise overview of lung cancer stages and treatment, with sections on communicating with the medical team, connecting with support systems, frequently asked questions, a glossary, and resources. Access at: www.cancercare.org/reading.html

➤ CancerCare. *Caring for Your Bones When You Have Lung Cancer.*
   This publication is aimed at people who have bone metastases as a result of lung cancer. Includes sections on treatment, pain control, sources of support, frequently asked questions, a glossary, and resources. Access at: www.cancercare.org/reading.html

➤ National Cancer Institute. *What You Need to Know about Lung Cancer.*
   A concise introduction to lung cancer covers staging and treatment options, emotional support, and a list of questions for the doctor. Access at: https://cissecure.nci.nih.gov/ncipubs/

➤ National Comprehensive Cancer Network (NCCN). *Lung Cancer: Treatment Guidelines for Patients.*
   This publication includes an overview of lung cancer as well as treatment decision "trees" explaining the treatment choices for different disease stages and conditions. Developed from the NCCN Clinical Practice Guidelines in Oncology—the standard for clinical policy in cancer care. A Spanish-language version is also available. Access at: www.nccn.org/patients/

➤ Ruckdeschel, John C. 2002. *Myths & Facts about Lung Cancer: What You Need to Know.* Melville, NY: PRR.
   This 80-page handbook with a detailed overview of lung cancer includes many color illustrations and photographs. The sidebar features facts that dispel common myths about lung cancer and repeat key points. Includes a list of resources and a glossary. The author is a lung cancer specialist from H. Lee Moffitt Cancer Center. To view online, download an Adobe Acrobat (.pdf) file or order access at: www.cancernetwork.com.

➤ The Wellness Community. *Frankly Speaking About Lung Cancer* (2d ed.).
   An overview of lung cancer includes sections about making treatment decisions, managing side effects, and integrating mind-body practices into

treatment. It also addresses psychological and practical concerns. Access at: www.thewellnesscommunity.org

Books

➤ Henschke, Claudia I. 2002. *Lung Cancer: Myths, Facts, Choices—and Hope.* New York: Norton.
This book was authored by Claudia Henschke, Ph.D., M.D., a radiologist specializing in chest imaging and lung cancer detection, with help from Peggy McCarty, M.B.A., a patient advocate. This comprehensive overview of lung cancer covers risk factors and diagnosis, the illness and its treatment, quality of life, and living with advanced disease. The authors stress that even for people facing limited time, life can still have hope, joy, and meaningful accomplishment. Includes a glossary.

➤ Parles, Karen. 2006. *100 Questions and Answers about Lung Cancer.* Updated Edition. Boston: Jones and Bartlett.
Detailed information about lung cancer is presented in an easy-to-read question-and-answer format. Terms are explained in the sidebar, and the book includes lists of Web sites, organizations, literature, and resources on general and specific topics related to lung cancer. This book was co-authored by Karen Parles, a librarian, lung cancer survivor, and advocate, and Joan H. Schiller, M.D., a lung cancer specialist from the University of Wisconsin.

➤ Scott, Walter. 2000. *Lung Cancer: A Guide to Diagnosis and Treatment.* Omaha, Nebraska: Addicus Books.
This overview of lung cancer is presented in an easy-to-read, clear, concise book. Author Walter Scott, M.D., specializes in lung cancer surgery. The text is accompanied by comments from patients and caregivers and includes an appendix of chemotherapy agents, a list of resources, and a glossary.

➤ St. John, Tina. 2004. *With Every Breath: A Lung Cancer Guidebook.* Vancouver, WA: T. M. St. John. E-book available at: www.lungcancerguidebook.org
The full-text of this book is available free online and can be downloaded chapter-by-chapter as Adobe Acrobat (.pdf) files. It is also possible to purchase the print version through the Lung Cancer Caring Ambassadors Program at: www.lungcancercap.org. The author is a physician whose husband was diagnosed with stage IV lung cancer at age 42. The text includes color illustrations and provides a detailed description of lung anatomy, lung cancer types, treatment, nutrition, supportive care, complementary therapies, and practical issues. Includes an appendix with chemotherapy side effects profiles and a glossary.

Audiovisual Resources

➤ Patient Education Institute. *Lung Cancer Interactive Tutorial.* Access at: www.
medlineplus.gov and click on "Interactive Tutorials," then select from a list.
This slideshow utilizes illustrations, sound, and animations to provide
basic, easy-to-understand explanations of lung anatomy, lung cancer
diagnosis, and treatment. It is possible to turn on a voice-over or print a
text version.

➤ The Wellness Community. *Frankly Speaking About Lung Cancer.* Access at:
www.thewellnesscommunity.org
A webcast of the publication described above features a lung cancer specialist who provides an overview of lung cancer and discusses making
treatment decisions, managing side effects, and integrating mind-body
practices into treatment.

Web Resources

Sites focusing on lung cancer

➤ CancerCare. *It's Time to Focus On Lung Cancer.* Access at: www.lung-
cancer.org
Easy-to-read information about lung cancer covers lung cancer 101,
women and lung cancer, clinical trials, and an extensive description of
support services provided by CancerCare specifically to lung cancer patients. Those include a hotline, individual counseling and support groups,
and financial assistance.

➤ Lung Cancer Alliance. *Lung Cancer Alliance.* Access at: www.lungcancer
alliance. org
The Lung Cancer Alliance is dedicated to advocating for people living with
lung cancer or for those at risk for the disease. The site provides information
on disease and treatment, clinical trials, and support resources; news about
lung cancer; and information about the organization's support services and
advocacy activities.

➤ Lung Cancer Online Foundation (LCOF). *Lung Cancer Online.* Access at:
www.lungcanceronline.org/
A comprehensive, annotated directory of Internet information and resources for patients and families, this site is edited by Karen Parles, a librarian and lung cancer survivor. The directory is divided into ten main
topics, such as finding the best medical care, services and support, treatment information, medical tests, and news. The main topics further
divide into subsections. This is an excellent starting point for any information search about lung cancer.

Detailed sections in general cancer sites

➤ American Cancer Society. *Learn about Lung Cancer—Non-small Cell* and *Learn about Lung Cancer—Small Cell.* Access at: www.cancer.org and select from the menu under "Choose a Cancer Topic." Disease-specific detailed guides can be printed as Adobe Acrobat (.pdf) files.

➤ Healthology. *Lung Cancer.* Access at: www.healthology.com and click on "Consumer Health Library." This site offers detailed articles, Webcasts, and transcripts featuring cancer professionals.

➤ National Cancer Institute. *Lung Cancer.* Access at: www.cancer.gov and click on "Types of Cancer." The top page of the section links to patient versions of PDQ® statements, clinical trial information, and other NCI publications on this topic.

➤ People Living with Cancer. *Lung Cancer.* Access at: www.plwc.org and click on "Cancer Type." The PLWC oncologist-approved lung cancer guide can be printed in its entirety or by subtopic.

Sections about lung cancer are also available at the following sites:

➤ Canadian Cancer Society. Access at: www.cancer.ca and click on "About Cancer."

➤ Cancerbackup. Access at: www.cancerbackup.org.uk/Home and click on "Cancer Types."

➤ Cancerconsultants.com. Access at: www.cancerconsultants.com and make a selection under "Links to Specific Cancer Type Information."

➤ CancerSource.com. Access at: www.cancersource.com/Patient.pg and make a selection from the "Diagnosis & Treatment" pull-down menu.

➤ OncologyChannel.com. Access at: www.oncologychannel.com and select a condition from the left sidebar.

Patient Support Organization

➤ Lung Cancer Alliance. Access at: www.lungcanceralliance.org
Phone: 800-298-2436

Melanoma

Anatomical facts: The skin is the largest organ in the body. Its main function is to cover and protect the internal organs against heat, sunlight, injury, and infection. Other functions are to regulate the body's temperature, store water and fat, and produce vitamin D. The skin has two main layers: the epidermis and the dermis. The outer layer, the epidermis, is made of three types of cells: squamous cells, basal cells, and melanocytes. The dermis, which lies underneath the epidermis, contains blood vessels, lymph vessels, hair follicles, and sweat glands.

Illustrations available at the Medical Illustrations Gallery of the People Living with Cancer Web site.

Access at: www.plwc.org and click on Library on the left sidebar.

Melanoma is a highly curable cancer if found early. The five-year survival rate for stage 1 melanoma is more than 90%, but these survival rates are dramatically reduced for melanoma diagnosed in later stages. The American Cancer Society estimates about 59,000 new cases of melanoma per year and about 8,000 deaths. Although we know how to prevent melanoma, incidence in the United States has been increasing. Half of all melanomas are found in people under age 57, and cases of melanoma in childhood, although very rare, are increasing.

There is a strong correlation between exposure to ultraviolet (UV) radiation and development of melanoma. The risk is relative to the level of exposure in a lifetime; as a result, people who live in areas that get large amounts of UV radiation from the sun and people who spend time under sunlamps and in tanning booths are at higher risk. Experts believe that avoiding UV radiation from artificial sources and taking precautions against UV radiation from the sun can greatly reduce melanoma incidence. Other risk factors include having moles, especially the ones called dysplastic nevi; having fair skin that burns or freckles easily; having a personal history of melanoma or other skin cancers; and having a family history of melanoma.

Most melanoma tumors develop in the melanocytes in the skin (cutaneous melanoma); however, this disease may develop in other organs that have melanocytes, such as the eye. Melanoma in the eye is called ocular melanoma or intraocular melanoma. Melanomas spread through the lymphatic system and may metastasize to lymph nodes and distant organs such as the liver, lungs, or brain.

Treatment of melanoma is complex and depends on the stage and extent of the disease; for that reason, proper staging is crucial. Oftentimes the lymph nodes near the tumor need to be examined under a microscope for the spread of cancer cells. When performing a lymph node dissection, the surgeon removes all the lymph nodes in the area of the tumor and sends them for analysis. A newer procedure called sentinel lymph node biopsy prevents the removal of healthy lymph nodes. With this method, the surgeon checks only the sentinel node, which is the node to which the tumor drains, for the presence of melanoma cells. The histological analysis is done during the surgery, and nodes are removed only if the sentinel node tests positive for cancer cells.

After surgery, doctors sometimes recommend treatment with biological therapies that work on the immune system. The drugs interferon and interleukin-2 have been shown to be effective against melanoma. Vaccine therapy is still in experimental stages. Patients with metastatic disease may be treated with chemotherapy, radiation therapy, and sometimes more surgery to remove metastatic tumors. Since melanoma spreads and progresses differently in each patient, treatment is tailored to the specific needs of the patient, and various drugs and treatment approaches may be used.

Melanoma survivors need to be diligent about performing skin self-exams and are monitored very closely by a physician. People with a history of skin cancer need to become knowledgeable about preventing UV exposure and about special products and clothing that protect from the sun.

Information Sources

Brochures, Booklets, and Other Short Print Publications

➤ National Cancer Institute. *What You Need to Know about Melanoma.*
This booklet on melanoma discusses possible causes, symptoms, diagnosis, treatment, emotional issues, and questions to ask the doctor. Includes glossary of terms and other resources. Access at: https://cissecure.nci.nih.gov/ncipubs/

➤ National Comprehensive Cancer Network (NCCN). *Melanoma: Treatment Guidelines for Patients.*
This publication includes an overview of melanoma as well as treatment decision "trees" explaining the treatment choices for different disease stages and conditions. Developed from the NCCN Clinical Practice Guidelines in Oncology—the standard for clinical policy in cancer care. A Spanish-language version also is available. Access at: www.nccn.org/patients/

Books

➤ Kaufman, Howard L. 2005. *The Melanoma Book: A Complete Guide to Prevention and Treatment.* New York: Gotham Books.
This comprehensive and detailed review of melanoma, written at a high reading level, is divided into four parts: preventing melanoma, diagnosing and staging melanoma, treating melanoma, and melanoma research. While readers will gain a deep understanding of the medical aspects of the disease, this book does not cover psychosocial and supportive-care issues. Each chapter ends with a description of a case study to illustrate the key points and a list of questions for the doctor.

➤ McClay, Edward F., Mary-Eileen T. McClay, and Jodie Smith. 2004. *100 Questions and Answers about Melanoma and Other Skin Cancers.* Boston: Jones and Bartlett.

Detailed information about skin cancer is presented in an easy-to-read question-and-answer format. Terms are explained in the sidebar, and the book includes lists of Web sites, organizations, literature, and resources on general and specific topics related to melanoma. This book was co–authored by two skin healthcare professionals and a melanoma survivor.

➤ Poole, Catherine M., with DuPont Guerry. 2005. *Melanoma: Prevention, Detection, and Treatment.* 2d ed. New Haven, CT: Yale University Press.
  This guidebook explains the disease and treatment in a well-organized and concise manner. It includes chapters about melanoma prevention, risk factors, early detection, treatment, and emotional support. Appendixes include a list of cancer centers and melanoma specialists, staging guidelines, and support services and resources.

Audiovisual Resources

➤ Patient Education Institute. *Melanoma Interactive Tutorial.* Access at: www.medlineplus.gov, click on "Interactive Tutorials" and select from a list.
  This slideshow utilizes illustrations, sound, and animations to provide basic, easy-to-understand explanations of skin anatomy and the diagnosis, staging, and treatment of melanoma. It is possible to turn on a voice-over or print a text version.

➤ Information Television Network. 2005. *Understanding Melanoma.* (30 min.). Boca Raton, FL: Information Television Network. Available in DVD and VHS formats. Access at: www.itvisus.com or Amazon.com
  Part of the public television series *Healthy Body/Healthy Mind*, this program features cancer specialists explaining melanoma risk factors and some of the early signs and symptoms to watch for. The program also features color graphics and animations that illustrate the scientific content.

Web Resources

Sites focusing on melanoma

➤ American Academy of Dermatology. *SkinCancerNet.* Access at: www. skincarephysicians.com/skincancernet/
  This site focuses on skin cancer prevention and screening. It includes visual guides describing the main skin cancer types and offers information about prevention and screening. The section on when to see a dermatologist includes access to a physician-finder database. The articles section includes more in-depth information about specific topics relating to melanoma, such as chemotherapy, immunotherapy, and more.

➤ *MelanomaCenter.org.* Access at: www.melanomacenter.org
This site includes detailed information about melanoma, from prevention to diagnosis, treatment, and follow-up care. It includes an interactive staging tool and information about clinical trials. The site focuses mainly on medical topics and has very little information about support, quality-of-life, and psychosocial issues.

➤ *Skin Cancer Foundation.* Access at: www.skincancer.org
The mission of the Skin Cancer Foundation is to increase awareness of the skin cancer epidemic. The site includes many educational materials about skin cancer prevention, including sun tanning, tanning beds, tanning in childhood, and more. It includes a short overview of melanoma treatment and a list of melanoma treatment centers.

Detailed sections in general cancer sites

➤ American Cancer Society. *Learn about Skin Cancer—Melanoma.* Access at: www.cancer.org and select from the menu under "Choose a Cancer Topic." A detailed guide about melanoma can be printed by section or as an Adobe Acrobat (.pdf) file.

➤ National Cancer Institute. *Melanoma.* Access at: www.cancer.gov and click on "Types of cancer." The top page of the section links to patient versions of PDQ® statements for specific melanoma types.

➤ People Living with Cancer. *Melanoma.* Access at: www.plwc.org and click on "Cancer Type." The PLWC oncologist-approved guide about melanoma can be printed in its entirety or by subtopic.

Sections about melanoma are also available at the following sites:

➤ Canadian Cancer Society. Access at: www.cancer.ca and click on "About Cancer."

➤ Cancerbackup. Access at: www.cancerbackup.org.uk/Home and click on "Cancer Types."

➤ Cancerconsultants.com. Access at: www.cancerconsultants.com and make a selection under "Links to Specific Cancer Type Information."

➤ CancerSource.com. Access at: www.cancersource.com/Patient.pg and make a selection from the "Diagnosis & Treatment" pull-down menu.

➤ OncologyChannel.com. Access at: www.oncologychannel.com and select a condition from the left sidebar.

Patient Support Organization

➤ American Melanoma Foundation. Access at: www.melanomafoundation.org
Phone: 619-448-0991

Multiple Myeloma

Anatomical facts: Plasma cells are white blood cells that make antibodies. Antibodies are part of the immune system and help protect the body from germs. The plasma cells are found mainly in the bone marrow—the soft, inner part of bones.

Illustrations available at the Medical Illustrations Gallery of the People Living with Cancer Web site.

Access at: www.plwc.org and click on Library on the left sidebar.

The American Cancer Society estimates approximately 20,000 new cases of multiple myeloma per year, and 11,000 deaths. Slightly more than half of new diagnoses occur in men and 80% of cases occur after age 60. Myeloma is very rare in people under age 45. This disease is twice as common in African Americans as in Caucasians.

Myeloma begins when a plasma cell becomes abnormal and produces more abnormal cells that form tumors in the bone marrow. If there is only one tumor, it is called a plasmacytoma. In most cases, tumors are formed in bones in many sites in the body; thus the disease is called multiple myeloma. Myeloma cells are very destructive. They crowd out normal blood cells and prevent them from functioning properly. This can result in a shortage of red blood cells, which may lead to fatigue; shortage of platelets, which may lead to excessive bleeding; and shortage of white blood cells, which interferes with the body's ability to fight infection. Myeloma cells also cause bones to dissolve; hence fractures and bone pain are a major problem in people with myeloma. Multiple myeloma is the most common type of plasma cell tumor.

People with other diseases that affect plasma cells—monoclonal gammopathy of undetermined significance (MGUS) or solitary plasmacytoma—will eventually develop multiple myeloma. Studies suggest that exposure to radioactivity, working in certain petroleum-related industries, and obesity may increase the risk of multiple myeloma.

The standard treatment for multiple myeloma in recent years is stem cell transplantation, especially in younger patients who do not have other health conditions. If stem cell transplantation is not possible, patients are treated with a few combinations of chemotherapy and steroids. The drug thalidomide induces temporary, partial, and even complete remissions in about 70% of patients. A class of drugs called bisphosphonates is effective in slowing down the process that causes bone damage.

Supportive-care issues for multiple myeloma patients include fatigue and bone pain.

Brochures, Booklets, and Other Short Print Publications

➤ The Leukemia & Lymphoma Society. *Myeloma.*
   A detailed overview of multiple myeloma covers normal blood and marrow, subtypes, diagnosis, treatment, complications, and social and emotional aspects. An easy-to-read version of this publication is titled *Myeloma: A Guide for Patients and Their Families.* Larger print and bullet points summarize the topic in a concise manner. Access at: www.leukemia-lymphoma.org

➤ Multiple Myeloma Research Foundation. *Multiple Myeloma: A Disease Overview.*
   A 32-page booklet on multiple myeloma covers symptoms, diagnostic tests, classification, prognostic indicators, genetic profiling, treatment options, questions for the doctor, and resources for patients. Access at: www. multiplemyeloma.org

➤ National Cancer Institute. *What You Need to Know about Multiple Myeloma.*
   This booklet on multiple myeloma discusses possible causes, symptoms, diagnosis, treatment, emotional issues, and questions to ask the doctor. Includes glossary of terms and other resources. Access at: https://cissecure. nci.nih.gov/ncipubs/

Books

➤ Bashey, Asad and Huston, James W. 2005. *100 Questions and Answers about Myeloma.* Sudbury, MA: Jones and Bartlett.
   Detailed information about myeloma is presented in an easy-to-read question-and-answer format covering treatment options, post–treatment quality of life, and sources of support. Terms are explained in the sidebar, and the book includes lists of Web sites, organizations, literature, and resources on general and specific topic related to myeloma. This book was co–authored by a hematologist-oncologist specializing in myeloma treatment and a myeloma survivor.

Audiovisual Resources

➤ Patient Education Institute. *Multiple Myeloma Interactive Tutorial.* Access at: www.medlineplus.gov, click on "Interactive Tutorials" and select from a list. This slide show utilizes illustrations, sound, and animations to provide basic, easy-to-understand explanations of blood cell types and the diagnosis, staging, and treatment of multiple myeloma. It is possible to turn on a voice-over or print a text version.

Web Resources

Sites focusing on multiple myeloma

➤ International Myeloma Foundation. Access at: www.myeloma.org
The site of the International Myeloma Foundation includes in-depth information about myeloma presented in text and video formats. Special features include a guide to new drugs in development, information and links to resources about clinical trials, and an overview of myeloma bone disease, with a caregiver's manual. The full text of the organization's publications and information about support services and educational events also are available on this site.

➤ The Leukemia and Lymphoma Society. Access at: www.leukemia-lymphoma.org
The site of the world's largest organization dedicated to blood cancers includes many sections and features for people with myeloma. Live and archived versions of educational teleconferences and Webcasts enable users to study complicated topics explained by top experts. The site also includes medical news about myeloma, short and longer overviews of the disease, and information about the organization's support services for patients.

➤ Leukaemia Research. Access at: www.lrf.org.uk
Leukaemia Research is a British research charity focusing on blood cancers and disorders. The "Information and Education" section offers printable booklets on adult and childhood blood cancers, including some on rare subtypes and conditions. The "News" section includes stories about research developments and other related articles.

➤ Multiple Myeloma Research Foundation. Access at: www.themmrf.org
The focus of this site is treatment and research. It provides an in-depth review for each of the various treatment options available to patients, as well as a comprehensive review of emerging therapies. The clinical trials database has a sophisticated search interface that enables searching by certain parameters, such as location and specific therapy. The "In the News" section keeps track of articles published in the scientific medical literature. The site also maintains a comprehensive list of links to other resources and sites of interest to myeloma patients and families.

Detailed sections in general cancer sites

➤ American Cancer Society. *Learn about Multiple Myeloma.* Access at: www.cancer.org and select from the menu under "Choose a Cancer Topic." A detailed guide about myeloma can be printed by section or as an Adobe Acrobat (.pdf) file.

➤ National Cancer Institute. *Multiple Myeloma/Other Plasma Cell Neo-plasms.* Access at: www.cancer.gov and click on "Types of Cancer." The top page of the section links to patient versions of PDQ® statements, clinical trial information, and other NCI publications on this topic.

➤ People Living with Cancer. *Multiple Myeloma.* Access at: www.plwc.org and click on "Cancer Type." The PLWC oncologist-approved guide for multiple myeloma can be printed in its entirety or by subtopic.

Sections about myeloma are also available at the following sites:

➤ Canadian Cancer Society. Access at: www.cancer.ca and click on "About Cancer."

➤ Cancerbackup. Access at: www.cancerbackup.org.uk/Home and click on "Cancer Types."

➤ Cancerconsultants.com. Access at: www.cancerconsultants.com and make a selection under "Links to Specific Cancer type Information."

➤ CancerSource.com. Access at: www.cancersource.com/Patient.pg and make a selection from the "Diagnosis & Treatment" pull-down menu.

➤ OncologyChannel.com. Access at: www.oncologychannel.com and select a condition from the left sidebar.

Patient Support Organizations

➤ International Myeloma Foundation. Access at: www.myeloma.org
Phone: 800-452-2873

➤ The Leukemia & Lymphoma Society. Access at: www.leukemia.org
Phone: 800-955-4572

Non-Hodgkin's Lymphoma

Anatomical facts: The lymphatic system is a network of vessels, similar to blood vessels, which carry the lymph fluid to different parts of the body. Lymph is a colorless fluid that contains infection-fighting white blood cells called lympho-cytes. Lymphocytes are made and stored in lymph nodes, small bean-shaped organs that cluster along the lymphatic system. There are two types of lympho-cytes: B lymphocytes (B cells) and T lymphocytes (T cells). Other parts of the lymphatic system include the spleen, thymus, tonsils, and bone marrow. Lym-phatic tissue is also found in other parts of the body, including the stomach, in-testines, and skin. The lymphatic system is part of the body's immune system.

Illustrations available at the Medical Illustrations Gallery of the People Living with Cancer Web site.

Access at: www.plwc.org and click on Library on the left sidebar.

The American Cancer Society estimates approximately 63,000 new cases of non-Hodgkin's lymphoma (NHL) per year. About 5% of cases are discovered in children; however, the type of non-Hodgkin's lymphoma seen in children is different from the adult type. Children's non-Hodgkin's lymphoma is discussed in Chapter 5 on p. 178.

NHL is the fifth most common cancer in the United States (excluding non-melanoma skin cancer), and more then half the cases are diagnosed in people older than 65. Non-Hodgkin's lymphoma is more common in men than in women and less common in African Americans and Asian Americans than in Caucasian Americans. The overall five-year survival rate is 60%, but survival rates vary considerably according to subtype and stage of the disease at the time of diagnosis.

People whose immune system is weakened as a result of an autoimmune disease, an organ transplant, or an human immunodeficiency virus (HIV) infection have a significant risk to develop NHL. It should be noted that most people diagnosed with NHL are not associated with a specific risk factor.

Non-Hodgkin's lymphoma develops from either B or T lymphocytes in the lymph nodes. NHL should not be confused with Hodgkin's disease, which is a different cancer that develops in the lymphatic tissue. Hodgkin's disease is discussed on page 89. The classification of NHL is very complex. It has changed and evolved frequently over the years to reflect an increased understanding of the chemical and generic characteristics of these cancers. NHLs are classified into close to 30 different types, each with its own unique appearance, pattern of growth, and immunologic and genetic features that determine how the cancer will progress and respond to treatment. Most lymphomas are usually designated as a "B cell" or "T cell" according to the type of the lymphocyte from which they originated. NHLs are also grouped according to their growth pattern and classified as an "indolent," or a "low grade," lymphoma which progresses very slowly, or an "aggressive" lymphoma which grows rapidly and requires immediate treatment. Ironically, aggressive lymphomas are easier to cure than indolent lymphomas that transform into more aggressive types.

The most common NHL type diagnosed in the United States is a diffuse large B cell lymphoma, which is a type of aggressive lymphoma that can start in the lymph nodes or in lymphatic tissue in the gastrointestinal tract, testicles, thyroid, skin, breast, central nervous system, or bones. The second most common type is follicular lymphoma, which is an indolent lymphoma that originates from B cells and occurs in many lymph node sites in the body as well as in the bone marrow.

Most people with NHL are treated with chemotherapy and radiation therapy. Bone marrow or stem cell transplantation may be used if standard therapy has failed. A new class of drugs, monoclonal antibodies, destroys NHL cells by targeting a specific substance that is found on the surface of some types of lymphoma cells. *Radioimmunotherapy* is a term referring to monoclonal antibody drugs that have radioactive molecules. Surgery is seldom used to treat NHL. Most patients have surgery only to obtain a biopsy. In rare cases, where a lymphoma started in an organ outside of the lymph system and has not spread, surgery is performed with a curative intent.

Some people live with NHL for many years and go on and off different treatment regimens a number of times. During remission periods, survivors and loved ones may experience anxiety and fear of relapse, which may be overwhelming, especially around times of checkups. A recurrence may cause strong feelings of devastation and disappointment. In addition, survivors may need to deal with long-term effects of treatment especially after a bone marrow or stem cell transplantation. Relevant topics include nutrition, fertility, sexuality, financial, insurance, and employment issues.

Information Sources

Brochures, Booklets, and Other Short Print Publications

> The Leukemia & Lymphoma Society. *The Lymphomas: A Guide for Patients and Their Families: Hodgkin and Non-Hodgkin Lymphoma Information.*
> This basic introduction to lymphoma starts with the anatomy of the lymphatic system and continues with a description of diagnostic tests, subtypes, and treatments for Hodgkin's and non-Hodgkin's lymphoma. An easy-to-read version of this publication is *The Lymphomas: A Guide for Patients and Their Families.* Larger print and bullet points summarize the topic in a concise manner. Access online at: www.leukemia-lymphoma.org

> Lymphoma Research Foundation. *Lymphoma Resource Guide.*
> A listing of organizations, online resources, audio- and videotapes, publications, and therapies that are of interest to lymphoma patients and families. Access online at: www.lymphoma.org

> Lymphoma Research Foundation. *Understanding Non-Hodgkin's Lymphoma: A Guide for Patients.*
> This 100-page booklet provides a comprehensive review of NHL, including diagnosis, treatment, coping with side effects, clinical trial experimental treatments, and living with cancer. Includes a glossary. Individual copies are free and can be obtained by calling the Lymphoma Research Foundation at: 800-500-9976

➤ National Comprehensive Cancer Network (NCCN). *Non-Hodgkin's Lymphoma: Treatment Guidelines for Patients.*
This publication includes an overview of non-Hodgkin's lymphoma as well as treatment decision "trees" explaining the treatment choices for different stages and conditions of NHL. This resource is developed from the NCCN Clinical Practice Guidelines in Oncology—the standard for clinical policy in cancer care. A Spanish-language version also is available. Access at: www.nccn.org/patients/

➤ National Cancer Institute. *What You Need to Know about Non-Hodgkin's Lymphoma.*
A concise introduction to non-Hodgkin's lymphoma covers staging, treatment options, and emotional support. Includes a glossary and a list of questions for the doctor. Access online at: https://cissecure.nci.nih.gov/ncipubs/

Books

➤ Adler, Elizabeth M. 2005. *Living with Lymphoma: A Patient's Guide.* Baltimore, MD: Johns Hopkins University Press.
Written by a neurobiologist and an NHL survivor, this book offers a detailed explanation of cell biology that helps understand the disease and treatment. While this book provides an in-depth look at the medical side of lymphoma and provides descriptions of specific drugs, drug combinations, and treatment approaches, psychosocial issues are not as meticulously covered. Sophisticated readers who are interested in learning the scientific aspects of lymphoma will appreciate this book.

➤ Holman, Peter, Jodi Garrett, and William D. Jansen. 2004. *100 Questions and Answers about Lymphoma.* Sudbury, MA: Jones and Bartlett.
Detailed information about lymphoma is presented in an easy-to-read question-and-answer format. Terms are explained in the sidebar, and the book includes lists of Web sites, organizations, literature, and resources on general and specific topics related to non-Hodgkin's lymphoma. This book was co–authored by a lymphoma specialist, an oncology nurse, and an NHL survivor.

Web Resources

Sites focusing on Non-Hodgkin's Lymphoma

➤ Leukaemia Research. Access at: www.lrf.org.uk
Leukaemia Research is a British research charity focusing on blood cancers and disorders. The "Information and Education" section offers printable

booklets on adult and childhood blood cancers, including some on rare subtypes and conditions. The "News" section includes stories about research developments and other related articles.

➤ The Leukemia & Lymphoma Society. Access at: www.leukemia-lymphoma. org

The site of the world's largest organization dedicated to blood cancers includes many sections and features for people with lymphoma. Live and archived versions of educational teleconferences and Webcasts enable users to study complicated topics explained by top experts. The site also includes medical news about lymphoma, short and longer overviews of the diseases, and information about the organization's support services for patients.

➤ Lymphoma Information Network. Access at: www.lymphomainfo.net/

This well-organized directory of lymphoma information sources presents short, concise introductions to many types of lymphoma. Each section has a list of references with links to other sites, PubMed abstracts, or books on Amazon. This site has been maintained for over ten years by an NHL survivor and is useful as a starting point for a search on specific or complex issues of lymphoma.

➤ Lymphoma Research Foundation. Access at: www.lymphoma.org

The Lymphoma Research Foundation is a patient-support and -advocacy organization providing support and education to lymphoma patients and families. Information about the disease, treatment, and research news are presented in fact sheets, Webcasts, newsletters, and other formats. This site also includes information about support programs and services for patients and families.

Detailed sections in general cancer sites

➤ American Cancer Society. *Learn about Lymphoma, Non-Hodgkin's Type.* Access at: www.cancer.org and select from the menu under "Choose a Cancer Topic." A detailed guide about NHL can be printed by section or as an Adobe Acrobat (.pdf) file.

➤ Healthology. *Lymphoma.* Access at: www.healthology.com and click on "Consumer Health Library." This site offers detailed articles, Webcasts, and transcripts featuring cancer professionals.

➤ National Cancer Institute. *Non-Hodgkin's Lymphoma, Adult.* Access at: www.cancer.gov and click on "Types of Cancer." The top page of the section links to patient versions of PDQ® statements, clinical trial information, and other NCI publications on this topic.

➤ People Living with Cancer. *Lymphoma, Non-Hodgkin.* Access at: www. plwc.org and click on "Cancer Type." The PLWC oncologist-approved non-Hodgkin's lymphoma guide can be printed in its entirety or by subtopic.

➤ The Wellness Community. *Frankly Speaking about Lymphoma*. Access at: www.thewellnesscommunity.org and click on "Cancer Information" on the left sidebar. This section explains lymphoma and its treatment, integrating mind-body practices into lymphoma treatment, and managing the personal impact of the illness.

Sections about non-Hodgkin's lymphoma are also available at the following sites:

➤ Canadian Cancer Society. Access at: www.cancer.ca and click on "About Cancer."

➤ Cancerbackup. Access at: www.cancerbackup.org.uk/Home and click on "Cancer Types."

➤ Cancerconsultants.com. Access at: www.cancerconsultants.com and make a selection under "Links to Specific Cancer Type Information."

➤ CancerSource.com. Access at: www.cancersource.com/Patient.pg and make a selection from the "Diagnosis & Treatment" pull-down menu.

➤ OncologyChannel.com. Access at: www.oncologychannel.com and select a condition from the left sidebar.

Patient Support Organizations

➤ The Leukemia & Lymphoma Society. Access at: www.leukemia.org
   Phone: 800-955-4572

➤ Lymphoma Research Foundation. Access at: www.lymphoma.org
   Phone: Los Angeles office 800-500-9976; New York office 800-235-6848

Ovarian Cancer

Anatomical facts: The ovaries are a pair of organs in the female reproductive system. They are located in the pelvis, one on each side of the uterus. Each ovary is about the size and shape of an almond. The ovaries have two functions: they produce eggs and the female hormone estrogen.

Illustrations available at the Medical Illustrations Gallery of the People Living with Cancer Web site.

Access at: www.plwc.org and click on Library on the left sidebar.

Ovarian cancer has the highest mortality rate of all gynecologic cancers. In the United States it ranks eighth in the number of new cases per year with 22,000, yet it ranks in fifth place in the number of deaths per year. The great majority of the 15,000 women who die from ovarian cancer each year could not be cured because their disease was not diagnosed early enough. With early diagnosis, when the tumor has not spread beyond the ovary, this cancer has a 95% survival rate after five years. Unfortunately, the symptoms of early-stage ovarian cancer are very vague, for example, gas, bloating, indigestion, back or leg pains, and other symptoms that mimic gastrointestinal and other conditions. For this reason, more than 70% of patients are diagnosed after their disease has already spread beyond the ovaries.

Although the exact causes of ovarian cancer are not fully understood, researchers have identified several risk factors. The most significant risk factor is having a genetic mutation in the BRCA1 or BRCA2 gene. These genetic mutations are more common among women of Ashkenazi Jewish ancestry and are also responsible for increased breast cancer risk. Other risk factors include age, obesity, early onset of menstruation and late onset of menopause, and never having children. Researchers are also studying the links between ovarian cancer and infertility, use of fertility drugs, use of estrogen replacement therapy, and use of talc, but so far none of these factors has been identified as a cause of ovarian cancer.

More then 90% of ovarian cancers are epithelial ovarian tumors; the remaining 10% are germ cell tumors and stromal tumors. Sometimes epithelial ovarian tumors develop outside of the ovaries, from the cells that line the pelvis or abdomen. These tumors are called primary peritoneal carcinoma and their symptoms and treatment are similar to ovarian epithelial tumors.

Early-stage ovarian cancer can be treated with surgery only. The surgery for ovarian cancer includes the removal of the ovaries, fallopian tubes, uterus, and other tissues or organs to which the disease has spread. The goal of the surgery is to remove as much of the cancer as possible. Women who have minimal tumor deposits after surgery generally experience longer remission periods and longer survival. Since more than 70% of patients are diagnosed with advanced disease, most ovarian cancer patients will be treated with chemotherapy in addition to surgery. Ovarian cancer that has recurred can be treated with radiation therapy and hormonal therapy in addition to more surgery and chemotherapy.

Newer and better drugs with fewer side effects are constantly being tested for ovarian cancer. Better drug regimens have improved the overall five-year survival rate from 30% in the 1960s to 50% today. This means that more women are living longer periods with ovarian cancer as a chronic disease. These women may ask for information on genetic testing, long-term side effects of cancer treatment, and practical issues of cancer survivorship.

Progress is also being made in developing a simple and effective screening method to enable the diagnosis of ovarian cancer when it is still in an early stage and curable.

Information Sources

Brochures, Booklets, and Other Short Print Publications

➤ National Cancer Institute. *What You Need to Know about Ovarian Cancer.* This booklet on ovarian cancer discusses possible causes, symptoms, diagnosis, treatment, emotional issues, and questions to ask the doctor. Includes resources for additional information. Access at: https://cissecure. nci.nih.gov/ncipubs/

➤ National Comprehensive Cancer Network (NCCN). *Ovarian Cancer: Treatment Guidelines for Patients.* This publication includes an overview of ovarian cancer as well as treatment decision "trees" explaining the treatment choices for different disease stages and conditions. Developed from the NCCN Clinical Practice Guidelines in Oncology—the standard for clinical policy in cancer care. A Spanish-language version also is available. Access at: www.nccn.org/patients/

➤ Piver, M. Steven, and Eltabbakh, Gamal. 2005. *Myths and Facts about Ovarian Cancer: What You Need to Know.* 5th ed. Manhasset, NY: Oncology Pub. Group of CMP Healthcare Media. This 64-page handbook, with a detailed overview of ovarian cancer, includes many color illustrations and photographs. The sidebar features facts that dispel common myths about ovarian cancer and repeat key points. Includes a list of resources and a glossary. The authors are ovarian cancer specialists. To view online, download an Adobe Acrobat (.pdf) file or access at: www.cancernetwork.com.

Books

➤ Conner, Kristine, and Lauren Langford. 2003. *Ovarian Cancer: Your Guide to Taking Control.* Sebastopol, CA: O'Reilly. This guide to ovarian cancer attempts to help women diagnosed with disease regain control over their lives and make informed decisions. The book starts with "Ten Things to Do Now"—tips to help women get through the time just before and just after diagnosis. The following chapters describe the disease's path from treatment to remission, covering medical as well as psychosocial issues. Recurring features include insights of ovarian cancer survivors, "pros and cons" tables, and lists of questions for the doctor for all decision points.

➤ Dizon, Don S., Nadeem R. Abu-Rustum, and Andrea Gibbs Brown. 2006. *100 Questions and Answers about Ovarian Cancer*. 2d ed. Boston: Jones and Bartlett.
Detailed information about ovarian cancer is presented in an easy-to-read question-and-answer format. Terms are explained in the sidebar, and the book includes lists of Web sites, organizations, literature, and resources on general and specific topics related to ovarian cancer. This book was co–authored by two gynecologic oncologists and includes the comments of an ovarian cancer survivor.

➤ Montz, Fredrick J., Robert E. Bristow, and Paula J. Anastasia. *A Guide to Survivorship for Women with Ovarian Cancer*. 2005. Baltimore: Johns Hopkins University Press.
This book, authored by two gynecologic oncologists and a gynecologic-oncology nurse, puts particular emphasis on the concept of survivorship. In addition to covering medical aspects of ovarian cancer, the authors address the emotional distress and worry that accompanies the disease. Chapters include controlling pain and suffering, complementary and alternative therapies, image recovery, taking care of social needs, end of life, and survivorship.

Book Chapters

➤ Hartmann, Lynn C., and Charles L. Loprinzi. 2005. *Mayo Clinic Guide to Women's Cancers*. Rochester, MN: Mayo Clinic.
This book was edited by two physicians from the Mayo Clinic with book chapters written and reviewed by Mayo Clinic experts. Part two of the book focuses on gynecologic cancer with a few chapters about ovarian cancer. The third part of the book, "Living with Cancer," provides supportive-care information that is relevant to all women with cancer. A unique feature of this book is the visual guide that includes color illustrations explaining the cancer process, anatomy surgery, and radiation. Other photos and illustrations, tables, and text boxes throughout the book help in understanding and comprehension.

➤ McGinn, Kerry Anne, and Pamela J. Haylock. 2003. *Women's Cancers: How to Prevent Them, How to Treat Them, How to Beat Them*. 3d ed., fully updated ed. Alameda, CA: Hunter House.
This book provides practical information for women with cancer and includes a chapter about cancer of the ovaries. Other chapters discuss working with the medical team, sources of support, complementary and alternative treatments, and feelings. The part called "Life after Cancer" focuses on the physical, emotional, and social challenges women may experience after treatment ends. The authors are oncology nurses.

Audiovisual Resources

➤ Patient Education Institute. *Ovarian Cancer Interactive Tutorial.* Access at: www.medlineplus.gov and click on "Interactive Tutorials," then select from a list.

This slideshow utilizes illustrations, sound, and animations to provide basic, easy-to-understand explanations of the anatomy, diagnosis, and treatment options of ovarian cancer. It is possible to turn on a voice-over or print a text version.

Web Resources

Sites focusing on ovarian cancer

➤ National Ovarian Cancer Association. Access at: www.ovariancanada. org

The site of this Canadian organization offers detailed information about ovarian cancer diagnosis, treatment, and survivorship, including physical and psychological aspects. The caregiver/partner section focuses on communication, quality-of-life concerns, and caring for the caregiver. A few fact sheets are provided in English, French, and other languages. The site also includes video files and a glossary.

➤ National Ovarian Cancer Resource Center. Access at: www.ovarian.org

This comprehensive site is maintained by the National Ovarian Cancer Coalition, a leading organization providing information and education. Special features include frequently asked questions, links to clinical trial sites relevant to ovarian cancer, and a breaking-news section. The site also includes the full text of the alliance's publications in English and Spanish, including a 24-page booklet on sexuality and intimacy.

➤ Women's Cancer Network. Access at: www.wcn.org

This site is provided by the Gynecologic Cancer Foundation, which is affiliated with the Society of Gynecologist Oncologists. Detailed information about cancer in women, including the reproductive cancer, is included. Special features are an extensive news section; a "Find a Doctor" database, which helps locate oncologists specializing in gynecologic cancers; and links to clinical trial databases.

Detailed sections in general cancer sites

➤ American Cancer Society. *Learn about Ovarian Cancer.* Access at: www. cancer.org and select from the menu under "Choose a Cancer Topic." A detailed guide about ovarian cancer can be printed as an Adobe Acrobat (.pdf) file.

➤ National Cancer Institute. *Ovarian Cancer*. Access at: www.cancer.gov and click on "Types of Cancer." The top page of the section links to patient versions of PDQ® statements, clinical trial information, and other NCI publications on this topic.

➤ People Living with Cancer. *Ovarian Cancer*. Access at: www.plwc.org and click on "Cancer Type." The PLWC oncologist-approved ovarian cancer guide can be printed in its entirety or by subtopic.

➤ The Wellness Community. *The Patient Active Guide to Living with Ovarian Cancer*. Access at: www.thewellnesscommunity.org and click on "Cancer Information" on the left sidebar. This section provides information about the diagnosis and treatment of ovarian cancer, side effects, lifestyle concerns, stress reduction, and strategies to approach ovarian cancer as a chronic disease.

Sections about ovarian cancer are also available at the following sites:

➤ Canadian Cancer Society. Access at: www.cancer.ca and click on "About Cancer."

➤ Cancerbackup. Access at: www.cancerbackup.org.uk/Home and click on "Cancer Types."

➤ Cancerconsultants.com. Access at: www.cancerconsultants.com and make a selection under "Links to Specific Cancer type Information."

➤ CancerSource.com. Access at: www.cancersource.com/Patient.pg and make a selection from the "Diagnosis & Treatment" pull-down menu.

➤ OncologyChannel.com. Access at: www.oncologychannel.com and select a condition from the left sidebar.

Patient-Support Organizations

➤ EyesOnThePrize.org. An online support group for gynecologic cancer survivors. Access at: www.eyesontheprize.org

➤ SHARE: Self-Help for Women with Breast or Ovarian Cancer. Access at: www.sharecancersupport.org
Phone: 212-719-0364

Pancreatic Cancer

Anatomical facts: The pancreas is located behind the stomach deep in the abdomen. This small, flat organ contains two types of glands: endocrine and exocrine. Endocrine cells are arranged in small clusters called islets and produce the hormones insulin and glucagon, which regulate the level of glucose (sugar) in the blood. Endocrine cells account for only 5% of cells in the pancreas. The rest are exocrine cells which make "juices" that contain enzymes necessary for food digestion. Pancreatic juice is delivered to the small intestine through a system of tiny tubes called ducts. The small ducts all lead to the pancreatic duct, which empties into the duodenum, the first section of the small intestine. The intersection of the pancreatic duct, the common bile duct that comes from the liver, and the duodenum is called ampulla of Vater.

Illustrations available at the Medical Illustrations Gallery of the People Living with Cancer Web site.

Access at: www.plwc.org and click on Library on the left sidebar.

Only 15% to 20% of pancreatic cancer patients are diagnosed while the cancer is still confined to the pancreas and surgery is feasible. This is the reason why only a quarter of the 37,000 people in the United States who are diagnosed with this cancer every year are still alive a year after the diagnosis. Cancer of the pancreas is the fourth leading cause of cancer deaths, with 33,000 deaths per year.

The reasons for the difficulty in diagnosing pancreatic cancer in the early stage are twofold: one is that tumors in this organ produce very vague symptoms, which are usually attributed to other digestive conditions, and the other is because the pancreas is located deep inside the abdomen and surrounded by other organs that interfere with the ability to see or feel tumors during a routine physical exam.

Several risk factors for pancreatic cancer have been identified. People who have diabetes or chronic pancreatitis are at increased risk. Smoking, obesity, and a diet high in meats and fat have been linked to the development of this cancer. Pancreatic cancer is more common among males, people over 60, people with a family history of pancreatic cancer, and African Americans.

Two distinct types of cancer originate from the exocrine cells and the endocrine cells in the pancreas. Tumors that develop from exocrine cells are mostly adenocarcinomas and are much more common than endocrine tumors. Many of the information sources about pancreatic cancer provide data relevant only to this tumor type. Tumors that arise from the endocrine cells of the pancreas, sometimes called islet cell tumors or neuroendocrine tumors, are very different from exocrine tumors with regard to symptoms, diagnosis, treatment, and prognosis. A third type of cancer called ampullary cancer develops in the ampulla of Vater. The treatment for this type of cancer is similar to that for exocrine pancreatic cancer, and sometimes it is included in pancreatic cancer information sources. When interacting with information seekers, the librarian should ask the patrons if they know the exact subtype. If this fact is unknown, the librarian should include information on the most common type and ask the patrons to verify with their health care provider that the information is relevant. (In many cases patients know if they are diagnosed with the rarer islet cell cancer.)

Pancreatic cancer can be cured if found early and surgery is possible. If the tumor is located in the "head" region of the pancreas, surgeons perform the Whipple procedure, where they cut out the diseased section and hook the remainder up to the small intestine. Sometimes it is necessary to remove the entire pancreas along with other tissues and organs, such as the spleen, bile duct, gallbladder, part of the small intestine, and lymph nodes. This procedure is called a pancreatectomy. If the entire pancreas is removed, patients will need to take insulin and oral enzymes to help with digestion. Unfortunately, even after surgery, pancreatic cancer tends to recur. Radiation therapy and chemotherapy are often prescribed after surgery to try and slow down the progression of the disease and improve symptoms. In recent years, the chemotherapy drug gemcitabine (Gemzar) has been shown to extend remission periods and improve survival rates of patients with inoperable pancreatic tumors.

Pancreatic cancer survivors suffer from many side effects caused by the disease and its treatment. One common problem is blockage of the bile duct, a condition that may cause pain and digestive problems. This blockage can be treated with open surgery or by inserting stents through an endoscope. Nutrition is a major issue for people with pancreatic cancer who may have trouble maintaining their body weight. Nutritional supplements or feeding tubes may improve the patient's nutrition and increase energy levels. Pain is another issue for patients with this cancer, and it is sometimes beneficial to ask the information seeker if he or she needs information about this topic. Patients and caregivers may also ask for information on end-of-life issues and advanced directives.

Information Sources

Brochures, Booklets, and Other Short Print Publications

➤ Abbruzzese, James L., and Ben Ebrahimi. 2002. *Myths and Facts about Pancreatic Cancer: What You Need to Know.* Melville, NY: PRR.
  This 64-page handbook with a detailed overview of pancreatic cancer includes many color illustrations and photographs. The sidebar features facts that dispel common myths about pancreatic cancer and

repeat key points. Includes a list of resources and a glossary. The authors are pancreatic cancer specialists from M. D. Anderson Cancer Center. To view online, download an Adobe Acrobat (.pdf) file or access at: www.cancernetwork.com.

➤ National Cancer Institute. *What You Need to Know about Cancer of the Pancreas.*
This booklet on pancreatic cancer discusses possible causes, symptoms, diagnosis, treatment, emotional issues, and questions to ask the doctor. Includes glossary of terms and other resources. Access at: https://cissecure. nci.nih.gov/ncipubs/

➤ PanCAN. *An Overview of Pancreatic Cancer.*
This booklet provides basic information about pancreatic cancer including anatomy, diagnostic tests, and treatment options. Has color photos, illustrations, and tables. Provided by the Pancreatic Cancer Action Network at 877-272-6226 or www.pancan.org

Books

➤ O'Reilly, Eileen, and Joanne Frankel Kelvin. 2003. *100 Questions and Answers about Pancreatic Cancer.* Sudbury, MA: Jones and Bartlett.
Detailed information about pancreatic cancer is presented in an easy-to-read question-and-answer format covering treatment options, post–treatment quality of life, and sources of support. Terms are explained in the sidebar, and the book includes lists of Web sites, organizations, literature, and resources on general and specific topics related to pancreatic cancer. This book was co–authored by a physician and a registered nurse and includes comments from two pancreatic cancer survivors.

Web Resources

Sites focusing on pancreatic cancer

➤ Pancreatic Cancer Action Network. Access at: www.pancan.org
One section of the site offers comprehensive information about pancreatic cancer including treatment option side effects, diet and nutrition, end of life, finding a health care professional, and clinical trials. The site also has information about patient-support programs and services and educational meetings and conferences with experts. It is possible to order the organization's publications and access the full text of the newsletter, which has articles about medical and supportive-care topics. The section for caregivers features tips and advice for the caregiver and for those helping the caregiver.

➤ Pancreas Cancer. Access at: http://pathology2.jhu.edu/pancreas/index.htm
Detailed information about pancreatic cancer is presented in a question-and-answer format with beautiful color illustrations. This site is provided by Johns Hopkins University and covers topics such as anatomy, causes, heredity, surgical and medical treatment, vaccine therapy, symptoms and side effects, pain management, diet, exercise, and end of life.

➤ Pancreatica.org. Access at: www.pancreatica.org
A searchable clinical trial registry and a list of abstracts and news stories about scientific developments in pancreatic cancer are at the heart of this site. Other useful features include a frequently-asked-questions section that provides a good summary of the disease and an annotated list of links to other resources.

Detailed sections in general cancer sites

➤ American Cancer Society. *Learn about Pancreatic Cancer*. Access at: www.cancer.org and select from the menu under "Choose a Cancer Topic." A detailed guide about pancreatic cancer can be printed as an Adobe Acrobat (.pdf) file.

➤ National Cancer Institute. *Pancreatic Cancer* and *Pancreatic Cancer: Islet Cell*. Access at: www.cancer.gov and click on "Types of Cancer." The top page of the sections links to patient versions of PDQ® statements, clinical trial information, and other NCI publications on this topic.

➤ People Living with Cancer. *Pancreatic Cancer*. Access at: www.plwc.org and click on "Cancer Type." The PLWC oncologist-approved guide for pancreatic cancer can be printed in its entirety or by subtopic.

Sections about pancreatic cancer are also available at the following sites:

➤ Canadian Cancer Society. Access at: www.cancer.ca and click on "About Cancer."

➤ Cancerbackup. Access at: www.cancerbackup.org.uk/Home and click on "Cancer Types."

➤ Cancerconsultants.com. Access at: www.cancerconsultants.com and make a selection under "Links to Specific Cancer type Information."

➤ CancerSource.com. Access at: www.cancersource.com/Patient.pg and make a selection from the "Diagnosis & Treatment" pull-down menu.

➤ OncologyChannel.com. Access at: www.oncologychannel.com and select a condition from the left sidebar.

Patient-Support Organizations

➤ Pancreatic Cancer Action Network. Access at: www.pancan.org
Phone: 877-272-6226

Prostate Cancer

Anatomical facts: The prostate gland is part of the male reproductive system. Its main function is the secretion of part of the seminal fluid that transports sperm through the penis during ejaculation. This walnut-shaped organ is located in front of the rectum and under the bladder. It encircles part of the urethra, the tube that carries urine from the bladder and semen out of the body through the penis.

Illustrations available at the Medical Illustrations Gallery of the People Living with Cancer Web site.

Access at: www.plwc.org and click on Library on the left sidebar.

Prostate cancer is the most common cancer in American men (excluding skin cancer). One in six American men is diagnosed with this disease during his lifetime. The American Cancer Society estimates about 218,000 new cases of prostate cancer per year. A little over 1.8 million men in the United States are survivors of prostate cancer. Of prostate cancer cases, 90% are diagnosed while the disease is either confined to the prostate or spread only to local lymph nodes. The five-year survival rate for these stages is nearly 100%. When prostate cancer is diagnosed after it has spread to distant organs, the five-year survival rate drops to 34%. Since 1992, the death rate has fallen about 3.6% every year, possibly because of better detection and treatment methods.

Prostate cancer occurs about 60% more often in African American men than in Caucasian American men. African American men are more likely to be diagnosed at an advanced stage and are more than twice as likely to die of prostate cancer than Caucasian American men. Prostate cancer incidence among Hispanic men is similar to that of white men, and it is lowest among Asian men. The reasons for the racial differences are unclear.

The likelihood of developing prostate cancer increases sharply with age. The majority of men diagnosed with prostate cancer are over 65 years old. It is very rare in men younger than 45. Autopsy reports of men over 60 reveal that more than 60% of them had undetected prostate cancer. This finding indicates that prostate cancer usually grows very slowly; however, some prostate cancers have the ability to grow and spread quickly.

Family history and a history of high-grade prostatic intraepithelial neoplasia also increase the risk. The role of diet, and especially the consumption of red meat, fruits, and vegetables, is still being evaluated in research studies.

Over 99% of prostate cancers are adenocarcinomas, and most information sources focus on this type. There are four main treatment approaches for prostate cancer: watchful waiting, surgery, radiation therapy, and hormonal therapy which may be given as single therapies or in combination. After diagnosis, most men will have to make a decision about which treatment approach to choose. Many men are overwhelmed by the different factors and data they have to consider and analyze in order to make an informed decision. Factors that influence the decision are age and overall health, the stage and grade of the cancer, and how likely it is to be cured with each one of the treatment modalities. Side effects are an important factor. Because of the prostate's location and function, surgery, radiation, and hormonal therapies are all associated with serious side effects that may affect sexual and urinary functions.

Watchful waiting means monitoring the cancer very closely without active treatment such as surgery hormonal therapy or radiation therapy. It is a reasonable option for older men whose cancer is small, not causing any symptoms, and is expected to grow very slowly.

The surgical procedure to remove the prostate, seminal vesicles, and part of the urethra is called prostatectomy. Sometimes it is possible to perform a nerve-sparing prostatectomy, where the surgeon avoids cutting or stretching the nerves and blood vessels that are needed for an erection. However, even with this technique, some men lose a degree of sexual function and may also suffer long-term urinary problems. The level of damage is influenced by the man's age, overall health, and sexual function before the surgery. In recent years a new technique called laparoscopic radical prostatectomy (LRP) has emerged. In this surgery, the prostate is removed with special long instruments that are inserted into the abdomen through small incisions. Several studies reported that patients require shorter hospital stays and experience less blood loss and pain with this approach. The rates of side effects are similar to those associates with open surgery. LRP is a complex procedure, and the surgeon's skill is crucial in determining the quality of life of patient after the operation. A variation on this technique is called the da Vinci system. The surgeon conducts the operation sitting at a panel near the operating table and utilizing several robotic arms to perform the surgery. For the patient, there is no difference between direct and remote (robotic) LRP. The most important factor in determining the clinical success of either type of LRP is the surgeon's experience and skill.

Cryosurgery is a less invasive procedure, which is sometimes used to treat very small prostate tumors that have not spread. With this method, long thin needles are inserted into the prostate and freeze the tumor. Cryosurgery is less invasive, so patients recover more quickly than after a radical prostatectomy, but it is still a relatively new technique, and doctors are still not sure of its long-term effectiveness.

Radiation therapy to the prostate is delivered either with external beam radiation or internally through radioactive seeds implanted in the prostate, a method called "brachytherapy." Both methods have the potential for negative effects on sexual and urinary function. Hormonal therapy blocks the supply of male hormones that promote prostate cancer growth. The drugs that induce hormone deprivation also cause side effects such as hot flashes, impotence, loss of sexual desire, and loss of bone density. Hormonal drug therapy can also cause breast enlargement and cardiovascular problems.

Chemotherapy is not used to treat early-stage prostate cancer because in most cases it can be cured with surgery or radiation therapy. This treatment option is mostly used to treat advanced-stage cancer that has stopped responding to hormonal therapy, with the goal of slowing down tumor growth and reducing pain. Treatment approaches combining chemotherapy or targeted therapies in combination with other treatments are being evaluated. Advanced-stage prostate cancer tends to spread to the bones. Metastatic disease can be treated with a class of drugs called bisphosphonates which slow down bone loss and strengthen bones. Bone pain can be controlled with drugs and/or radiation therapy.

When selecting information sources about prostate cancer, librarians and patrons should consider whether the author is a surgeon or a radiation oncologist. The author's background is important because it may bias the information: A urologist is likely to support surgery as the "best" option, while a radiation specialist may emphasize radiation oncology options.

Prostate cancer survivors face a number of difficulties with regard to their quality of life. Many of the sexual and urinary problems can be treated effectively by surgical procedures and/or drugs. Librarians should help survivors and their partners feel comfortable asking for information about these topics.

Information Sources

Brochures, Booklets, and Other Short Print Publications

➤ CancerCare. *Treatment Choices for Men Living with Advanced Prostate Cancer.*
A short booklet with color photographs and illustrations that help understand new hormonal therapies and chemotherapy available to men with advanced disease. Includes a discussion of side effects, pain control, and sources of support with a few frequently asked questions, a short glossary, and a list of resources. Access at: www.cancercare.org

➤ Institute for Continuing Healthcare Education. *Living with Advanced Prostate Cancer: When PSA Rises during Hormone Therapy.*

A 56-page glossy booklet with many color photographs and illustrations in friendly, easy-to-understand language. This publication covers a variety of topics of interest to men with advanced prostate cancer, including medical, support, and quality-of-life issues. This booklet can be ordered free at: www.iche.edu/advancedpca

➤ National Cancer Institute. *Treatment Choices for Men with Early Stage Prostate Cancer.*
This booklet is to help newly diagnosed men understand the treatment options available to them for prostate cancer found in the early stages (when cancer is confined to the prostate). It covers the risks and benefits of surgery, radiation, and watchful waiting and provides a comparison chart to give basic information about the three options. It discusses the importance of personal preference in weighing the risks and benefits of treatment and provides a list of questions to ask. Access at: https://cissecure.nci.nih.gov/ncipubs/

➤ National Cancer Institute. *Understanding Prostate Changes: A Health Guide for Men.*
This booklet discusses the spectrum of prostate conditions, both cancerous and noncancerous, that occur with age. It emphasizes that not all prostate changes mean prostate cancer and provides information about symptoms, treatment options, and tests to detect these conditions. Access at: https://cissecure.nci.nih.gov/ncipubs/

➤ National Cancer Institute. *What You Need to Know about Prostate Cancer.*
This booklet on prostate cancer discusses possible causes, symptoms, diagnosis, treatment, emotional issues, and questions to ask the doctor. Includes a glossary of terms and other resources. Access the full text at: https://cissecure.nci.nih.gov/ncipubs/

➤ National Comprehensive Cancer Network (NCCN). *Prostate Cancer: Treatment Guidelines for Patients.*
An overview of prostate cancer as well as treatment decision "trees" explaining the treatment choices for different stages and conditions of this disease. This resource is developed from the NCCN Clinical Practice Guidelines in Oncology—the standard for clinical policy in cancer care. A Spanish-language version also is available. Access at: www.nccn.org/patients/

Books

➤ Bostwick, David G., et al. 2005. *American Cancer Society's Complete Guide to Prostate Cancer.* Atlanta, GA: American Cancer Society, Health Promotions. A step-by-step guide through the emotional and physical aspects of the prostate cancer experience, from testing for prostate cancer, to diagnosis, to thinking about the future. The text includes quotes from men living with prostate cancer, tips on managing emotional reactions and side effects, and a section discussing life after treatment. Each chapter in this book was written by prostate cancer specialists, and the authors provide many tables and illustrations. An extensive resource section at the end of the book lists national and local organizations, and the glossary is very comprehensive.

➤ Centeno, Arthur, and Gary Onik. 2004. *Prostate Cancer: A Patient's Guide to Treatment*. Omaha, NE: Addicus Books.

Two prostate cancer specialists authored this easy-to-read, concise guide to prostate cancer. It covers the basics of prostate anatomy and diagnostic tests and offers detailed explanations of various treatment methods, including data on risks, complications, and side effects. Appendixes provide a summary of treatments for prostate cancer, resources, and a glossary.

➤ Ellsworth, Pamela, John A. Heaney, and Oliver Gill. 2003. *100 Questions and Answers about Prostate Cancer*. Boston: Jones and Bartlett.

Detailed information about prostate cancer is presented in an easy-to-read question-and-answer format. Terms are explained in the sidebar, and the book includes lists of Web sites, organizations, literature, and resources on topics that may be of interest to women with prostate cancer. This book was co–authored by two physicians and a prostate cancer survivor.

➤ Grimm, Peter D., John C. Blasko, and John E. Sylvester. 2004. *The Prostate Cancer Treatment Book: Advice from Leading Prostate Experts from the Nation's Top Medical Institutions*. New York: McGraw Hill.

This book is aimed at men during the first months after diagnosis, a time of momentous decisions and enormous emotional strain. Top prostate cancer experts from the nation's leading medical centers provide answers to questions about the best treatment options for fighting and beating prostate cancer. The focus of this book is treatment, and it provides in-depth explanations of surgery, hormonal treatment, external beam radiation, and radioactive seed implantation therapy. Real-life accounts of men treated for prostate cancer illustrate key points and provide insight.

➤ Klein, Eric A., Leah Jamnicky, and Robert Nam. 2003. *So You're Having Prostate Surgery*. Hoboken, NJ: Wiley.

Two surgeons and a nurse guide the reader through the tough decisions involving prostate surgery, from deciding whether surgery is really needed through the procedure itself and to the quickest routes to recovery. Surgery for both benign prostate enlargement and prostate cancer is covered in step-by-step detail, including medications and self-care steps. Real-life patient stories, extensive self-help sections, and detailed illustrations fully explain each procedure. Also provided are a comprehensive directory to Internet and other resources, a guide to complementary therapies, and a list of who's who of hospital staff.

➤ Lange, Paul H., and Christine A. Adamec. 2003. *Prostate Cancer for Dummies*. New York: Wiley.

This comprehensive and detailed book is rich in such graphical elements as bold headings, bullet points, icons, illustrations, and tables, which may help comprehension. Chapters include getting a diagnosis, making a treatment plan, changing lifestyle, coping with the side effects of prostate cancer, and handling work and family. The last chapter provides a list of ten myths and realities about prostate cancer, followed by must-dos for everyone battling prostate cancer and ten ways to beat the blues. The chief writer of this book is Paul Lange, M.D., chairman of urologic surgery at the University of Washington.

➤ Pienta, Kenneth J., and Mark A. Moyad. 2004. *Prostate Cancer from A to Z*. Ann Arbor, MI: J. W. Edwards.

The smart graphic design of this book and its many illustrations and photographs help present detailed, in-depth information about prostate cancer in a user-friendly manner. The text covers nutrition and supplements, diagnostic tests, treatment of localized disease, hormonal therapy, side effects of treatment, pain control, and therapies on the horizon. The authors are a surgeon and a researcher from the University of Michigan.

➤ Scardino, Peter T., and Judith Kelman. 2005. *Dr. Peter Scardino's Prostate Book: The Complete Guide to Overcoming Prostate Cancer, Prostatitis, and BPH*. New York: Avery.

Peter T. Scardino, M.D., a surgeon and head of the prostate cancer program at Memorial Sloan-Kettering Cancer, wrote this comprehensive book that includes information on benign and cancerous prostate conditions. Each chapter starts with a short synopsis and ends with a summary. The style is straightforward, clear, and concise, the book is long and rich in details that help the reader gain a thorough, in-depth understanding of the topic.

Audiovisual Resources

➤ Information Television Network. 2005. *Living with Prostate Cancer*. Boca Raton, FL: Information Television Network. (30 min.). Available in DVD and VHS formats. Access at: www.itvisus.com or Amazon.com.

Part of the public television series *Healthy Body/Healthy Mind*, this episode features cancer specialists discussing prostate cancer, treatment options, and potential side effects. The program also features prostate cancer patients discussing their experience with side effects and highlights new treatment approaches. Color graphics and animations illustrate the scientific content.

➤ Information Television Network. 2005. *Prostate Cancer.* Boca Raton, FL: Information Television Network. (30 min.). Available in DVD and VHS formats. Access at: www.itvisus.com or Amazon.com.
Part of the public television series *Healthy Body/Healthy Mind*, this program features cancer specialists explaining what the PSA test is and how it can be used to identify cancer at its earliest stage. The program also features patients who are helped by the test and color graphics and animations that illustrate the scientific content.

➤ Information Television Network. 2005. *Advanced Prostate Cancer.* Boca Raton, FL: Information Television Network. (30 min.). Available in DVD and VHS formats. Access at: www.itvisus.com or Amazon.com.
Part of the public television series *Healthy Body/Healthy Mind*, this program features cancer specialists discussing new breakthroughs in the care and treatment of advanced prostate cancer that enable patients to live longer without sacrificing their quality of life. The program also features patients living with advanced prostate cancer and color graphics and animations that illustrate the scientific content.

➤ Directed by Hyman, Herbert, Robert Nadler, and H. Gilbert Welch, et al. 2004. *Prostate Cancer.* Films for the Humanities. (29 min.). Available in DVD and VHS formats.
This program examines the importance of patient involvement in decisions concerning prostate cancer. It features two men who opted for surgery and a man who chose to wait before starting a treatment. Physicians from prominent cancer centers explain diagnosis and treatment.

➤ Directed by Zaritsky, John, Terence McKeown, and Point Grey Pictures Inc., et al. 2004. *Men Don't Cry: Prostate Cancer Stories.* Films for the Humanities & Sciences. (48 min.). Available in VHS and DVD formats.
This program explores intimate stories of prostate cancer survivors as they come to terms with the disease. Each, with the support of his spouse, chooses to fight it in his own way, balancing treatment options, rates of cure and survival, and quality-of-life concerns about impotence and incontinence.

➤ Patient Education Institute. *Prostate Cancer—What Is It? Interactive Tutorial.* Access at: www.medlineplus.gov, click on "Interactive Tutorials" and select from a list.
This slideshow utilizes illustrations, sound, and animations to provide basic, easy-to-understand explanations of the anatomy, diagnosis, and treatment options of prostate cancer. It is possible to turn on a voice-over or print a text version.

➤ Patient Education Institute. *Prostate Cancer—Radiation Therapy Interactive Tutorial.* Access at: www.medlineplus.gov, click on "Interactive Tutorials" and select from a list.

This slide show focuses on the different types of radiation therapy used to treat prostate cancer and the side effects of treatment.

Web Resources

Sites focusing on prostate cancer

➤ Prostate Cancer Foundation. Access at: www.prostatecancerfoundation.org
The Prostate Cancer Foundation (PCF) is the world's largest philanthropic source of support for prostate cancer research. The site provides a wealth of information about risk factors, screening, diagnosis, and treatment of prostate cancer. Especially useful is the ability to download the full text of the organization's publications, including *Report to the Nation on Prostate Cancer: A Guide for Men and Their Families, Nutrition and Prostate Cancer, New Therapies in Development,* and *Nobody Knows,* to raise awareness about prostate cancer. The section aimed at men living with prostate cancer includes information on bone metastases, nutrition, side effects, and issues to consider at various stages of the disease.

➤ Prostate Cancer Research Institute. Access at: www.prostate-cancer.org
This site is useful for patrons interested in comprehensive, highly detailed information. It includes articles that discuss and explain specific therapies, diagnostic tests, side effects, and nutritional factors. Tools for risk evaluation and self-assessment enable users to reach a deep understanding of their situation. Sophisticated users who have the ability to understand scientific concepts will benefit from this site.

➤ Us TOO International. Access at: www.ustoo.org
This site includes extensive information about support services for patients and families and about prostate cancer, including: treatment options, post–treatment issues, relapse, clinical trials, emerging treatments, and material relevant for African American men. Helpful features include an archive of audio and video files and downloadable files of publications providing in-depth information on topics such as bone health, self-care while living with cancer, hormonal therapy, and options when experiencing a rising PSA. The news section covers prostate cancer research and treatment advances.

Detailed sections in general cancer sites

➤ American Cancer Society. *Learn about Prostate Cancer.* Access at: www.cancer.org and select from the menu under "Choose a Cancer Topic." A disease-specific detailed guide can be printed by section or as an Adobe Acrobat (.pdf) file.

➤ Healthology. *Prostate Health.* Access at: www.healthology.com and click on "Consumer Health Library." This site offers detailed articles, Webcasts, and transcripts featuring cancer professionals.

➤ National Cancer Institute. *Prostate Cancer.* Access at: www.cancer.gov and click on "Types of Cancer." The top page of the section links to patient versions of PDQ® statements, clinical trial information, and other NCI publications on this topic.

➤ People Living with Cancer. *Prostate Cancer.* Access at: www.plwc.org and click on "Cancer Type." The PLWC oncologist-approved prostate cancer guide can be printed in its entirety or by subtopic.

Sections about prostate cancer are also available at the following sites:

➤ Canadian Cancer Society. Access at: www.cancer.ca and click on "About Cancer."

➤ Cancerbackup. Access at: www.cancerbackup.org.uk/Home and click on "Cancer Types."

➤ Cancerconsultants.com. Access at: www.cancerconsultants.com and make a selection under "Links to Specific Cancer type Information."

➤ CancerSource.com. Access at: www.cancersource.com/Patient.pg and make a selection from the "Diagnosis & Treatment" pull-down menu.

➤ OncologyChannel.com. Access at: www.oncologychannel.com and select a condition from the left sidebar.

Patient-Support Organizations

➤ Us TOO International. Access at: www.ustoo.org
Support hot line: 800-808-7866

Sarcoma

Anatomical facts: *The body's connective tissue consists of soft tissues and bones. Most bones are hollow and contain marrow, which is a mixture of fat cells and blood-forming cells. At each end of the bone is a zone of cartilage that acts as a cushion between bones and, together with ligaments and some other tissues, forms the joints between bones. Soft tissues include fat, blood vessels, nerves, muscles, deep skin tissues, tendons, and cartilage.*

Illustrations available at the Medical Illustrations Gallery of the People Living with Cancer Web site.

Access at: www.plwc.org and click on Library on the left sidebar.

Sarcoma is a general term that includes all tumors originating in the connective tissue. The American Cancer Society estimates about 9,200 new cases of soft tissue sarcomas and 2,300 new cases of primary bone sarcomas per year in the United States. Sarcoma tumors may also appear in children. Childhood sarcomas are described in Chapter 5 of this book. There are over a hundred distinct types of sarcoma tumors, which makes it impossible to give overall survival statistics.

Sarcoma tumors' names include the name of the tissue the tumor originated in. For example, liposarcoma starts in fatty cells, fibrosarcoma starts in the fibrous tissue that includes tendons and ligaments, leiomyosarcoma starts in the smooth muscle tissue, and chondrosarcoma starts in the cartilage. When a patron is inquiring about bone cancer, it is important to clarify that the topic in question is primary bone cancer, not a cancer that metastasized to the bone from a different site. Most tumors discovered in the bones are secondary, not primary, tumors.

About 40% of sarcomas occur in the legs, usually at or above the knee. About 15% develop in the hands and arms, another 15% in the head and neck, and 30% in the shoulders, chest, abdomen, or hips.

Most sarcomas do not have a strong link to a specific risk factor, although exposure to ionizing radiation and certain chemicals may be the cause for a small number of sarcomas. Several inherited genetic disorders, such as neurofibromatosis, increase the risk for specific types of sarcomas.

The treatment of choice for all types of sarcoma is surgery, with the goal of removing the tumor and a margin of about an inch of healthy tissue surrounding the tumor. When the tumor is in the abdomen or the pelvic bone, surgery is more difficult because the tumor may be next to vital organs that cannot be surgically removed. In rare cases an amputation is required. Most of the tumors in the arms and legs can be treated with limb-sparing surgery followed by radiation therapy. Surgery cannot cure a sarcoma after it has metastasized, unless there is only a single metastasis in either the lung or the brain. In that case the metastasis is removed with surgery, and the patient may still have long-term survival. Radiation therapy and chemotherapy are used to treat sarcomas as adjuvant therapy after surgery or as the main treatment if surgery is not feasible. One type of soft tissue sarcoma, gastrointestinal stromal tumor (GIST), responds well to the drug imatinib mesylate, a type of targeted therapy. The effectiveness of imatinib mesylate and other new drugs on different types of sarcoma is being evaluated in clinical trials.

Information seeking on sarcoma is especially challenging because of the large number of different tumors that are divided further into subtypes.

Each specific sarcoma is a completely distinct disease entity with its unique clinical behavior and outlook. In addition, the same histological entities behave differently in various body parts, and treatment of the same tumor type may be dissimilar in different locations. For example, treatment for leiyomyosarcoma that started in the uterus is completely different from treatment for leiyomyosarcoma that started in the gastrointestinal tract. Because these tumors are so rare, it is hard to find tumor-specific information in patient-friendly language. Most lay-language information sources offer separate overviews for soft tissue or bone sarcomas that contain small sections or paragraphs focusing on a few of the most common sarcomas. A good practice for librarians is to ask the information seeker for the medical name of the cancer, determine (with the help of a good reference source) if the tumor is considered a soft tissue or a bone sarcoma, and provide the corresponding overview. For more specific information the librarian needs to know the primary tumor site in addition to the medical name. Tumor-specific information can sometimes be found by utilizing the sources described in Chapter 3 that discuss locating advanced cancer information in patient-friendly language.

Quality-of-life issues for sarcoma survivors differ greatly because of the large variety of tumors and affected body parts. The few sarcoma survivors who receive amputation as part of the treatment may need information on limb loss.

Information Sources

Brochures, Booklets, and Other Short Print Publications

➤ National Cancer Institute. *Soft Tissue Sarcomas: Questions and Answers* and *Bone Cancer: Questions and Answers.*
   These are short publications that cover risk factors, diagnosis, and treatment of soft tissue and bone sarcomas. Access at: www.cancer.gov

Web Resources

Sites focusing on sarcoma

➤ Sarcoma Alliance. Access at: www.sarcomaalliance.org
   The site of this patient-support organization offers a comprehensive list of links to other Web sites and articles about soft tissue and bone sarcomas. The section "The First Thing You Should Know" offers advice to newly diagnosed patients on how to get quality medical care and support. This site also includes a list of sarcoma centers, specialists, and clinical trial registries.

➤ The NW Sarcoma Foundation. Access at: www.nwsarcoma.org
The mission of this organization is to provide education and support to patients and families living with this cancer. The site includes explanations of sarcoma, its biology, and pathology, and treatment options, with color illustrations that help understand the complex anatomy of the skeletal system. The section on support provides links to many organizations and resources that may be of help. The section "Where to Go for Treatment" contains a list of sarcoma treatment centers in the United States.

Detailed sections in general cancer sites

➤ American Cancer Society. *Learn about Bone Cancer* and *Learn about Sarcoma—Adult Soft Tissue Cancer*. Access at: www.cancer.org and select from the menu under "Choose a Cancer Topic." Detailed guides about sarcoma can be printed by section or as Adobe Acrobat (.pdf) files.

➤ National Cancer Institute. *Bone Cancer* and *Soft Tissue Sarcoma*. Access at: www.cancer.gov and click on "Types of Cancer." The top page of the section links to patient versions of PDQ® statements, clinical trial information, and other NCI publications on this topic.

➤ People Living with Cancer. *Sarcoma*. Access at: www.plwc.org and click on "Cancer Type." The PLWC oncologist-approved sarcoma guide can be printed in its entirety or by subtopic.

Sections about sarcoma cancer are also available at the following sites:

➤ Cancerbackup. Access at: www.cancerbackup.org.uk/Home and click on "Cancer Types."

➤ Cancerconsultants.com. Access at: www.cancerconsultants.com and make a selection under "Links to Specific Cancer type Information."

➤ CancerSource.com. Access at: www.cancersource.com/Patient.pg and make a selection from the "Diagnosis & Treatment" pull-down menu.

Patient-Support Organization

➤ Sarcoma Alliance. Access at: www.sarcomaalliance.com
Phone: 415-381-7236

Skin Cancer, Non-Melanoma

Anatomical facts: The skin is the largest organ in the body. Its main function is to cover and protect the internal organs against heat, sunlight, injury, and infection. Other functions are to regulate the body's temperature, store water and fat, and produce vitamin D. The skin has two main layers: the epidermis and dermis. The outer layer, the epidermis, is made of three types of cells: squamous cells, basal cells, and melanocytes. The dermis, which lies underneath the epidermis, contains blood vessels, lymph vessels, hair follicles, nerves, and sweat glands.

Illustrations available at the Medical Illustrations Gallery of the People Living with Cancer Web site.

Access at: www.plwc.org and click on Library on the left sidebar.

Skin cancer is the most common type of cancer in the United States. The American Cancer Society does not provide an annual projection of skin cancer diagnoses because most non-melanoma cases are not reported. It is estimated that 40% to 50% of Americans are diagnosed with non-melanoma skin cancer by the time they reach age 65. Fortunately, the majority of cancers that develop in the skin are either basal cell carcinoma or squamous cell carcinoma. Both of these cancers are usually diagnosed in the early stages and are highly curable. Although it is very common, only 1,000–2,000 deaths per year are attributed to non-melanoma skin cancer, and most deaths occur when people do not receive treatment soon enough or when a person has a suppressed immune system.

The cause for both basal cell carcinoma and squamous cell carcinoma is exposure to ultraviolet (UV) radiation from the sun or artificial sources such as sunlamps and tanning booths. Occurrence of skin cancer is correlated to the level of UV exposure in a lifetime, resulting in a higher incidence among people who live in areas that get high levels of UV radiation and people over the age of 50.

Most non-melanoma skin cancers can be completely cured by a fairly minor surgical procedure performed in the physician's office as outpatient surgery. One of these procedures, Mohs surgery, can be performed only by physicians who have had special training. This is a multistep procedure that consists of removing a thin layer of the growth and examining it under the microscope before moving on to the next one. The goal of this surgery is to remove only cancerous tissue, with a very small margin of healthy tissue. With this method, it is possible to achieve a better cosmetic result. This is an important advantage, especially when treating tumors on the face.

Chemotherapy and radiation therapy are used sometimes to treat non-melanoma skin cancer. Chemotherapy can be applied directly to the affected part of the skin with a lotion or cream, thereby avoiding the exposure of healthy organs and tissues to chemotherapy. Although this treatment frequently causes inflammation and sensitivity, this side effect is only temporary.

Although most non-melanoma skin cancers can be completely cured, survivors need to perform skin self-exams and be monitored very closely by a physician. People with a history of skin cancer must become knowledgeable about preventing UV exposure and about special products and clothing that protect from the sun.

Information Sources

Brochures, Booklets, and Other Short Print Publications

➤ American Academy of Dermatology.
  ➤ *Actinic Keratoses*
  ➤ *Basal Cell Carcinoma*
  ➤ *Skin Cancer*
  ➤ *Squamous Cell Carcinoma*
  These short publications contain brief overviews of the conditions with pictures. To read or order access at: www.aad.org.
➤ National Cancer Institute. *What You Need to Know about Skin Cancer.*
  This booklet on skin cancer discusses possible causes, symptoms, diagnosis, treatment, emotional issues, and questions to ask the doctor. Includes a glossary of terms and other resources. Access at: https://cissecure.nci.nih.gov/ncipubs/

Books

➤ McClay, Edward F., Mary-Eileen T. McClay, and Jodie Smith. 2004. *100 Questions and Answers about Melanoma and Other Skin Cancers*. Boston: Jones and Bartlett.
  Detailed information about skin cancer is presented in an easy-to-read question-and-answer format. Terms are explained in the sidebar, and the book includes lists of Web sites, organizations, literature, and resources on general and specific topics related to skin cancer. This book was co-authored by two skin health care professionals and a melanoma survivor.

Audiovisual Resources

➤ Patient Education Institute. *Skin Cancer Interactive Tutorial*. Access at: www.medlineplus.gov and click on "Interactive Tutorials," then select from a list.
  This slideshow utilizes illustrations, sound, and animations to provide basic, easy-to-understand explanations of skin anatomy and the diagnosis and treatment options of skin cancer. It is possible to turn on a voice-over or print a text version.

Web Resources

Sites focusing on skin cancer

➤ American Academy of Dermatology. *SkinCancer.Net*. Access at: www. skincarephysicians.com/skincancernet/
This site focuses on skin cancer prevention and screening. It includes visual guides describing the main skin cancer types and offers information about prevention and screening. The section on when to see a dermatologist provides access to a physician-finder database. The articles section includes more in-depth information about specific topics relating to skin cancer.

➤ Skin Cancer Foundation. Access at: www.skincancer.org
The mission of the Skin Cancer Foundation is to increase awareness of the skin cancer epidemic. The site includes many educational materials about skin cancer prevention including sun tanning, tanning beds, tanning in childhood, and more. The site provides a short overviews of basal cell carcinoma, squamous cell carcinoma, and actinic keratosis.

Detailed sections in general cancer sites

➤ American Cancer Society. *Learn about Skin Cancer—Nonmelanoma*. Access at: www.cancer.org and select from the menu under "Choose a Cancer Topic." A detailed guide about non-melanoma skin cancer can be printed by section or as an Adobe Acrobat (.pdf) file.

➤ National Cancer Institute. *Skin Cancer*. Access at: www.cancer.gov and click on "Types of cancer." The top page of the section links to patient versions of PDQ® statements for specific skin cancer types.

➤ People Living With Cancer. *Skin Cancer (Non-Melanoma)*. Access at: www. plwc.org and click on "Cancer Type." The PLWC oncologist-approved guide about non-melanoma skin cancer can be printed in its entirety or by subtopic.

Sections about skin cancer are also available at the following sites:

➤ Canadian Cancer Society. Access at: www.cancer.ca and click on "About Cancer."

➤ Cancerbackup. Access at: www.cancerbackup.org.uk/Home and click on "Cancer Types."

➤ Cancerconsultants.com. Access at: www.cancerconsultants.com and make a selection under "Links to Specific Cancer Type Information."

➤ CancerSource.com. Access at: www.cancersource.com/Patient.pg and make a selection from the "Diagnosis & Treatment" pull-down menu.

➤ OncologyChannel.com. Access at: www.oncologychannel.com and select a condition from the left sidebar.

Stomach Cancer

Anatomical facts: The stomach is a saclike organ located in the left upper abdomen under the ribs. It receives food from the esophagus that has been chewed and swallowed, and starts the digestive process in the body. The stomach muscles create a rippling motion that mixes and mashes the food along with juices made by glands located in the lining of the stomach. After about three hours, the food turns into semi-liquid form, which is then delivered to the small intestine.

Illustrations available at the Medical Illustrations Gallery of the People Living with Cancer Web site.

Access at: www.plwc.org and click on Library on the left sidebar.

The American Cancer Society estimates about 21,000 new cases of stomach cancer (sometimes called gastric cancer) per year and 11,000 deaths. This cancer is the 13th most common cause of cancer deaths in the United States, with an estimated 14,000 deaths per year. In developing countries, however, the incidence of gastric cancer is much higher. The reasons for this difference are not completely known, but they may be linked to less use of refrigeration for food storage and more use of salted and smoked foods. Some experts suspect that the use of antibiotics to treat childhood infections helps prevent gastric cancer because these drugs can kill *Helicobacter pylori* bacteria, which may be the major cause of this disease.

Stomach cancer is a lot more common among males, and incidence increases sharply after age 50. Hispanics and African Americans are more likely to get it than non-Hispanic whites. It is most common in the Asian/Pacific Islander population. This disease has been linked to infection with the *Helicobacter pylori* bacteria, which may also cause stomach ulcers. Obesity, smoking, and alcohol consumption have been identified as risk factors, as well as diets rich in smoked foods, salted fish and meat, and pickled vegetables. Other medical conditions affecting the stomach and family history also increase the risk.

Most cancers of the stomach are adenocarcinomas that start in the innermost lining of this organ, called the mucosa. The term *stomach cancer*, or *gastric cancer*, almost always refers to adenocarcinoma-type cancer of the stomach. Other cancers that may grow in the stomach are lymphomas, gastrointestinal stromal tumors (GISTs), and carcinoid tumors. These are completely different disease entities and should not be confused with gastric cancer. Information on these types should be found in separate information sources.

The main treatment for stomach cancer is surgery. An endoscopic mucosal resection is sometimes possible for very early-stage tumors. This is a less invasive procedure, where the surgeon removes the diseased part of the innermost layer of the stomach through an endoscope, which is a hollow tube inserted into the stomach. Most stomach cancers are treated either with a subtotal gastrectomy, where only part of the stomach is removed, or a total gastrectomy, where the entire organ is removed. A gastrectomy is a major surgical procedure that is likely to cause short- and long-term complications. Some gastric cancer patients are also treated with radiation therapy and/or chemotherapy in addition to surgery. If the cancer has spread, the goal of treatment is to palliate symptoms rather than cure the cancer.

After stomach surgery, patients will have to adapt to a new way of eating. Removal of the stomach may cause heartburn; abdominal pain, especially after eating; and shortages of some vitamins. The severity of the problems depends on the extent of the surgery. Most people will need to change their diets; eat smaller, more frequent meals; and take essential vitamins, some of which are available only by injection. Severe weight loss and malnutrition can occur after a partial or a total gastrectomy, and some patients may need high-calorie food supplements, feeding tubes, or artificial nutrition via infusion.

Information Sources

Brochures, Booklets, and Other Short Print Publications

➤ National Cancer Institute. *What You Need to Know about Stomach Cancer.* This booklet on stomach cancer discusses possible causes, symptoms, diagnosis, treatment, emotional issues, and questions to ask the doctor. Includes a glossary of terms and other resources. Access at: https://cissecure. nci.nih.gov/ncipubs/

Web Resources

Detailed sections in general cancer sites

➤ American Cancer Society. *Learn about Stomach Cancer.* Access at: www. cancer.org and select from the menu under "Choose a Cancer Topic." A detailed guide about stomach cancer can be printed by section or as an Adobe Acrobat (.pdf) file.

➤ National Cancer Institute. *Stomach Cancer.* Access at: www.cancer.gov and click on "Types of cancer." The top page of the section links to patient versions of PDQ® statements, clinical trial information, and other NCI publications on this topic.

➤ People Living with Cancer. *Stomach Cancer.* Access at: www.plwc.org and click on "Cancer Type." The PLWC oncologist-approved stomach cancer guide may be printed in its entirety or by subtopic.

Sections about stomach cancer are also available at the following sites

➤ Canadian Cancer Society. Access at: www.cancer.ca and click on "About Cancer."

➤ Cancerbackup. Access at: www.cancerbackup.org.uk/Home and click on "Cancer Types."

➤ Cancerconsultants.com. Access at: www.cancerconsultants.com and make a selection under "Links to Specific Cancer type Information."

➤ CancerSource.com. Access at: www.cancersource.com/Patient.pg and make a selection from the "Diagnosis & Treatment" pull-down menu.

➤ OncologyChannel.com. Access at: www.oncologychannel.com and select a condition from the left sidebar.

Patient-Support Organizations

➤ American Cancer Society. Access at: www.cancer.org
Phone: 800-ACS-2345

Testicular Cancer

Anatomical facts: The testicles are a pair of male sex glands located under the penis in a saclike pouch called the scrotum. The testicles have two main functions: to produce and store sperm and to produce the male hormone testosterone, which controls the development of the reproductive organs, sexual function, and other male physical characteristics.

Illustrations available at the Medical Illustrations Gallery of the People Living with Cancer Web site.

Access at: www.plwc.org and click on Library on the left sidebar.

Testicular cancer occurs most often in men between the ages of 20 and 39. It accounts for only 1% of all cancers in men, with just about 8,000 new cases diagnosed per year in the United States. Testicular cancer is one of the most curable forms of cancer, with only 350–400 deaths per year. It is more prevalent in white men than in African American or Asian American males.

It is unknown what causes testicular cancer; however, several risk factors have been identified. The main risk factor is one or two undescended testicles. In this condition the testicles, which normally develop in the belly and then move down (descend) into the scrotum before birth, descend only partially or remain in the belly. This condition affects about 3% of boys and is usually corrected by surgery soon after birth. About 14% of testicular cancer cases are diagnosed in men who had this condition. Having a history of testicular cancer increases a person's risk of developing the disease in his other testicle. Another factor is having a brother or father diagnosed with testicular cancer.

The most common type of testicular cancer is germ cell tumors, which account for 90% of all tumors. Germ cell tumors grow in the cells that make sperm and are divided into two major subtypes.

➤ Seminomas occur mostly in men between their late 30s and early 50s.

➤ Nonseminomas occur in younger men between their late teens and early 40s. There are four main subtypes of nonseminomas, and most tumors are mixed, having at least two different types; however, all nonseminoma germ cell cancers are treated the same.

Tumors may contain both seminoma and nonseminoma cells. In that case they will be treated as nonseminoma.

Stromal tumors account for less than 10% of testicular cancers. The two main types are leydig cell tumors and sertoli cell tumors. These tumors usually do not spread beyond the testicle and can be cured by surgery. If they do metastasize, they have a worse prognosis than germ cell tumors because they do not respond well to chemotherapy or radiation.

Lymphoma and childhood leukemia may spread to the testicles, but these tumors are not considered testicular cancer but rather a metastatic form of the primary cancer.

Since the mid-1970s, cure and survival rates for testicular cancer have changed dramatically. This change is attributed to the use of the chemotherapy drug cisplatin, which is particularly effective against this cancer. Today, patients with early-stage testicular cancer have a five-year survival rate of 90%, and patients with advanced disease have a 70% chance to be alive five years after diagnosis.

Surgery is the primary treatment for this type of cancer. Removal of the testicle is called orchiectomy and is done through an incision in the groin. Sometimes lymph nodes from the retroperitoneum (an area in the abdomen near the back) need to be removed and tested for the presence of tumor cells. This procedure, called retroperitoneal lymph node dissection, may be done at the same time as the orchiectomy or during a second operation. Radiation therapy may also be used in addition to chemotherapy. Men whose cancer has recurred after treatment with chemotherapy sometimes receive high-dose chemotherapy followed by an autologous stem cell transplantation.

Treatment for testicular cancer may sometimes impair sexual function and fertility. Since most testicular cancer patients are young men, these issues affect almost all of them. Infertility may be caused by damage to nerves during a retroperitoneal lymph node dissection or if the both testicles are removed in surgeries. It is very important that patients discuss the options of a nerve-sparing surgery (to maintain erection) and sperm banking before treatment. Men who lose only one testicle usually retain normal sexual function; however, the loss of a testicle causes a change in the look and feel of the scrotum. A prosthesis implanted at the time of surgery restores a more natural look.

Information Sources

Brochures, Booklets, and Other Short Print Publications

➤ National Cancer Institute. *Testicular Cancer: Questions and Answers.* This is a short publication that covers risk factors, diagnosis and treatment of testicular cancer. Access at: www.cancer.gov

Web Resources

Sites focusing on testicular cancer

➤ Testicular Cancer Resource Center. Access at: http://tcrc.acor.org This comprehensive Web site is provided by a testicular cancer survivor and a medical advisory board of well-known testicular cancer physicians. In addition to information about diagnosis and treatment options, it also contains sections on sexuality, fertility, and testicular implants. Useful features include a list of specialists, explanation of the pathology report, and questions-and-answers by two testicular cancer experts.

Detailed sections in general cancer sites

➤ American Cancer Society. *Learn about Testicular Cancer.* Access at: www.cancer.org and select from the menu under "Choose a Cancer Topic." A detailed guide about testicular cancer can be printed by section or as an Adobe Acrobat (.pdf) file.

➤ National Cancer Institute. *Testicular Cancer.* Access at: www.cancer.gov and click on "Types of Cancer." The top page of the section links to patient versions of PDQ® statements, clinical trial information, and other NCI publications on this topic.

➤ People Living with Cancer. *Testicular Cancer.* Access at: www.plwc.org and click on "Cancer Type." The PLWC oncologist-approved testicular cancer guide can be printed in its entirety or by subtopic.

Sections about testicular cancer are also available at the following sites:

➤ Canadian Cancer Society. Access at: www.cancer.ca and click on "About Cancer."

➤ Cancerbackup. Access at: www.cancerbackup.org.uk/Home and click on "Cancer Types."

➤ Cancerconsultants.com. Access at: www.cancerconsultants.com and make a selection under "Links to Specific Cancer Type Information."

➤ CancerSource.com. Access at: www.cancersource.com/Patient.pg and make a selection from the "Diagnosis & Treatment" pull-down menu.

➤ OncologyChannel.com. Access at: www.oncologychannel.com and select a condition from the left sidebar.

Patient-Support Organizations

➤ American Cancer Society. Access at: www.cancer.org
Phone: 800-ACS-2345

Thyroid Cancer

Anatomical facts: The thyroid is a gland that lies at the front of the neck, beneath the voice box (larynx). It has two lobes and is shaped like a butterfly. The thyroid produces a hormone that regulates the body's metabolism. In order to produce the thyroid hormone, the thyroid gland absorbs iodine from the blood.

Illustrations available at the Medical Illustrations Gallery of the People Living with Cancer Web site.

Access at: www.plwc.org and click on Library on the left sidebar.

Thyroid nodules, which are benign tumors that develop on the thyroid gland, are very common and occur in one-third of all adults. Only 10% to 15% of these nodules are cancerous. About 33,000 new cases of thyroid cancer each year are diagnosed in the United States. Thyroid cancer may occur in people of all ages; however, 75% of cases are discovered in women. Most thyroid cancers can be successfully treated and cured. The number of deaths per year is approximately 1,500.

Several risk factors for thyroid cancer have been identified. A number of inherited syndromes increase the risk to develop thyroid cancer. Low iodine in the diet increases the incidence of follicular carcinomas. People who were exposed to radiation in the head and neck area or were exposed to radioactive fallout from nuclear weapons or power plant accidents also have a higher risk.

Thyroid cancers are divided into a number of main types, and these are divided further into subtypes. There are significant differences in the natural history, treatment principles, and prognosis between these types. For this reason, it is important to find out the specific type the client is inquiring about. A number of information sources offer separate sections for the specific types of thyroid cancer.

➤ Eighty to ninety percent of thyroid cancers are papillary carcinomas or follicular carcinomas. (Subtypes of papillary carcinomas include the follicular variant, tall cell variant, columnar cell variant, and diffuse sclerosing variant.) Most of these tumors tend to grow slowly and can be treated successfully. One subtype of follicular carcinoma, hurthle cell carcinoma, carries a worse prognosis.

➤ Five to ten percent of thyroid cancers are medullary thyroid carcinomas (MTCs). These tumors have a worse prognosis than papillary and follicular carcinomas. About 20% of MTCs are inherited and run in families.

➤ The rarest type of thyroid cancer, anaplastic carcinoma, is an aggressive cancer that spreads quickly to the neck and other parts of the body. Fortunately, less than 2% of thyroid cancers are of the anaplastic type.

Information on treatment of thyroid lymphomas should be found in non-Hodgkin's lymphoma information sources.

Most thyroid cancer patients are treated with surgery to remove the tumor. Thyroidectomy is the name of the surgical procedure used to remove the entire thyroid. Sometimes it is possible to remove only one lobe of the thyroid. If the cancer has spread to nearby tissues, more neck tissue and lymph nodes will be removed. People who have had their thyroid removed will have to take thyroid hormone replacement pills for the rest of their life.

Radioactive iodine therapy capitalizes on the fact that the thyroid gland absorbs all the iodine in the body. The radioactive iodine given to the patient concentrates in the thyroid gland and destroys thyroid cells without damaging other parts of the body. Tumors that do not take up iodine, such as medullary carcinomas, may be treated with conventional external beam radiation therapy. Chemotherapy, sometimes in combination with radiation therapy, is frequently used to treat anaplastic-type tumors. It is hardly ever used to treat other types of thyroid cancer.

Cure rates for thyroid cancer are very high, and the great majority of patients can expect full recovery and high quality of life after treatment. Although they have to take thyroid hormone replacement pills for the rest of their lives, this therapy has very few side effects.

Information Sources

Brochures, Booklets, and Other Short Print Publications

➤ National Cancer Institute. *What You Need to Know about Thyroid Cancer.* This concise introduction to thyroid cancer discusses symptoms, diagnosis, treatment, and emotional issues. Includes a list of questions for the doctor and a short glossary. Access at https://cissecure.nci.nih.gov/ncipubs/

➤ Thyroid Foundation of America and the American Thyroid Association. *Cancer of the Thyroid.*
A one-page summary of the major facts regarding thyroid cancer. Access at: www.thyroid.org/patients/brochures/ThyroidCancerFAQ.pdf

Books

➤ Rosenthal, M. Sara. 2003. *The Thyroid Cancer Book.* 2d ed. Victoria, BC: Trafford.
A comprehensive overview of thyroid cancer with separate chapters focusing on specific types such as papillary and follicular, medullary, and anaplastic thyroid cancer. This book also covers radioactive iodine therapy, follow-up care, and complementary therapies. A list of resources in the United States and the world and the low-iodine recipes are helpful.

➤ Van Nostrand, Douglas, Gary Bloom, and L. Wartofsky. 2004. *Thyroid Cancer: A Guide for Patients.* Baltimore, MD: Keystone Press.
This book was edited by two physicians and a patient advocate, with each chapter written by a medical specialist. It covers the different types of thyroid cancer, diagnostic procedures, and various treatment methods including surgery, radiation, and radioiodine therapy. Essays written by five thyroid cancer survivors discuss living with thyroid cancer and emotional coping with the disease. The high reading level and focus on the medical/scientific aspects make this book suitable for the sophisticated reader who is interested in understanding the science behind the disease and the treatment. Includes photographs, illustrations and a glossary. Portions of this are available at: www.thyca.org

Web Resources

Sites focusing on thyroid cancer

➤ Light of Life Foundation. Access at: www.lightoflifefoundation.org
This site offers concise and easy-to-read information about thyroid cancer and a sampling of a few low-iodine recipes from the foundation cookbook. Information about the organization's advocacy and support activities can also be found here.

➤ Thyroid-Cancer.net. Access at: www.thyroid-cancer.net
Developed by physicians at the Johns Hopkins Thyroid Tumor Center, this site offers up-to-date information on thyroid cancer in a question-and-answer format. The "patient tools" area enables users to personalize the site, organize medications and pharmacy information, track lab results, prepare questions for their doctor, and more. This site is well organized and easy to use but may lack detail.

➤ ThyCa: Thyroid Cancer Survivors' Association. Access at: www.thyca.org
The site of the Thyroid Cancer Survivors' Association maintains current information about thyroid cancer and support services available to people at any stage of testing, treatment, or lifelong monitoring for thyroid cancer, as well as to their caregivers. This is a very large site with detailed information on diagnostic tests, anaplastic thyroid cancer, and various treatment methods. Special features include a downloadable low-iodine cookbook, access to both patient-to-patient and group support networks, and information about educational conferences and events.

Detailed sections in general cancer sites

➤ American Cancer Society. *Learn about Thyroid Cancer*. Access at: www. cancer.org and select from the menu under "Choose a Cancer Topic." A detailed guide about thyroid cancer can be printed by section or as an Adobe Acrobat (.pdf) file.

➤ National Cancer Institute. *Thyroid Cancer*. Access at: www.cancer.gov and click on "Types of Cancer." The top page of the section links to patient versions of PDQ® statements, clinical trial information, and other NCI publications on this topic.

➤ People Living with Cancer. *Thyroid Cancer*. Access at: www.plwc.org and click on "Cancer Type." The PLWC oncologist-approved thyroid cancer guide can be printed in its entirety or by subtopic.

Sections about thyroid cancer are also available at the following sites:

➤ Canadian Cancer Society. Access at: www.cancer.ca and click on "About Cancer."

➤ Cancerbackup. Access at: www.cancerbackup.org.uk/Home and click on "Cancer Types."

➤ Cancerconsultants.com. Access at: www.cancerconsultants.com and make a selection under "Links to Specific Cancer type Information."

➤ CancerSource.com. Access at: www.cancersource.com/Patient.pg and make a selection from the "Diagnosis & Treatment" pull-down menu.

➤ OncologyChannel.com. Access at: www.oncologychannel.com and select a condition from the left sidebar.

Patient-Support Organizations

➤ Light of Life Foundation. Access at: www.lightoflifefoundation.org
Phone: 877-565-6325

➤ ThyCa:Thyroid Cancer Survivors' Association, Inc. Access at: www.thyca.org
Phone: 877-588-7904

Uterine Cancer

Anatomical facts: *The uterus is a hollow organ where the baby grows during pregnancy. It is similar to a pear in shape and size and is located in the pelvis. The uterus is connected to the vagina through the cervix. The fallopian tubes extend from either side of the top of the uterus to the ovaries.*

Illustrations available at the Medical Illustrations Gallery of the People Living with Cancer Web site.

Access at: www.plwc.org and click on Library on the left sidebar.

Cancer of the uterus is one for the few cancers that gives a warning sign early in the development of disease: abnormal vaginal bleeding. This is the reason why 75% of the 39,000 women diagnosed with this cancer every year in the United States discover the disease in an early stage. Early diagnosis means that the cancer can be cured with surgery alone. The majority of cases are diagnosed in women between the ages of 45 and 74. Only 5% of patients are diagnosed before age 40.

The first question in the reference interview with a client looking for information about cancer of the uterus is whether she is interested in information about endometrial cancer or uterine sarcoma. Of tumors in the uterus, 95% start in its inner lining, called the endometrium. Endometrial cancer is very different from uterine sarcomas, which include endometrial stromal sarcomas, uterine leiomyosarcomas, and uterine carcinosarcomas. Many information sources have separate sections for endometrial cancer and uterine sarcomas.

The development of endometrial cancer is linked to female hormones. Increased production of estrogen, for example, in women who began menstruation early, entered menopause late, have never been pregnant, or use hormone replacement therapy, raises the risk of developing endometrial cancer. Obese women produce higher levels of estrogen and are also at increased risk.

Most women diagnosed with uterine cancer are treated with surgery. Removal of the uterus (hysterectomy) is usually sufficient to cure endometrial cancer that has not spread beyond the first few millimeters of the endometrium. A radical hysterectomy that includes removal of the cervix, uterus, ovaries, and fallopian tubes is needed for tumors that invade deeper into the endometrium and for uterine sarcomas. According to stage and age, patients can also be treated with radiation therapy, chemotherapy, and hormonal therapy, separately or in combination. The goal of hormonal therapy is to reduce the amount of estrogen in the body.

Removal of the ovaries induces the onset of menopause, and women with uterine cancer may be interested in information on treating menopausal symptoms and side effects such as osteoporosis, hot flashes, vaginal dryness, insomnia, mood swings, and heart disease.

Information Sources

Brochures, Booklets, and Other Short Print Publications

➤ Gynecologic Cancer Foundation. *Understanding Endometrial Cancer: A Woman's Guide.*
This is an overview of endometrial cancer covering mainly treatment options and quality-of-life issues, including fatigue, work life, relationships, and intimacy. Offers tips for talking with the treatment team and a resource list. Access at: www.thegcf.org.

➤ National Cancer Institute. *What You Need to Know about Cancer of the Uterus.*
A concise introduction to uterine cancer covering staging, treatment options, and emotional issues. Includes a glossary and a list of questions for the doctor. Access at: https://cissecure.nci.nih.gov/ncipubs/

Books Chapters

➤ Hartmann, Lynn C., and Charles L. Loprinzi. 2005. *Mayo Clinic Guide to Women's Cancers.* Rochester, MN: Mayo Clinic.
This book was edited by two physicians from Mayo Clinic, and book chapters are written and reviewed by Mayo Clinic experts. Part two of the book focuses on gynecologic cancer, with a few chapters about endometrial cancer and uterine sarcoma. The third part of the book, "Living with Cancer," provides supportive-care information relevant to all women with cancer. A unique feature of this book is the visual guide that includes color illustrations explaining the cancer process, anatomy surgery, and radiation. Other photos and illustrations, tables, and text boxes throughout the text help in understanding and comprehension.

➤ McGinn, Kerry Anne, and Pamela J. Haylock. 2003. *Women's Cancers: How to Prevent Them, How to Treat Them, How to Beat Them.* 3d ed., fully updated ed. Alameda, CA: Hunter House.
This book provides practical information for women with cancer and includes a chapter about cancer of the uterus. Other chapters discuss working with the medical team, sources of support, complementary and alternative treatments, and feelings. The part titled "Life after Cancer" focuses on the physical, emotional, and social challenges women may experience after treatment ends. The authors are oncology nurses.

Web Resources

Sites focusing on uterine cancer

➤ Women's Cancer Network. Access at: www.wcn.org
This site is provided by the Gynecologic Cancer Foundation, which is affiliated with the Society of Gynecologic Oncologists. Detailed information about cancer in women, including reproductive cancer, is provided. Special features include an extensive news section; a "Find a Doctor" database, which helps locate oncologists specializing in gynecologic cancers; and links to clinical trial databases.

Detailed sections in general cancer sites

➤ American Cancer Society. *Learn about Endometrial Cancer* and *Learn about Uterine Sarcoma*. Access at: www.cancer.org and select from the menu under "Choose a Cancer Topic." Disease-specific detailed guides can be printed by section or as Adobe Acrobat (.pdf) files.
➤ National Cancer Institute. *Uterine Cancer, Endometrial* and *Uterine Sarcoma*. Access at: www.cancer.gov and click on "Types of Cancer." The top page of the section links to patient versions of PDQ® statements, clinical trial information, and other NCI publications on this topic.
➤ People Living with Cancer. *Uterine Cancer*. Access at: www.plwc.org and click on "Cancer Type." The PLWC oncologist-approved uterine cancer guide may be printed in its entirety or by subtopic.

Sections about uterine cancer are also available at the following sites:

➤ Canadian Cancer Society. Access at: www.cancer.ca and click on "About Cancer."
➤ Cancerbackup. Access at: www.cancerbackup.org.uk/Home and click on "Cancer Types."
➤ Cancerconsultants.com. Access at: www.cancerconsultants.com and make a selection under "Links to Specific Cancer Type Information."
➤ CancerSource.com. Access at: www.cancersource.com/Patient.pg and make a selection from the "Diagnosis & Treatment" pull-down menu.
➤ OncologyChannel.com. Access at: www.oncologychannel.com and select a condition from the left sidebar.

Patient-Support Organizations

➤ EyesOnThePrize.org. An online support group for gynecologic cancer survivors. Access at: www.eyesontheprize.org

Chapter 5

Main Types of Childhood Cancer

Childhood Brain and Central Nervous System Tumors

Anatomical facts: The brain is the center of thought, memory, emotion, and speech, as well as the coordinator of the body's voluntary and involuntary actions and processes. A network of nerves located in the brain itself and in the spinal cord exchanges messages between the brain and the rest of the body. These messages tell our muscles how to move, transmit information gathered by our senses, and help coordinate our internal organs. The soft, spongy mass of brain tissue located in the head is protected by the bones of the skull and three thin membranes called meninges. Watery fluid called cerebrospinal fluid cushions the brain. This fluid flows through spaces between the meninges and through spaces within the brain called ventricles. The brain and the spinal cord compose the central nervous system.

Illustration available in the Pediatric Brain Tumor Foundation publication *Basic Facts About Pediatric Brain and Spinal Cord Tumors.* Access at: www.pbtfus.org and click on "Family Support."

Tumors in the brain and spinal cord are the second most common cancers in children (after leukemia). Approximately 3,200 children and adolescents are diagnosed with a central nervous system (CNS) tumor every year in the United States. While the overall five-year survival rate for all childhood CNS tumors is over 50%, prognosis varies greatly according to tumor type. The location of these tumors within the brain, in close proximity to areas responsible for vital functions in the body, presents a difficult challenge in treatment. Even benign tumors, which make up about one-fourth of all childhood brain tumors, can cause significant damage and even death. Unlike adult CNS tumors, almost all brain tumors in children are primary tumors, not metastases of cancers that start in other parts of the body and spread to the brain.

The great majority of childhood CNS tumors are not caused by any known risk factor. Children who received radiation directed at the head have a slightly higher risk to develop a brain tumor ten and more years after the original treatment. Other environmental factors, such as exposure to certain chemicals or to cellular phones, have been suggested as risk factors, but studies have not found any evidence to support these claims. A few rare genetic disorders are associated with a higher risk for developing a childhood brain tumor.

The classification of brain tumors is very complex, and librarians may be presented with many terms and medical names. The term *glioma* is often used when discussing brain tumors. It is not a specific type of cancer but rather a general term that includes all tumors that arise from glial cells surrounding and supporting nerve cells in the brain.

Glioma tumors include astrocytomas, primitive neuroectodermal tumors, oligodendrogliomas, ependymomas, brain stem gliomas, optic gliomas, and others. Since these tumors are completely different disease entities, the librarian should ask for a more specific name in order to find relevant information. Many information sources offer separate overviews for specific types of childhood brain tumors.

The most common types of brain tumors in children are astrocytomas, accounting for about one-half of all childhood brain tumors. Many astrocytomas cannot be cured because they infiltrate the surrounding normal brain tissue and therefore cannot be completely removed. Astrocytomas are divided into many subtypes, each with its distinct clinical features and speed of progression.

Primitive neuroectodermal tumors (PNETs) are tumors that occur almost exclusively in children. Most tumors of this type arise in the cerebellum part of the brain and are called medulloblastomas. These are fast-growing tumors that have the ability to spread along the spinal cord and the meninges, but they can be effectively treated; over 50% of these tumors can be cured by surgery, radiation therapy, and chemotherapy.

Ependymoma is another tumor type that can sometimes be cured, because these tumors do not usually infiltrate the normal brain tissue like other glioma tumors.

The first step in treating CNS tumors is usually surgery. The surgery to open the skull and enable access to the brain is called craniotomy. During surgery the neurosurgeon makes the decision as to how much of the tumor can be removed. Complete removal is not possible if the tumor has infiltrated normal brain tissue or if the tumor's removal will cause an unacceptable injury to structures that control essential functions. Many children need the placement of a shunt if the tumor causes an obstruction to the flow of cerebrospinal fluid. A shunt lowers the pressure caused by the blockage and alleviates symptoms.

Radiation therapy is effective against many brain tumors, but it may cause severe cognitive disabilities in children younger than three years old. The child's age, tumor type, and extent of tumor removal during surgery are the determining factors in making a decision about treatment with radiation therapy. In some cases children are treated with chemotherapy first in order to prevent tumor growth and delay therapy with radiation as much as possible.

Chemotherapy is less effective against CNS cancers because of its difficulty in penetrating through the blood-brain barrier. The blood-brain barrier is a system of thin membranes that filter chemical molecules from the blood, including many drugs, in order to protect the sensitive brain tissue. Some chemotherapy drugs have the ability to penetrate the blood-brain barrier and be active against brain tumors. The cure rates for medulloblastoma have dramatically improved as a result of treatment with chemotherapy.

Most children with brain tumors are treated with steroids to reduce the brain swelling caused by the tumor or its treatment. Some patients are also treated with drugs that prevent seizures.

Tumors in the brain and spinal cord and their treatment may cause difficulties in speech, movement, memory and cognitive ability. Rehabilitative services such as speech therapy, physical therapy, and occupational therapy can greatly improve or even restore function. Survivors of childhood CNS tumors receive therapy and services from many specialists for many years in order to become as active and independent as possible. The brain tumor patient organizations listed below provide information and referrals for rehabilitation services and providers.

Information Sources

Brochures, Booklets, and Other Short Print Publications

➤ National Brain Tumor Foundation. *Understanding and Coping with Your Child's Brain Tumor.*
This 54-page publication provides parents with the information they need when their child is diagnosed with a brain tumor. It covers diagnostic tests, choosing a treatment team, tumor types, treatment methods, social and emotional support, and returning to school. Special features include a glossary and a resource guide. To access a printable version go to: www.braintumor.org

➤ National Cancer Institute. *What You Need to Know about Brain Tumors.*
This booklet covers adult and childhood brain tumors. It discusses possible causes, symptoms, diagnosis, treatment, emotional issues, and questions

to ask the doctor. Includes a glossary of terms and other resources. Access at: https://cissecure.nci.nih.gov/ncipubs/
➤ Pediatric Brain Tumor Foundation.
  ➤ *Questions for Your Medical Care Team When Your Child Has a Brain Tumor*
  ➤ *Basic Facts about Pediatric Brain and Spinal Cord Tumors*
  ➤ *Basic Facts about Medulloblastoma/PNET*
  ➤ *Basic Facts about Juvenile Pilocytic Astrocytoma*
  ➤ *Basic Facts about Astrocytoma*
  ➤ *Basic Facts about Glioma*
  ➤ *Basic Facts about Ependymoma*
  Short publications with facts about specific tumor types and other brochures for parents of children with brain tumors are available at: www. pbtfus.org.

Books

Brain tumors–specific books

➤ Children's Brain Tumor Foundation. 2003. *A Resource Guide for Parents of Children with Brain or Spinal Cord Tumors*. 3d ed. New York: Children's Brain Tumor Foundation.
  This resource book provides information necessary for families facing the challenge of a childhood brain tumor. The medical overview includes information about the cells and structure of the brain and spinal cord. Other sections address hospitalization, returning home, and school issues. The book contains an extensive list of resource organizations that offer assistance to families of children with brain tumors.
➤ Segal, Gail. 2002. *Dictionary for Brain Tumor Patients*. Des Plaines, IL: American Brain Tumor Association.
  This dictionary contains short definitions to terms the patient with a brain tumor is likely to hear or read. In addition to medical terms, the dictionary includes lists of medical abbreviations, prefixes, roots, and suffixes that can help a layperson understand medical lingo, as well as useful measurement tables. Available online at the ABTA site, www.abta.org
➤ Shiminski-Maher, Tania, et al. 2002. *Childhood Brain and Spinal Cord Tumors: A Guide for Families, Friends and Caregivers*. Cambridge, MA: O'Reilly.
  This book offers detailed medical information about both benign and malignant brain and spinal cord tumors that strike children and adolescents. In addition, it offers day-to-day practical advice on how to cope with

procedures, hospitalization, family and friends, school, social and financial issues, communication, feelings about failed therapy, and the difficult issues of death and bereavement. Woven among the medical details and the practical advice are the voices of parents and children who have lived with cancer and its treatments.

➤ Zeltzer, Paul M. 2004. *Brain Tumors: Leaving the Garden of Eden: A Survival Guide to Diagnosis, Learning the Basics, Getting Organized and Finding Your Medical Team.* Encino, CA: Shilysca Press.

This 400-page comprehensive reference guide covering adult and childhood brain tumors was authored by a renowned neuro-oncologist. The book starts with the basics about brain tumors and advises readers on finding a good medical team, getting a second opinion, and using the Internet to search for information. The text includes chapters on all major types of brain tumors, including those diagnosed mostly in children. The chapter about medications explains how to deal with side effects and avoid dangerous interactions of drugs used for pain control, seizures, fatigue, and brain swelling.

Relevant childhood cancer books

➤ Carroll, William L., and Jessica B. Reisman. 2005. *100 Questions and Answers about Your Child's Cancer.* Sudbury, MA: Jones and Bartlett Publishers.

This book presents practical answers to questions about childhood cancer, treatment options, post–treatment quality of life, and coping strategies for both patients and parents. Two child cancer experts authored this book and incorporated comments from parents of children with cancer. The book provides detailed information on diagnostic tests, supportive-care issues, and side effects and complications of treatment that are common to all children treated for cancer. The text is easy to read, and definitions for key terms are provided in the sidebar.

➤ Keene, Nancy. 2003. *Educating the Child with Cancer: A Guide for Parents and Teachers.* Kensington, MD: Candlelighters Childhood Cancer Foundation.

This book was developed with the intent of promoting understanding and communication among parents, educators, and medical professionals so that together they can provide an appropriate education for children who have been treated for cancer. Learning issues that face children treated for cancer from infancy through adulthood are covered in depth, with some chapters written by experts and others by parents. Topics include gaining access to special education services, helping siblings in the classroom, treatment-related late effects that may cause learning difficulties, and grief in the classroom. Each chapter ends with a list of key points.

➤ Woznick, Leigh A., and Carol D. Goodheart. 2002. *Living with Childhood Cancer: A Practical Guide to Help Parents Cope.* Washington, DC: American Psychological Association.

The focus of this book is the psychological impact of childhood cancer. It provides guidance and advice to parents on managing the emotional and practical challenges of the disease and treatment. The book describes how adults, children, teenagers, and families may cope with illness and stress and offers strategies for successful coping. Topics include communication, stress, trauma, pain, side effects, encouraging child development, building self-esteem, dying and grieving, and long-term survivorship. Specific information is provided for different age groups and various types of families. The authors are a psychologist and her daughter who is the mother of a child with cancer.

Web Resources

Sites focusing on childhood brain tumors

➤ The Childhood Brain Tumor Foundation. Access at: www.childhoodbrain tumor.org

A collection of articles about childhood brain tumors and supportive-care issues is available on this site. The articles were written by health care professionals and childhood brain tumor specialists. The site also offers the full text of the organization's newsletter and information about the services offered to families.

➤ Children's Brain Tumor Foundation. Access at: www.cbtf.org

This site features a medical overview and information on supporting the child with a brain tumor at the hospital, at school, and at home. A detailed section on various organizations offering patient support services is very useful for childhood brain tumor patients and families.

Sites focusing on adult and childhood brain tumors

➤ American Brain Tumor Association. Access at: www.abta.org

This organization offers information and support services for people diagnosed with brain tumors. The "Tumor Information" section offers tumor-specific information as well as Adobe Acrobat (.pdf) files of two premier publications: *A Primer of Brain Tumors: A Patient's Reference Manual* and *Dictionary for Brain Tumor Patients.* Both publications are updated periodically and sent to patients and family free of charge. The "Care and Support" section provides information about living with a brain tumor and coping with the emotional and physical challenges.

➤ The Brain Tumor Society Online. Access at: www.tbts.org
This site is provided for the entire brain tumor community, from newly diagnosed patients to survivors, families, and health care professionals. The "Patients Resources" section includes detailed medical information for topics such as pathology, nutrition, and lay-language summaries of published professional articles. This site also includes information about support services for patients and families and downloadable files of brochures and fact sheets published by the Brain Tumor Society.

➤ Musella Foundation for Brain Tumor Research Information. *Clinical Trials and Noteworthy Treatments For Brain Tumors.* Access at: www.virtual trials.com
At the heart of this site is a comprehensive database of clinical trials for brain tumors. The site also includes a 48-page brain tumor guide for the newly diagnosed, which is downloadable as Adobe Acrobat (.pdf) files; lay-term summaries of published studies; medical news; an online dictionary; and many interactive features. The extensive video library featuring brain tumor experts discussing various treatments is especially interesting.

➤ National Brain Tumor Foundation (NBTF). Access at: www.braintumor.org
This site presents information regarding treatment options and community resources for brain tumor patients and families. Features include a database of questions answered by health care professionals, a link library arranged by topic, and a treatment-center database. Adobe Acrobat (.pdf) files of publications such as fact sheets and brochures are available.

Detailed sections in childhood cancer sites

➤ CureSearch. Access at: www.curesearch.org
This site has a detailed section about brain tumors, and the information is presented separately to parents and patients in different age groups: preschool, ages 5–10, 10–14, and 14–22. Topics covered include diagnostic tests, treatment methods, impact on the patient and family, navigating the health care system, and school issues. The interactive section of the site provides a clinical trial matching service, discussion boards, and a resource directory for national and local support groups and services. Provided by the Children's Cancer Group and the National Childhood Cancer Foundation.

➤ Penn State Hershey Medical Center. *Home Care Guide.* Access at: www. hmc.psu.edu/hematology/homeguide/
Nurses and physicians from the children's hematology/oncology team at Penn State Hershey Medical Center developed this guide for caregivers of children with childhood cancer. The guide provides treatment plans for a variety of supportive-care and psychosocial issues that may occur while a

child is undergoing treatment. Each plan gives caregivers the information they need in order to solve problems, including understanding the problem, when to get professional help, what caregivers can do on their own, possible obstacles, and how to carry out and adjust the plan.

Detailed sections in general cancer sites

➤ American Cancer Society. *Learn about Brain/CNS Tumors in Children.* Access at: www.cancer.org and select from the menu under "Choose a Cancer Topic." A detailed guide about childhood brain tumors can be printed as an Adobe Acrobat (.pdf) file.

➤ Cancerbackup. *Brain Tumors in Children.* Access at: www.cancerbackup. org.uk/Home and click on "Cancer Type."

➤ National Cancer Institute. *Childhood Cancers.* Access at: www.cancer.gov and click on "Types of Cancer." The top page of the section links to patient versions of PDQ® statements about different types of childhood brain tumors, clinical trial information, and other relevant NCI publications.

➤ People Living with Cancer. *Central Nervous System, Childhood.* Access at: www.plwc.org and click on "Cancer Type." The PLWC oncologist-approved guides on different types of childhood brain tumors can be printed in their entirety, or by subtopic.

Patient-Support Organizations

➤ American Brain Tumor Association. Access at: www.abta.org
Patient line: 800-886-2282

➤ The Brain Tumor Society. Access at: www.tbts.org
Phone: 800-770-8287

➤ Candlelighters. Access at: www.candlelighters.org
Phone: 800-366-2223

➤ Childhood Brain Tumor Foundation. Access at: www.childhoodbraintumor.org
Phone: 301-515-2900

➤ Children's Brain Tumor Foundation. Access at: http://www.cbtf.org
Phone: 212-367-9000

➤ National Brain Tumor Foundation (NBTF). Access at: www.braintumor.org
Phone: 800-934-CURE

➤ The National Children's Cancer Society. Access at: http://nationalchildrens cancersociety.com
Phone: 800-5-FAMILY

➤ Pediatric Brain Tumor Foundation of the United States. Access at: http:// www.pbtfus.org
Phone: 800-253-6530

Childhood Hodgkin's Disease

Anatomical facts: The lymphatic system is a network of vessels, similar to blood vessels, that carry the lymph fluid to different parts of the body. Lymph is a colorless fluid that contains infection-fighting white blood cells called lymphocytes. Lymphocytes are made and stored in lymph nodes, small bean-shaped organs that cluster along the lymphatic system. There are two types of lymphocytes: B lymphocytes (B cells) and T lymphocytes (T cells). Other parts of the lymphatic system include the spleen, thymus, tonsils, and bone marrow. Lymphatic tissue also is found in other parts of the body, including the stomach, intestines, and skin. The lymphatic system is part of the body's immune system.

Illustration available at the Medical Illustrations Gallery of the People Living with Cancer Web site .

Access at: www.plwc.org and click on Library on the left sidebar.

Hodgkin's disease is one of the most curable cancers. Improvements in treatment contributed to a 60% drop in death rates since the 1970s. The overall five-year survival rate is 85%. The National Cancer Institute reports approximately 850–900 cases of Hodgkin's disease diagnosed in children and adolescents under 20 years per year in the United States. Hodgkin's disease is very rarely diagnosed in children younger than 5.

Hodgkin's disease is one of two cancers that start in the lymphatic system. Non-Hodgkin's lymphoma can also occur in children. It is discussed in this chapter on page 178.

The cause of Hodgkin's disease is unknown. People with a weakened immune system, such as people infected with HIV; people who have received an organ transplant; or people with other immunodeficiency disorders have a slightly increased risk. Infection with the Epstein-Barr virus, which causes mononucleosis, somewhat increases the risk for developing Hodgkin's disease, but the virus's exact role in this process is not fully understood. There does not appear to be a connection between lifestyle factors or environmental exposures and Hodgkin's disease.

Hodgkin's disease is characterized by the development of unique abnormal B lymphocytes called Reed-Sternberg cells. These cells are much larger than normal lymphocytes and also look different from the cells of non-Hodgkin's lymphoma and other cancers. The disease may affect one or more lymph nodes in any part of the body, but it usually starts in the upper part of the body, most typically in the chest, neck, or under the arms. Hodgkin's disease spreads through the lymphatic vessels in an orderly manner from one lymph node cluster to the other, from nearby clusters to distant ones. The enlargement of the lymphatic tissue may put pressure on healthy structures and cause pain.

The majority of newly diagnosed Hodgkin's disease patients can be cured with a combination of chemotherapy and radiation therapy. Even though radiation therapy works well to cure localized Hodgkin's disease, it can significantly impair growth and cause severe long-term effects in children. For this reason most children with Hodgkin's are treated with a combination of chemotherapy and lower-dose radiation therapy or with chemotherapy alone. Treatment usually consists of chemotherapy lasting four to six months, sometimes followed by radiation therapy.

Treatment with bone marrow or stem cell transplantations is used in the rare cases of patients who relapsed after first-line treatment with chemotherapy and radiation. Most patients do not undergo surgery, except for biopsy and to implant a catheter to administer chemotherapy.

Treatment for Hodgkin's disease has the potential to cause infertility in boys and girls. Information about options for fertility preservation can help parents prepare for a discussion with the doctor or a cancer fertility expert before starting treatment.

It is estimated that 123,000 long-term survivors of Hodgkin's disease live in the United States, many of whom where treated as children. Long-term effects of treatment are weighty concerns for this population. Young women and girls who were treated with radiation therapy to the chest area are at increased risk to develop breast cancer. Treatment may also cause thyroid dysfunction or heart damage and increase the risk for secondary cancers. Long-term survivors need to be watched very closely for the development of any of those conditions. Information sources about late effects of treatment are presented in the section about childhood cancer survivors on page 36.

Information Sources
Brochures, Booklets, and Other Short Print Publications
Lymphoma specific
➤ The Leukemia & Lymphoma Society.
  ➤ *The Lymphomas.*
    This booklet offer a general overview of Hodgkin's and non-Hodgkin's lymphomas that is relevant to adults and children. Topics covered include blood and marrow components, the lymphatic system, and classification of lymphomas. An easy-to-read version of this publication is titled *The Lymphomas: A Guide for Patients and Their Families.* Larger print and bullet points summarize the topic in a concise manner.

➤ *Emotional Aspects of Childhood Blood Cancers.*
This addresses psychosocial issues concerning children with blood cancers. Access at: www.leukemia-lymphoma.org

➤ Lymphoma Research Foundation.

➤ *Lymphoma Resource Guide.*
A listing of organizations, online resources, audio and videotapes, publications, and therapies that are of interest to lymphoma patients and families. Access at: www.lymphoma.org

➤ *Understanding Hodgkin's Lymphoma: A Guide for Patients.*
This 84-page booklet provides a comprehensive review of Hodgkin's lymphoma including diagnosis, treatment, coping with side effects, clinical trial experimental treatments, and living with cancer. Includes a glossary. Relevant for adults and children. Individual copies are free and can be obtained by calling the Lymphoma Research Foundation at 800-500-9976.

➤ National Cancer Institute. *What You Need to Know about Hodgkin's Disease.*
A concise introduction to Hodgkin's disease covering staging, treatment options, and emotional support. Includes a glossary and a list of questions for the doctor.

Relevant childhood cancer publications

➤ National Cancer Institute. *Young People with Cancer: A Handbook for Parents.*
This publication discusses the most common types of childhood cancer, treatments, and side effects, as well as issues that may arise when a child is diagnosed with cancer. Offers medical information and practical tips gathered from parents. Access at: https://cissecure.nci.nih.gov/ncipubs/

➤ National Childhood Cancer Foundation. *The Children's Oncology Group (COG) Family Handbook.*
This 80-page handbook was written by nurses, doctors, and other childhood cancer professionals. The information is relevant to all types of childhood cancer and covers medical and psychosocial issues. The publication includes illustrations and has several areas that may be customized for a specific child. To download access, go to www.curesearch.org.

➤ National Children's Cancer Society. *The Mountain You've Climbed: A Parent's Guide to Childhood Cancer Survivorship.*
This guide is designed to answer parents' questions regarding childhood cancer and offer suggestions on how to integrate the cancer experience into all areas of the family's life. It addresses issues beginning from the time of diagnosis through the completion of treatment and beyond. Order at: http://nationalchildrenscancersociety.com

Books

Lymphoma-specific books (for adults and childhood lymphomas)

➤ Adler, Elizabeth M. 2005. *Living with Lymphoma: A Patient's Guide.* Baltimore, MD: Johns Hopkins University Press.

Written by a neurobiologist and a lymphoma survivor, this book offers a detailed explanation of cell biology that helps readers understand the disease and treatment. While this book provides an in-depth look at the medical side of lymphoma and detailed descriptions of specific drugs, drug combinations, and treatment approaches, psychosocial issues are not as meticulously covered. Sophisticated readers who are interested in learning the scientific aspects of lymphoma will appreciate this book.

➤ Holman, Peter, Jodi Garrett, and William D. Jansen. 2004. *100 Questions and Answers about Lymphoma.* Sudbury, MA: Jones and Bartlett.

Detailed information about lymphoma is presented in an easy-to-read question-and-answer format. Terms are explained in the sidebar, and the book includes lists of Web sites, organizations, literature, and resources on general and specific topics related to Hodgkin's lymphoma. This book was co–authored by a lymphoma specialist, an oncology nurse, and a lymphoma survivor.

Relevant childhood cancer books

➤ Carroll, William L., and Jessica B. Reisman. 2005. *100 Questions and Answers about Your Child's Cancer.* Sudbury, MA: Jones and Bartlett.

This book presents practical answers to questions about childhood cancer, treatment options, post-treatment quality of life, and coping strategies for both patients and parents. Two child cancer experts authored this book and incorporated comments from parents of children with cancer. The book provides detailed information about diagnostic tests, supportive-care issues, and side effects and complications of treatment that are common to all children treated for cancer. The text is easy to read, and definitions for key terms are provided in the sidebar.

➤ Keene, Nancy. 2003. *Educating the Child with Cancer: A Guide for Parents and Teachers.* Kensington, MD: Candlelighters Childhood Cancer Foundation.

This book was developed with the intent of promoting understanding and communication among parents, educators, and medical professionals so that together they can provide an appropriate education for children who have been treated for cancer. Learning issues that face children treated for cancer from infancy through adulthood are covered in depth, with some chapters written by experts and others by parents. Topics include gaining access to special education services, helping siblings in the classroom, physical activity in school, treatment-related late effects that may cause learning difficulties, and grief in the classroom. Each chapter ends with a list of key points.

➤ Woznick, Leigh A., and Carol D. Goodheart. 2002. *Living with Childhood Cancer: A Practical Guide to Help Parents Cope*. Washington, DC: American Psychological Association.

The focus of this book is the psychological impact of childhood cancer. It provides guidance and advice to parents on managing the emotional and practical challenges of the disease and its treatment. The book describes how adults, children, teenagers, and families may cope with illness and stress and offers strategies for successful coping. Topics include communication, stress, trauma, pain, side effects, encouraging child development, building self-esteem, dying and grieving, and long-term survivorship. Specific information is provided for different age groups and different types of families. The authors are a psychologist and her daughter who is the mother of a child with cancer.

Web Resources

Sites focusing on lymphoma

➤ Leukaemia Research. Access at: www.lrf.org.uk/
Leukaemia Research is a British research charity focusing on blood cancers and disorders. The "Information and Education" section offers printable booklets on adult and childhood blood cancers, including some on rare subtypes and conditions. The "News" section includes stories about research developments and other related articles.

➤ The Leukemia & Lymphoma Society. Access at: www.leukemia-lymphoma. org
The site of the world's largest organization dedicated to blood cancers includes many sections and features relevant to childhood Hodgkin's disease. Live and archived versions of educational teleconferences and Webcasts enable users to study complicated topics explained by top experts. The site also includes medical news about lymphoma, short and longer overviews of the diseases, and information about the organization's support services for patients.

➤ Lymphoma Information Network. Access at: www.lymphomainfo.net/
This well-organized directory of lymphoma information sources presents short, concise introductions to many types of lymphoma. Each section has a list of references with links to other sites, PubMed abstracts, or books on Amazon. This site has been maintained for over ten years by an

NHL survivor and is useful as a starting point for a search on specific or complex issues in lymphoma.

➤ Lymphoma Research Foundation. Access at: www.lymphoma.org
The Lymphoma Research Foundation is a patient-support and –advocacy organization providing support and education to lymphoma patients and families. Information about the disease and its treatment and research news are presented in fact sheets, Webcasts, newsletters, and other formats. This site also includes information about support programs and services for patients and families.

Detailed sections in childhood cancer sites

➤ CureSearch. Access at: www.curesearch.org
This site has a detailed section about Hodgkin's disease, and the information is presented separately to parents and patients in different age groups: preschool, ages 5–10, 10–14, and 14–22. Topics covered include diagnostic tests, treatment methods, impact on the patient and family, navigating the health care system, and school issues. The interactive section of the site includes a clinical trial matching service, discussion boards, and a resource directory for national and local support groups and services. Provided by the Children's Cancer Group and the National Childhood Cancer Foundation.

➤ Penn State Hershey Medical Center. *Home Care Guide*. Access at: www. hmc.psu.edu/hematology/homeguide/
Nurses and physicians from the children's hematology/oncology team at Penn State Hershey Medical Center developed this guide for caregivers of children with childhood cancer. The guide provides treatment plans for a variety of supportive-care and psychosocial issues that may occur while a child is undergoing treatment. Each plan provides caregivers with the information they need in order to solve problems, including understanding the problem, when to get professional help, what caregivers can do on their own, possible obstacles, and how to carry out and adjust the plan.

Detailed sections in general cancer sites

➤ American Cancer Society. *Learn about Hodgkin Disease*. Access at: www. cancer.org and select from the menu under "Choose a Cancer Topic."
A detailed guide about Hodgkin's disease can be printed by section or as an Adobe Acrobat (.pdf) file.

➤ Cancerbackup. *Hodgkin Lymphoma in Children*. Access at: www.cancer backup.org.uk/Home and click on "Cancer Type."

➤ National Cancer Institute. *Childhood Cancers.* Access at: www.cancer.gov and click on "Types of Cancer."
The top page of the section links to a patient version of a PDQ® statement on clinical trial information, and other NCI publications on this topic.
➤ People Living with Cancer. *Lymphoma, Hodgkin, Childhood Cancer.* Access at: www.plwc.org and click on "Cancer Type."
The PLWC oncologist-approved guides on childhood Hodgkin's disease can be printed in their entirety or by subtopic.

Patient-Support Organizations

➤ Candlelighters. Access at: www.candlelighters.org
Phone: 800-366-2223
➤ Leukemia & Lymphoma Society. Access at: www.leukemia-lymphoma.org
Phone: 914-949-5213
➤ Leukemia Research Foundation. Access at: www.leukemia-research.org
Phone: 847-424-0600
➤ Lymphoma Research Foundation. Access at: www.lymphoma.org
Phone: (Los Angeles office) 800-500-9976
➤ The National Children's Cancer Society. Access at: http://nationalchildrens cancersociety.com
Phone: 800-5-FAMILY

Childhood Leukemia

Anatomical facts: Bone marrow is the soft material in the center of most bones. It contains blood-forming cells called stem cells that mature in the marrow and then move into the blood vessels. Stem cells mature into different types of blood cells. Each type has a special function. Red blood cells carry oxygen from the lungs to all other tissues of the body and carry away carbon dioxide, a waste product of cell activity. Platelets help form blood clots, which controls bleeding. White blood cells help fight infection. The three main types of white blood cells are granulocytes, monocytes, and lymphocytes.

Illustration available at the National Cancer Institute publication What You Need to Know about Leukemia.
Access at: https://cissecure.nci.nih.gov/ncipubs.

Leukemia is the most common cancer in children and adolescents, with 3,800 new diagnoses per year. It accounts for about one-third of all cancers in children under age 15 and one-fourth of cancers occurring before age 20.

As in other childhood cancers, lifestyle factors do not cause leukemia. Children with specific genetic diseases and conditions such as Down's syndrome have a higher risk of developing leukemia. Exposure to high doses of radiation, such as the radiation resulting from the 1986 Chernobyl accident, also increases the risk for leukemia in children.

Leukemia is a cancer that originates in the bone marrow and involves mostly white blood cells that transform into malignant cells. The large number of malignant cells prevents the bone marrow from functioning properly and causes a decline in the number of normal blood cells. The great majority of leukemias in children are of acute kind, meaning that they develop rapidly. Chronic leukemias, which grow slowly, are extremely rare in children. Of children with leukemia, 80% have acute lymphocytic leukemia (ALL), which develops in lymphocytes and has a five-year survival rate of 85%. Most of the remaining children have acute myelogenous leukemia (AML), which develops from other types of blood cells and has a five-year survival rate of 50%. Leukemia cells travel through the bloodstream; therefore, the disease affects the entire body and not just a specific body part like other cancers.

The main treatment for childhood leukemia is chemotherapy. Children with ALL are classified into low-risk, standard-risk, high-risk, or very-high-risk categories. The level of risk determines the aggressiveness of therapy and enables doctors to treat low- and standard-risk patients with less toxic therapy. Treatment for ALL lasts from two to three years depending on the risk level. Children with AML are treated with higher doses of chemotherapy over a shorter period of time than are children with ALL.

Many children with leukemia can be cured with chemotherapy alone. Children whose disease has spread to the brain or testicles usually receive radiation therapy. Stem cell transplantation is sometimes used to treat very-high-risk ALL or children with relapsed ALL. Children with AML may receive a stem cell transplant after achieving remission, with the goal of preventing relapse.

All children with leukemia receive an implantable catheter that can be used to administer chemotherapy, draw blood, and infuse fluids or blood products. A catheter reduces the number of needle sticks needed during treatment. Parents learn how to care for and maintain the device.

Information Sources

Brochures, Booklets, and Other Short Print Publications

Leukemia-specific

➤ The Leukemia & Lymphoma Society.
  ➤ *Acute Lymphocytic Leukemia (ALL)*

> ➤ *Acute Myelogenous Leukemia (AML)*
>   These booklets offer detailed overviews including anatomy, subtypes, diagnosis, treatment, side effects of treatment, and social and emotional aspects. They are relevant for adult and childhood leukemias. Easy-to-read versions of these publications are titled:
> ➤ *Acute Lymphocytic Leukemia: A Guide for Patients and Their Families*
> ➤ *Acute Myelogenous Leukemia : A Guide for Patients and Their Families*
>   Larger print and bullet points summarize the topic in a concise manner.
> ➤ *Emotional Aspects of Childhood Blood Cancers*
>   Addresses psychosocial issues concerning children with blood cancers. Access online at: www.leukemia-lymphoma.org

➤ National Cancer Institute. *What You Need to Know about Leukemia.*
A concise introduction to leukemia covers staging, treatment options, and emotional support. Includes a glossary and a list of questions for the doctor.

Relevant childhood cancer publications

➤ National Childhood Cancer Foundation. *The Children's Oncology Group (COG) Family Handbook.*
This 80-page handbook was written by nurses, doctors, and other childhood cancer professionals. The information is relevant for all types of childhood cancer and covers medical and psychosocial issues. The publication includes illustrations and has several areas that may be customized for a specific child. Access online at: www.curesearch.org.

➤ National Cancer Institute. *Young People with Cancer: A Handbook for Parents.*
This publication discusses the most common types of childhood cancer, treatments, and side effects, as well as issues that may arise when a child is diagnosed with cancer. Offers medical information and practical tips gathered from parents. Access at: https://cissecure.nci.nih.gov/ncipubs/

➤ National Children's Cancer Society. *The Mountain You've Climbed: A Parents' Guide to Childhood Cancer Survivorship.*
This guide is designed to answer parents' questions regarding childhood cancer and offer suggestions on how to integrate the cancer experience into all areas of the family's life. It addresses issues beginning from the time of diagnosis through the completion of treatment and beyond. Order online at: http://nationalchildrenscancersociety.com

Books

Books focusing on childhood leukemia

➤ Keene, Nancy. 2002. *Childhood Leukemia: A Guide for Families, Friends and Caregivers.* 3d ed. Sebastopol, CA: O'Reilly.

This parent guide has detailed medical information about leukemia and the various treatment options, as well as day-to-day practical advice on how to cope with procedures, hospitalization, family and friends, school, social and financial issues, communication, feelings, and, if therapy is not successful, the difficult issues of death and bereavement. Woven among the medical details and the practical advice are the voices of parents and children who have lived with leukemia and its treatments.

Relevant childhood cancer books

➤ Carroll, William L., and Jessica B. Reisman. 2005. *100 Questions and Answers about Your Child's Cancer*. Sudbury, MA: Jones and Bartlett.
  This book presents practical answers to questions about childhood cancer, treatment options, post–treatment quality of life, and coping strategies for both patients and parents. Two child-cancer experts authored this book and incorporated comments from parents of children with cancer. The book provides detailed information about diagnostic tests, supportive-care issues, and side effects and complications of treatment that are common to all children treated for cancer. The text is easy to read, and definitions for key terms are provided in the sidebar.

➤ Keene, Nancy. 2003. *Educating the Child with Cancer: A Guide for Parents and Teachers*. Kensington, MD: Candlelighters Childhood Cancer Foundation, 2003.
  This book was developed with the intent of promoting understanding and communication among parents, educators, and medical professionals so that together they can provide an appropriate education for children who have been treated for cancer. Learning issues that face children treated for cancer from infancy through adulthood are covered in depth, with some chapters written by experts and others by parents. Topics include gaining access to special education services, helping siblings in the classroom, physical activity in school, treatment-related late effects that may cause learning difficulties, and grief in the classroom. Each chapter ends with a list of key points.

➤ Woznick, Leigh A., and Carol D. Goodheart. 2002. *Living with Childhood Cancer: A Practical Guide to Help Parents Cope*. Washington, DC: American Psychological Association.
  The focus of this book is the psychological impact of childhood cancer. It provides guidance and advice to parents on managing the emotional and practical challenges of the disease and its treatment. The book describes how adults, children, teenagers, and families may cope with illness and stress and offers strategies for successful coping. Topics include

communication, stress, trauma, pain, side effects, encouraging child development, building self-esteem, dying and grieving, and long-term survivorship. Specific information is provided for different age groups and various types of families. The authors are a psychologist and her daughter who is the mother of a child with cancer.

Web Resources

Sites focusing on leukemia

➤ The Leukemia & Lymphoma Society. Access at: www.leukemia-lymphoma.org
The site of the world's largest organization dedicated to blood cancers includes many sections and features relevant to childhood leukemia. Live and archived versions of educational teleconferences and Webcasts enable users to study complicated topics explained by top experts. The site also includes medical news about leukemia, short and longer overviews of the diseases, and information about the organization's support services for patients.
➤ Leukaemia Research. Access at: www.lrf.org.uk/
Leukaemia Research is a British research charity focusing on blood cancers and disorders. The "Information and Education" section offers printable booklets on adult and childhood blood cancers, including some on rare subtypes and conditions. The "News" section includes stories about research developments and other related articles.

Detailed sections in childhood cancer sites

➤ CureSearch. Access at: www.curesearch.org
This site has a detailed section about leukemia, and the information is presented separately to parents and patients in different age groups: preschool, ages 5–10, 10–14, and 14–22. Topics covered include diagnostic tests, treatment methods, impact on the patient and family, navigating the health care system, and school issues. The interactive section of the site includes a clinical trial matching service, discussion boards, and a resource directory for national and local support groups and services. Provided by the Children's Cancer Group and the National Childhood Cancer Foundation.
➤ Penn State Hershey Medical Center. *Home Care Guide.* Access at: www. hmc.psu.edu/hematology/homeguide/
Nurses and physicians from the children's hematology/oncology team at Penn State Hershey Medical Center developed this guide for caregivers of children with childhood cancer. The guide provides treatment plans for a variety of supportive-care and psychosocial issues that may occur while a child is undergoing treatment. Each plan gives caregivers the information

they need in order to solve problems, including understanding the problem, when to get professional help, what caregivers can do on their own, possible obstacles, and how to carry out and adjust the plan.

Detailed sections in general cancer sites

➤ American Cancer Society. *Learn about Leukemia—Children's.* Access at: www.cancer.org and select from the menu under "Choose a Cancer Topic."
A detailed guide about childhood leukemia can be printed by section or as an Adobe Acrobat (.pdf) file.

➤ National Cancer Institute. *Childhood Cancers.* Access at: www.cancer.gov and click on "Types of Cancer."
The top page of the section links to patient versions of PDQ® statements, clinical trial information, and other NCI publications on this topic.

➤ People Living with Cancer. *Leukemia, Acute Lymphoblastic (ALL), Childhood Cancer* and *Leukemia, Acute Myeloid (AML), Childhood Cancer.* Access at: www.plwc.org and click on "Cancer Type."
The PLWC oncologist-approved guides on childhood leukemias can be printed in their entirety or by subtopic.

➤ Cancerbackup. *Acute lymphoblastic leukaemia (ALL) in children.* Access at: www.cancerbackup.org.uk/Home and click on "Cancer Type."

Patient-Support Organizations

➤ Candlelighters. Access at: www.candlelighters.org
Phone: 800-366-2223

➤ Leukemia & Lymphoma Society. Access at: www.leukemia-lymphoma.org
Phone: 914-949-5213

➤ Leukemia Research Foundation. Access at: www.leukemia-research.org
Phone: 847-424-0600

➤ The National Children's Cancer Society. Access at: http://nationalchildrens cancersociety.com
Phone: 800-5-FAMILY

➤ National Children's Leukemia Foundation. Access at: www.leukemia foundation.org
Phone: 800-448-3467

Childhood Non-Hodgkin's Lymphoma

Anatomical facts: The lymphatic system is a network of vessels, similar to blood vessels, that carry the lymph fluid to different parts of the body. Lymph is a colorless fluid that contains infection-fighting white blood cells called lymphocytes. Lymphocytes are made and stored in lymph nodes, small bean-shaped organs that cluster along the lymphatic system. There are two types of lymphocytes: B lymphocytes (B cells) and T lymphocytes (T cells). Other parts of the lymphatic system include the spleen, thymus, tonsils, and bone marrow. The lymphatic system is part of the body's immune system.

Illustration available at the Medical Illustrations Gallery of the People Living with Cancer Web site.

Access at: www.plwc.org and click on Library in the left sidebar.

Approximately 450 cases of non-Hodgkin's lymphoma (NHL) diagnosed in children and adolescents younger then 20 in the United States per year. The five-year survival rate has substantially improved, from 45% for the years 1974 to 1976 to 86% for the period of 1995–2001. NHL can be diagnosed in children of all ages, with 70% of cases occurring in boys; it is twice as common in white children as in African American children.

Non-Hodgkin's lymphoma is one of two cancers that start in the lymphatic system. Hodgkin's disease can also occur in children. It is discussed in this chapter on page 169.

Children whose immune system is weakened as a result of an immunodeficiency syndrome or medications given after organ transplantation have a significant risk to develop NHL, but most children diagnosed with NHL do not have a known risk factor.

Non-Hodgkin's lymphomas of children are a heterogeneous group of tumors distinctly different from the adult NHL types. While most adult NHLs are low or intermediate grades, almost all the NHLs in children are high grade, meaning that they develop rapidly, but respond well to chemotherapy. The type most frequently diagnosed in children from ages 5 to 14 is Burkitt's or Burkitt-like lymphoma, also called small noncleaved cell lymphoma (SNCL). Diffuse large B cell lymphoma is the most common type among those aged 15 to 19. Other types are lymphoblastic lymphoma and anaplastic large-cell lymphoma.

Childhood NHLs grow very rapidly and require treatment urgently. It is important to perform the diagnostic tests as soon as possible in order to determine the exact subtype and stage of the disease. Therapy is determined by the extent of disease, whether it is restricted to one part of the body or has spread to distant areas. The main treatment for childhood NHL is a combination of several chemotherapy agents. The exact regimen and duration of treatment are determined by the subtype and stage. Treatment for lymphoblastic lymphoma, which is histologically similar to T cell acute lymphoblastic leukemia (T cell ALL), may last two to three years, while treatment of other types of NHL may last just a few months. Bone marrow or stem cell transplantations are used to treat children whose disease has relapsed.

Chemotherapy is the mainstay of treatment for NHL. Radiation therapy is not typically used to treat childhood NHL. Most patients do not undergo surgery, apart from a biopsy and/or to implant a central venous catheter to administer chemotherapy, draw blood, and infuse fluids or blood products.

Information Sources

Brochures, Booklets, and Other Short Print Publications

Lymphoma specific

➤ The Leukemia & Lymphoma Society.
  ➣ *The Lymphomas.*
    This booklet offers a general overview of Hodgkin's and non-Hodgkin's lymphomas that is relevant to adults and children. Topics covered include blood and marrow components, the lymphatic system, and classification of lymphomas. An easy-to-read version of this publication is titled *The Lymphomas: A Guide for Patients and Their Families.* Larger print and bullet points summarize the topic in a concise manner.
  ➣ *Emotional Aspects of Childhood Blood Cancers.*
    This addresses psychosocial issues concerning children with blood cancers. Access at: www.leukemia-lymphoma.org
➤ Lymphoma Research Foundation.
  ➣ *Lymphoma Resource Guide.*
    A listing of organizations, online resources, audio and videotapes, publications, and therapies that are of interest to Lymphoma patients and families. Access at: www.lymphoma.org
  ➣ *Understanding Non-Hodgkin's Lymphoma: A Guide for Patients.*
    This 100-page booklet provides a comprehensive review of NHL, including diagnosis, treatment, coping with side effects, clinical trial experimental treatments, and living with cancer. Includes a glossary. Individual copies are free and can be obtained by calling the Lymphoma Research Foundation at: 800-500-9976.
➤ National Cancer Institute. *What You Need to Know about Non Hodgkin's Lymphoma.*
    A concise introduction to non-Hodgkin's lymphoma covering staging, treatment options, and emotional support. Includes a glossary and a list of questions for the doctor.

Relevant childhood cancer publications

➤ National Cancer Institute. *Young People with Cancer: A Handbook for Parents.* This publication discusses the most common types of childhood cancer, treatments, and side effects, as well as issues that may arise when a child is diagnosed with cancer. Offers medical information and practical tips gathered from parents. Access at: https://cissecure.nci.nih.gov/ncipubs/

➤ National Childhood Cancer Foundation. *The Children's Oncology Group (COG) Family Handbook.* This 80-page handbook was written by nurses, doctors, and other childhood cancer professionals. The information is relevant to all types of childhood cancer and covers medical and psychosocial issues. The publication includes illustrations and has several areas that may be customized for a specific child. Access at: www.curesearch.org.

➤ National Children's Cancer Society. *The Mountain You've Climbed: A Parent's Guide to Childhood Cancer Survivorship.* This guide is designed to answer parents' questions regarding childhood cancer and offer suggestions on how to integrate the cancer experience into all areas of the family's life. It addresses issues beginning from the time of diagnosis through the completion of treatment and beyond. Order at: http://nationalchildrenscancersociety.com.

Books

Lymphoma-specific books (for adult and childhood lymphomas)

➤ Adler, Elizabeth M. 2005. *Living with Lymphoma: A Patient's Guide.* Baltimore, MD: Johns Hopkins University Press. Written by a neurobiologist and a lymphoma survivor, this book offers a detailed explanation of cell biology that helps readers understand the disease and its treatment. While this book provides an in-depth look at the medical side of lymphoma and provides detailed descriptions of specific drugs, drug combinations, and treatment approaches, psychosocial issues are not as meticulously covered. Sophisticated readers who are interested in learning the scientific aspects of lymphoma will appreciate this book.

➤ Holman, Peter, Jodi Garrett, and William D. Jansen. 2004. *100 Questions and Answers about Lymphoma.* Sudbury, MA: Jones and Bartlett. Detailed information about lymphoma is presented in an easy-to-read question-and-answer format. Terms are explained in the sidebar, and the book includes lists of Web sites, organizations, literature, and resources on general and specific topics related to non-Hodgkin's lymphoma. This book was co–authored by a lymphoma specialist, an oncology nurse, and a lymphoma survivor.

Relevant childhood cancer books

➤ Carroll, William L., and Jessica B. Reisman. 2005. *100 Questions and Answers about Your Child's Cancer*. Sudbury, MA: Jones and Bartlett.
This book presents practical answers to questions about childhood cancer, treatment options, post–treatment quality of life, and coping strategies for both patients and parents. Two child cancer experts authored this book and incorporated comments from parents of children with cancer. The book provides detailed information about diagnostic tests, supportive-care issues, and side effects and complications of treatment that are common to all children treated for cancer. The text is easy to read and definitions for key terms are provided in the sidebar.

➤ Keene, Nancy. 2003. *Educating the Child with Cancer: A Guide for Parents and Teachers*. Kensington, MD: Candlelighters Childhood Cancer Foundation.
This book was developed with the intent of promoting understanding and communication among parents, educators, and medical professionals so that together they can provide an appropriate education for children who have been treated for cancer. Learning issues that face children treated for cancer from infancy through adulthood are covered in depth, with some chapters written by experts and others by parents. Topics include gaining access to special education services, helping siblings in the classroom, physical activity in school, treatment-related late effects that may cause learning difficulties, and grief in the classroom. Each chapter ends with a list of key points.

➤ Woznick, Leigh A., and Carol D. Goodheart. 2002. *Living with Childhood Cancer: A Practical Guide to Help Parents Cope*. Washington, DC: American Psychological Association.
The focus of this book is the psychological impact of childhood cancer. It provides guidance and advice to parents on managing the emotional and practical challenges of the disease and its treatment. The book describes how adults, children, teenagers, and families may cope with illness and stress and offers strategies for successful coping. Topics include communication, stress, trauma, pain, side effects, encouraging child development, building self-esteem, dying and grieving, and long-term survivorship. Specific information is provided for different age groups and various types of families. The authors are a psychologist and her daughter who is the mother of a child with cancer.

Sites Focusing on Lymphoma

➤ Leukaemia Research. Access at: www.lrf.org.uk/
Leukaemia Research is a British research charity focusing on blood cancers and disorders. The "Information and Education" section offers printable booklets on adult and childhood blood cancers, including some on rare subtypes and conditions. The "News" section includes stories about research developments and other related articles.

➤ The Leukemia & Lymphoma Society. Access at: www.leukemia-lymphoma. org
The site of the world's largest organization dedicated to blood cancers includes many sections and features relevant to childhood non-Hodgkin's lymphoma. Live and archived versions of educational teleconferences and Webcasts enable users to study complicated topics explained by top experts. The site also includes medical news about lymphoma, short and longer overviews of the diseases, and information about the organization's support services for patients.

➤ Lymphoma Information Network. Access at: www.lymphomainfo.net
This well-organized directory of lymphoma information sources presents short, concise introductions to many types of lymphoma. Each section has a list of references with links to other sites, PubMed abstracts, or books on Amazon. This site has been maintained for over ten years by an NHL survivor and is useful as a starting point for a search on specific or complex issues in lymphoma.

➤ Lymphoma Research Foundation. Access at: www.lymphoma.org
The Lymphoma Research Foundation is a patient-support and –advocacy organization providing support and education to lymphoma patients and families. Information about the disease and its treatment and research news are presented in fact sheets, Webcasts, newsletters, and other formats. This site also includes information about support programs and services for patients and families.

Detailed sections in childhood cancer sites

➤ CureSearch. Access at: www.curesearch.org
This site has a detailed section about lymphoma, and the information is presented separately to parents and patients in different age groups: preschool, ages 5–10, 10–14, and 14–22. Topics covered include diagnostic tests, treatment methods, impact on the patient and family, navigating the health care system, and school issues. The interactive section of the site includes a clinical trial matching service, discussion boards, and a resource directory for national and local support groups and services.

Provided by the Children's Cancer Group and the National Childhood Cancer Foundation.

➤ Penn State Hershey Medical Center. *Home Care Guide*. Access at: www. hmc.psu.edu/hematology/homeguide/
Nurses and physicians from the children's hematology/oncology team at Penn State Hershey Medical Center developed this guide for caregivers of children with childhood cancer. The guide provides treatment plans for a variety of supportive-care and psychosocial issues that may occur while a child is undergoing treatment. Each plan provides caregivers with the information they need in order to solve problems, including understanding the problem, when to get professional help, what caregivers can do on their own, possible obstacles, and how to carry out and adjust the plan.

Detailed sections in general cancer sites

➤ American Cancer Society. *Childhood Non-Hodgkin's Lymphoma*. Access at: www.cancer.org and select from the menu under "Choose a Cancer Topic."
A detailed guide about non-Hodgkin's lymphoma in children can be printed as an Adobe Acrobat (.pdf) file.

➤ Cancerbackup. *Non-Hodgkin's Lymphoma (NHL) in Children*. Access at: www.cancerbackup.org.uk/Home and click on "Cancer Type."

➤ National Cancer Institute. *Childhood Cancers*. Access at: www.cancer.gov and click on "Types of Cancer."
The top page of the section links to a patient version of a PDQ® statement, clinical trial information, and other NCI publications on this topic.

➤ People Living with Cancer. *Lymphoma, Non-Hodgkin, Childhood Cancer*. Access at: www.plwc.org and click on "Cancer Type."
The PLWC oncologist-approved guides on childhood non-Hodgkin's lymphoma can be printed in their entirety or by subtopic.

Patient-Support Organizations

➤ Candlelighters. Access at: www.candlelighters.org
Phone: 800-366-2223

➤ Leukemia & Lymphoma Society. Access at: www.leukemia-lymphoma.org
Phone: 914-949-5213

➤ Leukemia Research Foundation. Access at: www.leukemia-research.org
Phone: 847-424-0600

➤ Lymphoma Research Foundation. Access at: www.lymphoma.org
Phone: (Los Angeles office) 800-500-9976

➤ The National Children's Cancer Society. Access at: http://nationalchildrens
cancersociety.com
Phone: 800-5-FAMILY

Ewing's Family of Tumors

The Ewing's family of tumors is a class of tumors that share common features. The exact origin of these tumors is unknown; although they are found mostly in bones or soft tissues, they do not originate in these cell types. The majority of Ewing's tumors are diagnosed in children between the ages of 10 and 20, but they may also occur in adulthood or in children younger than 10. Approximately 250 children and adolescents are diagnosed with the Ewing's family of tumors in the United States each year. Ewing's tumors affect mostly Caucasians; they are rare among African Americans and Asian Americans. The five-year survival rate for children and adolescents who do not have visible metastases at diagnosis is approximately 70%. The outlook for patients with metastases at diagnoses is not as good.

More than half of all Ewing's tumors develop in the bones, and the rest appear in soft tissues. These tumors are often referred to as Ewing's sarcoma. Primitive neuroectodermal tumor (PNET) is included in the Ewing's family of tumors because its cells have the same DNA abnormalities as Ewing's sarcoma, as well as similar proteins that are rarely found in other types of cancer. PNETs can occur in bones or soft tissues. Ewing's sarcomas and PNETs are treated similarly; therefore information on these tumors is presented together.

The majority of Ewing's tumors occur in the pelvis, and some occur in the middle of the long bones in the legs. The next most common sites are the ribs and the spine. Ewing's tumors that develop in the soft tissues are called extraosseous sarcomas, and they can occur almost anywhere in the body.

Ewing's tumors can develop metastases, for this reason the majority of patients are treated with chemotherapy in addition to surgery or radiation therapy. Treatment typically starts with chemotherapy, followed by either surgery or radiation therapy. The type and extent of surgery are determined by the location and size of the tumor. If the tumor is located in the femur, which is the long bone of the upper leg, it may be possible to utilize limb-sparing surgery instead of amputation. Chemotherapy may be given again after surgery or radiation therapy, and in cases of metastatic disease very high doses of chemotherapy are given, followed by a stem cell transplant.

Children and adolescents with Ewing's tumors receive chemotherapy for an extended period of time. Some children suffer long-term effects, depending on the specific therapies they received. Surgery may cause deformities, and children who were treated with limb-sparing surgery or amputation have a long and difficult rehabilitation process.

Information Sources

Brochures, Booklets, and Other Short Print Publications

➤ National Cancer Institute. *Young People with Cancer: A Handbook for Parents.* This publication discusses the most common types of childhood cancer, treatments, and side effects as well as issues that may arise when a child is diagnosed with cancer. Offers medical information and practical tips gathered from parents. Access at: https://cissecure.nci.nih.gov/ncipubs/

➤ National Childhood Cancer Foundation. *The Children's Oncology Group (COG) Family Handbook.*
This 80-page handbook was written by nurses, doctors, and other childhood cancer professionals. The information is relevant to all types of childhood cancer and covers medical and psychosocial issues. The publication includes illustrations and has several areas that may be customized for a specific child. Access at: www.curesearch.org.

➤ National Children's Cancer Society. *The Mountain You've Climbed: A Parent's Guide to Childhood Cancer Survivorship.*
This guide is designed to answer parents' questions regarding childhood cancer and to offer suggestions on how to integrate the cancer experience into all areas of the family's life. It addresses issues beginning from the time of diagnosis through the completion of treatment and beyond. Order at: http://nationalchildrenscancersociety.com

Books

Book chapters

➤ Janes-Hodder, Honna, and Nancy Keene. 2002. *Childhood Cancer: A Parent's Guide to Solid Tumor Cancers.* 2d ed. Sebastopol, CA: O'Reilly.
This book provides a detailed overview of Ewing's sarcoma as well as other childhood solid tumors. Chapters offer practical advice on how to cope with procedures, hospitalization, family and friends, school, social and financial issues, communications, feelings, and, if treatment is not successful, issues of grief and bereavement. The text includes stories from children and parents who have experienced childhood cancer. Appendixes include ones for blood counts and what they mean and an extensive resource list.

Relevant childhood cancer books

➤ Carroll, William L., and Jessica B. Reisman. 2005. *100 Questions and Answers about Your Child's Cancer.* Sudbury, MA: Jones and Bartlett.

This book presents practical answers to questions about childhood cancer, treatment options, post–treatment quality of life, and coping strategies for both patients and parents. Two child cancer experts authored this book and incorporated comments from parents of children with cancer. The book provides detailed information about diagnostic tests, supportive-care issues, and side effects and complications of treatment that are common to all children treated for cancer. The text is easy to read, and definitions for key terms are provided in the sidebar.

➤ Keene, Nancy. 2003. *Educating the Child with Cancer: A Guide for Parents and Teachers*. Kensington, MD: Candlelighters Childhood Cancer Foundation. This book was developed with the intent of promoting understanding and communication among parents, educators, and medical professionals so that together they can provide an appropriate education for children who have been treated for cancer. Learning issues that face children treated for cancer from infancy through adulthood are covered in depth, with some chapters written by experts and others by parents. Topics include gaining access to special education services, helping siblings in the classroom, physical activity in school, treatment-related late effects that may cause learning difficulties, and grief in the classroom. Each chapter ends with a list of key points.

➤ Woznick, Leigh A., and Carol D. Goodheart. 2002. *Living with Childhood Cancer: A Practical Guide to Help Parents Cope*. Washington, DC: American Psychological Association. The focus of this book is the psychological impact of childhood cancer. It provides guidance and advice to parents on managing the emotional and practical challenges of the disease and treatment. The book describes how adults, children, teenagers, and families may cope with illness and stress and offers strategies for successful coping. Topics include communication, stress, trauma, pain, side effects, encouraging child development, building self-esteem, dying and grieving, and long-term survivorship. Specific information is provided for different age groups and various types of families. The authors are a psychologist and her daughter who is the mother of a child with cancer.

Web Resources

Detailed sections in childhood cancer sites

➤ CureSearch. Access at: www.curesearch.org This site has a detailed section about Ewing's sarcoma, and the information is presented separately to parents and patients in different age groups: preschool, ages 5–10, 10–14, and 14–22. Topics covered include diagnostic tests, treatment methods, impact on the patient and family, navigating the health care system, and school issues. The interactive section of the site includes a clinical trial matching service, discussion boards, and a resource directory for national and local support groups and services. Provided by the Children's Cancer Group and the National Childhood Cancer Foundation.

➤ Penn State Hershey Medical Center. *Home Care Guide*. Access at: www. hmc.psu.edu/hematology/homeguide/
Nurses and physicians from the children's hematology/oncology team at Penn State Hershey Medical Center developed this guide for caregivers of children with childhood cancer. The guide provides treatment plans for a variety of supportive-care and psychosocial issues that may occur while a child is undergoing treatment. Each plan offers caregivers the information they need in order to solve problems including understanding the problem, when to get professional help, what caregivers can do on their own, possible obstacles, and how to carry out and adjust the plan.

Detailed sections in general cancer sites

➤ American Cancer Society. *Learn about Ewing's Family of Tumors*. Access at: www.cancer.org and select from the menu under "Choose a Cancer Topic." A detailed guide about Ewing's family of tumors can be printed by section or as an Adobe Acrobat (.pdf) file.

➤ Cancerbackup. *Ewing's Sarcoma in Children*. Access at: www.cancer backup.org.uk/Home and click on "Cancer Type."

➤ National Cancer Institute. *Ewing's Family of Tumors*. Access at: www. cancer.gov and click on "Types of Cancer."
The top page of the section links to patient versions of PDQ® statements, clinical trial information, and other NCI publications on this topic.

➤ People Living with Cancer. *Ewing's Sarcoma, Childhood Cancer*. Access at: www.plwc.org and click on "Cancer Type."
The PLWC oncologist-approved guide on Ewing's sarcoma can be printed in its entirety, or by subtopic.

Patient-Support Organizations

➤ Candlelighters. Access at: www.candlelighters.org
Phone: 800-366-2223

➤ The National Children's Cancer Society. Access at: http://nationalchildrenscancersociety.com
Phone: 800-5-FAMILY

➤ Sarcoma Alliance. Access at: www.sarcomaalliance.org
Phone: 415-381-7236

Neuroblastoma

Anatomical facts: The sympathetic nervous system is the part of the nervous
system that controls involuntary body functions, such as heart rate, blood
pressure, and body temperature. It includes nerve fibers that run alongside
the spinal cord, clusters of nerve cells called ganglia (plural of ganglion) at
certain points along the path of the nerve fibers, and nervelike cells found in
the center of the adrenal glands. The adrenals are two small triangular-
shaped organs located in the abdomen on top of each kidney.

Illustration available at the Medical Illustrations Gallery of the People
Living with Cancer Web site.
Access at: www.plwc.org and click on Library in the left sidebar.

Neuroblastoma is a cancer that develops most often in young children. It
is very rare in people older than ten, and 90% of diagnoses occur in children
younger than five years old. About 650 new cases of neuroblastoma are diagnosed in the United States each year. Most tumors originate in the abdomen:
one–third in the adrenal glands and another third in the ganglia of the abdomen. The remaining start in ganglia of the chest, neck, pelvis, or spinal cord.
More than half the cases are not diagnosed until after the disease has already
spread from the primary site to lymph nodes, bone marrow, and other distant organs. Survival rates for neuroblastoma have improved in the past
three decades, especially for early-stage tumors diagnosed in infants. The
majority of children who are diagnosed in early stages or before their first
birthday are cured.

Patients with neuroblastoma are divided into risk categories according to
their age and the disease's stage at diagnosis and certain biologic features of
the tumor cells. The majority of children are treated with chemotherapy
and/or radiation therapy. Many children also receive surgery to remove
tumors and/or metastases. In cases where complete surgical removal is possible, surgery alone is enough to cure the disease. Even in cases where complete removal is not possible, cure may still be achieved sometimes with the
combination of the three treatment methods.

Children with high-risk or relapsed neuroblastoma are sometimes treated
with very-high-dose chemotherapy followed by an autologous stem cell transplant. A number of new therapies for neuroblastoma are being investigated

in clinical trials, including retinoids, substances that are chemically related to vitamin A; monoclonal antibodies; and other biological therapies.

Information Sources

Brochures, Booklets, and Other Short Print Publications

➤ National Cancer Institute. *Young People with Cancer: A Handbook for Parents.*
This publication discusses the most common types of childhood cancer, treatments, and side effects, as well as issues that may arise when a child is diagnosed with cancer. Offers medical information and practical tips gathered from parents. Access at: https://cissecure.nci.nih.gov/ncipubs/

➤ National Childhood Cancer Foundation. *The Children's Oncology Group (COG) Family Handbook.*
This 80-page handbook was written by nurses, doctors, and other childhood cancer professionals. The information is relevant to all types of childhood cancer and covers medical and psychosocial issues. The publication includes illustrations and has several areas that may be customized for a specific child. Access at: www.curesearch.org.

➤ National Children's Cancer Society. *The Mountain You've Climbed: A Parent's Guide to Childhood Cancer Survivorship.*
This guide is designed to answer parents' questions regarding childhood cancer and offer suggestions on how to integrate the cancer experience into all areas of the family's life. It addresses issues beginning from the time of diagnosis through the completion of treatment and beyond. Order at: http://nationalchildrenscancersociety.com

Books

Book chapters

➤ Janes-Hodder, Honna, and Nancy Keene. 2002. *Childhood Cancer: A Parent's Guide to Solid Tumor Cancers.* 2d ed. Sebastopol, CA: O'Reilly.
This book provides a detailed overview of neuroblastoma as well as other childhood solid tumors. Chapters offer practical advice on how to cope with procedures, hospitalization, family and friends, school, social and financial issues, communications, feelings, and, if treatment is not successful, issues of grief and bereavement. The text provides stories from children and parents who have experienced childhood cancer. Appendixes include blood counts and what they mean and an extensive resource list.

Relevant childhood cancer books

➤ Carroll, William L., and Jessica B. Reisman. 2005. *100 Questions and Answers about Your Child's Cancer*. Sudbury, MA: Jones and Bartlett.

This book presents practical answers to questions about childhood cancer, treatment options, post–treatment quality of life, and coping strategies for both patients and parents. Two child cancer experts authored this book and incorporated comments from parents of children with cancer. The book provides detailed information about diagnostic tests, supportive-care issues, and side effects and complications of treatment that are common to all children treated for cancer. The text is easy to read, and definitions for key terms are provided in the sidebar.

➤ Keene, Nancy. 2003. *Educating the Child with Cancer: A Guide for Parents and Teachers*. Kensington, MD: Candlelighters Childhood Cancer Foundation.

This book was developed with the intent of promoting understanding and communication among parents, educators, and medical professionals so that together they can provide an appropriate education for children who have been treated for cancer. Learning issues that face children treated for cancer from infancy through adulthood are covered in depth, with some chapters written by experts and others by parents. Topics include gaining access to special education services, helping siblings in the classroom, physical activity in school, treatment-related late effects that may cause learning difficulties, and grief in the classroom. Each chapter ends with a list of key points.

➤ Woznick, Leigh A., and Carol D. Goodheart. 2002. *Living with Childhood Cancer: A Practical Guide to Help Parents Cope*. Washington, DC: American Psychological Association.

The focus of this book is the psychological impact of childhood cancer. It provides guidance and advice to parents on managing the emotional and practical challenges of the disease and its treatment. The book describes how adults, children, teenagers, and families may cope with illness and stress and offers strategies for successful coping. Topics include communication, stress, trauma, pain, side effects, encouraging child development, building self-esteem, dying and grieving, and long-term survivorship. Specific information is provided for different age groups and various types of families. The authors are a psychologist and her daughter who is the mother of a child with cancer.

Web Resources

Sites focusing on neuroblastoma

➤ Children's Neuroblastoma Cancer Foundation. Access at: www.cncf-child cancer.org

The site of this advocacy and support organization for people affected by neuroblastoma offers a parents' handbook, news about research advances, video files of educational conferences, and information about the organization's activities.

➤ NANT—New Approaches to Neuroblastoma Therapy. Access at: www.nant.org
NANT is a collaborative research group of 14 universities and childrens' hospitals with strong research and treatment programs for neuroblastoma. The site provides information about clinical trials conducted by the group, contact information of treatment centers, and downloadable files of publications related to the NANT study.

Detailed sections in childhood cancer sites

➤ CureSearch. Access at: www.curesearch.org
This site has a detailed section about neuroblastoma, and the information is presented separately to parents and patients in different age groups: preschool, ages 5–10, 10–14, and 14–22. Topics covered include diagnostic tests, treatment methods, impact on the patient and family, navigating the health care system, and school issues. The interactive section of the site includes a clinical trial matching service, discussion boards, and a resource directory for national and local support groups and services. Provided by the Children's Cancer Group and the National Childhood Cancer Foundation.

➤ Penn State Hershey Medical Center. *Home Care Guide.* Access at: www.hmc.psu.edu/hematology/homeguide/
Nurses and physicians from the children's hematology/oncology team at Penn State Hershey Medical Center developed this guide for caregivers of children with childhood cancer. The guide provides treatment plans for a variety of supportive-care and psychosocial issues that may occur while a child is undergoing treatment. Each plan gives caregivers the information they need in order to solve problems including understanding the problem, when to get professional help, what caregivers can do on their own, possible obstacles, and how to carry out and adjust the plan.

Detailed sections in general cancer sites

➤ American Cancer Society. *Learn about Neuroblastoma.* Access at: www.cancer.org and select from the menu under "Choose a Cancer Topic."
A detailed guide about neuroblastoma can be printed by section or as an Adobe Acrobat (.pdf) file.

➤ Cancerbackup. *Neuroblastoma in Children.* Access at: www.cancerbackup.org.uk/Home and click on "Cancer Type."

➤ National Cancer Institute. *Neuroblastoma.* Access at: www.cancer.gov and click on "Types of Cancer."
The top page of the section links to patient versions of PDQ® statements, clinical trial information, and other NCI publications on this topic.

➤ People Living with Cancer. *Neuroblastoma, Childhood Cancer.* Access at: www.plwc.org and click on "Cancer Type."
The PLWC oncologist-approved guide on neuroblastoma can be printed in its entirety, or by subtopic.

Patient-Support Organizations

➤ Candlelighters. Access at: www.candlelighters.org
Phone: 800-366-2223

➤ Children's Neuroblastoma Cancer Foundation. Access at: www.cncf-child cancer.org
Phone: 866-671-2623

➤ The National Children's Cancer Society. Access at: http://nationalchild-renscancersociety.com
Phone: 800-5-FAMILY

Osteosarcoma

Anatomical facts: The bones are living, growing tissues that form the body's skeleton. Throughout life, bone tissue changes constantly; bits of old bone are removed and replaced by new bone cells. The process of bone growth consists of resorption and formation. During resorption old bone tissue is broken down and removed by special cells called osteoclasts. During bone formation new bone tissue is laid down to replace the old. Special cells called osteoblasts perform this task. During childhood and adolescence much more bone is deposited than withdrawn as the skeleton grows in both size and density.

Illustration available at the Medical Illustrations Gallery of the People Living with Cancer Web site.

Access at: www.plwc.org and click on Library on the left sidebar.

Osteosarcoma is the most common primary bone tumor and can occur in people of all ages. The peak incident is during the second decade of life, during the adolescent growth spurt. About 400 cases are diagnosed each year in children and adolescents younger than 20 in the United States. Boys are more likely to develop osteosarcoma than are girls. The five-year survival rate in children and adolescents has significantly improved in the past three decades and is now at 65%.

Osteosarcoma can occur in any bone, but in children and adolescents the most common site is around the knee in the femur, which is the long bone in the upper leg. The long bone of the lower leg, the tibia, is the second most common site, followed by the humerus, the long bone of the upper arm that connects to the shoulder. Osteosarcoma tumors most often develop in the growth plates, which are located at the end of the long bones.

The presence of metastases at diagnosis is a determining factor in planning treatment for osteosarcoma. Children whose tumors can be completely removed with surgery have a better prognosis.

The primary treatment method for osteosarcoma is surgery to remove the tumor. In the past, patients were treated with amputation, but today 50% to 80% of patients are eligible for a limb-salvage surgery instead of amputation. In a limb-sparing procedure, the diseased part of the bone is removed and replaced by a metal prosthesis. Limb salvage can be done to treat tumors in the legs and arms. Surgery can also be used to remove metastases in distant organs, such as the lungs or brain. Chemotherapy is also a standand treatment for osteosarcoma and is given to all patients either before or after surgery. The great advances in survival rates since the 1960s are attributed to the utilization of chemotherapy in the treatment of osteosarcoma. Radiation therapy has a more limited role in the treatment of osteosarcoma and is used mostly for the purpose of reducing swelling and relieving pain.

Children with osteosarcoma have a long and difficult rehabilitation process, and in many cases the rehabilitation phase is the most difficult part of all the treatments. The rehabilitation after limb-salvage surgery is more intense than after amputation. It takes an average of one year for patients to learn to walk after limb-salvage involving a leg. Children and teenagers that were treated with amputation may be able to walk three-to-six month after surgery. Body image and psychological adjustment to life after amputation or a limb-sparing surgery are major issues for osteosarcoma survivors, many of whom are teenagers.

Information Sources

Brochures, Booklets, and other Short Print Publications

➤ National Cancer Institute. *Young People with Cancer: A Handbook for Parents.* This publication discusses the most common types of childhood cancer, treatments, and side effects, as well as issues that may arise when a child is diagnosed with cancer. Offers medical information and practical tips gathered from parents. Access at: https://cissecure.nci.nih.gov/ncipubs/

➤ National Childhood Cancer Foundation. *The Children's Oncology Group (COG) Family Handbook.*
This 80-page handbook was written by nurses, doctors, and other childhood cancer professionals. The information is relevant to all types of childhood cancer and covers medical and psychosocial issues. The publication includes illustrations and has several areas that may be customized for a specific child. Access at: www.curesearch.org.

➤ National Children's Cancer Society. *The Mountain You've Climbed: A Parent's Guide to Childhood Cancer Survivorship.*
This guide is designed to answer parents' questions regarding childhood cancer and offer suggestions on how to integrate the cancer experience into all areas of the family's life. It addresses issues beginning from the time of diagnosis through the completion of treatment and beyond. Order at: http://nationalchildrenscancersociety.com

Books

Book chapters

➤ Janes-Hodder, Honna, and Nancy Keene. 2002. *Childhood Cancer: A Parent's Guide to Solid Tumor Cancers.* 2d ed. Sebastopol, CA: O'Reilly.
This book provides a detailed overview of osteosarcoma as well as other childhood solid tumors. Chapters offer practical advice on how to cope with procedures, hospitalization, family and friends, school, social and financial issues, communications, feelings, and, if treatment is not successful, issues of grief and bereavement. The text provides stories from children and parents who have experienced childhood cancer. Appendixes include blood counts and what they mean, and an extensive resource list.

Relevant childhood cancer books

➤ Carroll, William L., and Jessica B. Reisman. 2005. *100 Questions and Answers about Your Child's Cancer.* Sudbury, MA: Jones and Bartlett.
This book presents practical answers to questions about childhood cancer, treatment options, post–treatment quality of life, and coping strategies for both patients and parents. Two child cancer experts authored this book and incorporated comments from parents of children with cancer. The book provides detailed information about diagnostic tests, supportive-care issues, and side effects and complications of treatment that are common to all children treated for cancer. The text is easy to read, and definitions for key terms are provided in the sidebar.

➤ Keene, Nancy. 2003. *Educating the Child with Cancer: A Guide for Parents and Teachers.* Kensington, MD: Candlelighters Childhood Cancer Foundation.

This book was developed with the intent of promoting understanding and communication among parents, educators, and medical professionals so that together they can provide an appropriate education for children who have been treated for cancer. Learning issues that face children treated for cancer from infancy through adulthood are covered in depth, with some chapters written by experts and others by parents. Topics include gaining access to special education services, helping siblings in the classroom, physical activity in school, treatment-related late effects that may cause learning difficulties, and grief in the classroom. Each chapter ends with a list of key points.

➤ Woznick, Leigh A., and Carol D. Goodheart. 2002. *Living with Childhood Cancer: A Practical Guide to Help Parents Cope.* Washington, DC: American Psychological Association.

The focus of this book is the psychological impact of childhood cancer. It provides guidance and advice to parents on managing the emotional and practical challenges of the disease and its treatment. The book describes how adults, children, teenagers, and families may cope with illness and stress and offers strategies for successful coping. Topics include communication, stress, trauma, pain, side effects, encouraging child development, building self-esteem, dying and grieving, and long-term survivorship. Specific information is provided for different age groups and various types of families. The authors are a psychologist and her daughter who is the mother of a child with cancer.

Web Resources

Detailed sections in childhood cancer sites

➤ CureSearch. Access at: www.curesearch.org
This site has a detailed section about osteosarcoma, and the information is presented separately to parents and patients in different age groups: preschool, ages 5–10, 10–14, and 14–22. Topics covered include diagnostic tests, treatment methods, impact on the patient and family, navigating the health care system, and school issues. The interactive section of the site includes a clinical trial matching service, discussion boards, and a resource directory for national and local support groups and services. Provided by the Children's Cancer Group and the National Childhood Cancer Foundation.

➤ Penn State Hershey Medical Center. *Home Care Guide.* Access at: www.hmc.psu.edu/hematology/homeguide/
Nurses and physicians from the children's hematology/oncology team at Penn State Hershey Medical Center developed this guide for caregivers of

children with childhood cancer. The guide provides treatment plans for a variety of supportive-care and psychosocial issues that may occur while a child is undergoing treatment. Each plan gives caregivers the information they need in order to solve problems, including understanding the problem, when to get professional help, what caregivers can do on their own, possible obstacles, and how to carry out and adjust the plan.

Detailed sections in general cancer sites

➤ American Cancer Society. *Learn about Osteosarcoma.* Access at: www. cancer.org and select from the menu under "Choose a Cancer Topic." A detailed guide about osteosarcoma can be printed as an Adobe Acrobat (.pdf) file.

➤ Cancerbackup. *Osteosarcoma in Children.* Access at: www.cancerbackup. org.uk/Home and click on "Cancer Type."

➤ National Cancer Institute. *Osteosarcoma/Malignant Fibrous Histiocytoma of Bone.* Access at: www.cancer.gov and click on "Types of Cancer." The top page of the section links to patient versions of PDQ® statements, clinical trial information, and other NCI publications on this topic.

➤ People Living with Cancer. *Osteosarcoma, Childhood Cancer.* Access at: www.plwc.org and click on "Cancer Type." The PLWC oncologist-approved guide on osteosarcoma can be printed in its entirety, or by subtopic.

Patient-Support Organizations

➤ Candlelighters. Access at: www.candlelighters.org Phone: 800-366-2223

➤ The National Children's Cancer Society. Access at: http://nationalchildrens cancersociety.com Phone: 800-5-FAMILY

➤ Sarcoma Alliance. Access at: www.sarcomaalliance.org Phone: 415-381-7236

Retinoblastoma

Anatomical facts: The eye operates like a camera: light enters the eye through a small hole called the pupil and is focused on the retina, which can be compared to a camera's film. The retina is the nerve tissue that lines the inside of the back of the eye. The retina is connected to the brain by the optic nerve. The pattern of light appearing on the retina is transmitted to the brain through the optic nerve. Retinoblasts are the cells from which mature retinal cells develop in a process that takes place while the baby is still in the uterus.

Illustrations available at the Medical Illustrations Gallery of the People Living with Cancer Web site .

Access at: www.plwc.org and click on Library on the left sidebar.

Retinoblastoma is a type of eye cancer that occurs in very young children. There are approximately 250 new diagnosed cases each year in the United States. The highest incidence of this tumor is among infants, and almost all cases are diagnosed before age four. The five-year survival rate for this tumor is 95%.

Retinoblastoma is the only childhood cancer in which heredity plays a significant role. In about 25% to 40% of cases, the disease is caused by an inherited genetic mutation. Children born with the genetic defect may develop more than one tumor, usually in both eyes (bilateral or multifocal retinoblastoma). Children with the noninherited form of the disease usually develop only one tumor (unilateral or unifocal retinoblastoma). These two forms are treated very differently.

Proper staging of retinoblastoma tumors is crucial for a successful outcome and preservation of vision. The key factors in devising a treatment strategy are whether the tumor is present in just one eye or both, how good the vision is in the affected eye(s), and whether the tumor has metastasized beyond the eyeball. In general, the treatment for unilateral retinoblastoma is usually enucleation, which is surgical removal of the eye. If the diseased eye still has good potential for vision, enucleation is avoided and the tumor is treated with minor surgical procedures that preserve the eye. By contrast, most children with bilateral retinoblastoma are not treated with enucleation unless the tumors are very advanced. In addition to surgery, chemotherapy and/or radiation therapy are often utilized in the treatment strategy of both unilateral and bilateral retinoblasotomas.

Nine out of ten children with retinoblastoma become long-term survivors. The majority of these children have at least one eye with good vision. About 20% suffer a vision loss, but complete blindness is rare. Children with the inherited form of retinoblastoma have a high risk of developing other cancers, such as pinealoma, which is a type of brain tumor; osteosarcoma; soft-tissue sarcomas; and melanoma. Families of children diagnosed with retinoblastoma are advised to undergo genetic testing and counseling. If the inherited mutation is found, children and family members are carefully observed and screened for the development of these cancers.

Information Sources

Brochures, Booklets, and Other Short Print Publications

➤ National Cancer Institute. *Young People with Cancer: A Handbook for Parents.*
This publication discusses the most common types of childhood cancer, treatments, and side effects, as well as issues that may arise when a child is diagnosed with cancer. Offers medical information and practical tips gathered from parents. Access at: https://cissecure.nci.nih.gov/ncipubs/

➤ National Childhood Cancer Foundation. *The Children's Oncology Group (COG) Family Handbook.*
This 80-page handbook was written by nurses, doctors, and other childhood cancer professionals. The information is relevant to all types of childhood cancer and covers medical and psychosocial issues. The publication includes illustrations and has several areas that may be customized for a specific child. Access at: www.curesearch.org.

➤ National Children's Cancer Society. *The Mountain You've Climbed: A Parent's Guide to Childhood Cancer Survivorship.*
This guide is designed to answer parents' questions regarding childhood cancer and offer suggestions on how to integrate the cancer experience into all areas of the family's life. It addresses issues beginning from the time of diagnosis through the completion of treatment and beyond. Order at: http://nationalchildrenscancersociety.com

Books

Book chapters

➤ Janes-Hodder, Honna, and Nancy Keene. 2002. *Childhood Cancer: A Parent's Guide to Solid Tumor Cancers.* 2d ed. Sebastopol, CA: O'Reilly.
This book provides a detailed overview of retinoblastomas as well as other childhood solid tumors. Chapters offer practical advice on how to cope with procedures, hospitalization, family and friends, school, social and financial issues, communications, feelings, and, if treatment is not successful, issues of grief and bereavement. The text provides stories from children and parents who have experienced childhood cancer. Appendixes include blood counts and what they mean, and an extensive resource list.

Relevant childhood cancer books

➤ Carroll, William L., and Jessica B. Reisman. 2005. *100 Questions and Answers about Your Child's Cancer.* Sudbury, MA: Jones and Bartlett.

This book presents practical answers to questions about childhood cancer, treatment options, post–treatment quality of life, and coping strategies for both patients and parents. Two child cancer experts authored this book and incorporated comments from parents of children with cancer. The book provides detailed information about diagnostic tests, supportive-care issues, and side effects and complications of treatment that are common to all children treated for cancer. The text is easy to read, and definitions for key terms are provided in the sidebar.

➤ Keene, Nancy. 2003. *Educating the Child with Cancer: A Guide for Parents and Teachers.* Kensington, MD: Candlelighters Childhood Cancer Foundation. This book was developed with the intent of promoting understanding and communication among parents, educators, and medical professionals so that together they can provide an appropriate education for children who have been treated for cancer. Learning issues that face children treated for cancer from infancy through adulthood are covered in depth, with some chapters written by experts and others by parents. Topics include gaining access to special education services, helping siblings in the classroom, physical activity in school, treatment-related late effects that may cause learning difficulties, and grief in the classroom. Each chapter ends with a list of key points.

➤ Woznick, Leigh A., and Carol D. Goodheart. 2002. *Living with Childhood Cancer: A Practical Guide to Help Parents Cope.* Washington, DC: American Psychological Association. The focus of this book is the psychological impact of childhood cancer. It provides guidance and advice to parents on managing the emotional and practical challenges of the disease and its treatment. The book describes how adults, children, teenagers, and families may cope with illness and stress and offers strategies for successful coping. Topics include communication, stress, trauma, pain, side effects, encouraging child development, building self-esteem, dying and grieving, and long-term survivorship. Specific information is provided for different age groups and various types of families. The authors are a psychologist and her daughter who is the mother of a child with cancer.

Web Resources

Sites focusing on retinoblastoma

➤ EyeCancerNetwork. Access at: http://eyecancer.com The content of this site is provided by Dr. Paul T. Finger, an ophthalmologist from New York University School of Medicine. The site includes detailed descriptions, images, and information about the diagnosis and treatment for various eye tumors, including retinoblastoma. It features color illustrations, articles about various treatments, frequently asked questions, and an international physician list.

➤ *Retinoblastoma.com*. Access at: www.retinoblastoma.com
This site is provided by Dr. David H. Abramson, chief of the Ophthalmic Oncology Service at Memorial Sloan-Kettering Cancer Center in New York City. For parents, the most useful section of the site is the "Parent's Guide to Understanding Retinoblastoma." This is a detailed overview, with color illustrations, that includes an explanation of the eye's anatomy, genetics of retinoblastoma, treatment, and long-term consequences of the illness. In addition to the guide, which may be printed as a 12-page Adobe Acrobat (.pdf) file, the site has video files of various treatment procedures, information on genetic counseling, and links to other sites of interest.

Detailed sections in childhood cancer sites

➤ CureSearch. Access at: www.curesearch.org
This site has a detailed section about retinoblastoma, and the information is presented separately to parents and patients in different age groups: preschool, ages 5–10, 10–14, and 14–22. Topics covered include diagnostic tests, treatment methods, impact on the patient and family, navigating the health care system, and school issues. The interactive section of the site includes a clinical trial matching service, discussion boards, and a resource directory for national and local support groups and services. Provided by the Children's Cancer Group and the National Childhood Cancer Foundation.

➤ Penn State Hershey Medical Center. *Home Care Guide*. Access at: www. hmc.psu.edu/hematology/homeguide/
Nurses and physicians from the children's hematology/oncology team at Penn State Hershey Medical Center developed this guide for caregivers of children with childhood cancer. It provides treatment plans for a variety of supportive-care and psychosocial issues that may occur while a child is undergoing treatment. Each plan gives caregivers the information they need in order to solve problems including understanding the problem, when to get professional help, what caregivers can do on their own, possible obstacles, and how to carry out and adjust the plan.

Detailed sections in general cancer sites

➤ American Cancer Society. *Learn about Retinoblastoma (An Eye Cancer)*. Access at: www.cancer.org and select from the menu under "Choose a Cancer Topic."

A detailed guide about retinoblastoma can be printed by section or as an Adobe Acrobat (.pdf) file.

➤ Cancerbackup. *Retinoblastoma in Children.* Access at: www.cancer backup.org.uk/Home and click on "Cancer Type."

➤ National Cancer Institute. *Retinoblastoma.* Access at: www.cancer.gov and click on "Types of Cancer."
The top page of the section links to patient versions of PDQ® statements, clinical trial information, and other NCI publications on this topic.

➤ People Living with Cancer. *Retinoblastoma, Childhood Cancer.* Access at: www.plwc.org and click on "Cancer Type."
The PLWC oncologist-approved guide on retinoblastoma can be printed in its entirety or by subtopic.

Patient-Support Organizations

➤ Candlelighters. Access at: www.candlelighters.org
Phone: 800-366-2223

➤ The National Children's Cancer Society. Access at: http://nationalchildrens cancersociety.com
Phone: 800-5-FAMILY

➤ Retinoblastoma International. Access at: www.retinoblastoma.net
Phone: 323-669-2299

Rhabdomyosarcoma

Anatomical facts: The body's connective tissue consists of soft tissues such as muscles, fat, cartilage, and blood vessels. Rhabdomyoblasts are embryonic cells that eventually develop into the body's voluntary muscles. These cells start to form in fetuses at about seven weeks after conception.

Illustration available at the Medical Illustrations Gallery of the People Living With Cancer Web site.

Access at: www.plwc.org and click on Library on the left sidebar.

Rhabdomyosarcoma (RMS) is the sixth most common type of childhood cancer, with 350 new cases diagnosed each year in the United States. RMS develops when rhabdomyoblasts become malignant and form a tumor. Because this type of cancer develops from embryonic cells, it is extremely rare in adulthood. Over 90% of rhabdomyosarcomas are diagnosed in people under 25 years old, and about 60% of these cases are diagnosed in children under the age of 10. The overall five-year survival rate for children with rhabdomyosarcoma is about 66%, but prognosis is dependent on many factors, including the location and size of the tumor, the results of surgery, and whether the cancer has metastasized (spread).

The incidence of rhabdomyosarcoma has not changed very much over the past few decades. This disease is not associated with any known risk factors, and there is no particular geographic location or ethnic group that has an unusually high rate of RMS.

Rhabdomyosarcoma tumors can occur in any part of the body. Embryonal rhabdomyosarcoma (ERMS) is the most common type and usually affects infants and young children. The most common site where ERMS develops are the head and neck area, bladder, vagina, and in or around the prostate and testes. The second main type, alveolar rhabdomyosarcoma (ARMS), occurs more often in the large muscles of the trunk, arms, and legs and is most likely to be diagnosed among older children or teenagers.

The main treatment option for rhabdomyosarcoma is surgery. The goal of surgery is to remove the tumor along with a margin of normal tissue. A complete removal is not always possible and depends on the tumor's location. If a tumor is in close proximity to important structures and organs, like in the head and neck region, the surgeon removes as much of the tumor as he or she can without causing damage to essential functions. All patients are also treated with chemotherapy. Radiation therapy is used in some, but not all, cases. Treatment plans for rhabdomyosarcoma are individualized and tailored according to the size and location of the tumor and the child's developmental stage.

Information Sources

Brochures, Booklets, and Other Short Print Publications

➤ National Cancer Institute. *Young People with Cancer: A Handbook for Parents.*
This publication discusses the most common types of childhood cancer, treatments, and side effects as well as issues that may arise when a child is diagnosed with cancer. Offers medical information and practical tips gathered from parents. Access at: https://cissecure.nci.nih.gov/ncipubs/

➤ National Childhood Cancer Foundation. *The Children's Oncology Group (COG) Family Handbook.*
This 80-page handbook was written by nurses, doctors, and other childhood cancer professionals. The information is relevant to all types of childhood cancer and covers medical and psychosocial issues. The publication includes illustrations and has several areas that may be customized for a specific child. Access at: www.curesearch.org.

➤ National Children's Cancer Society. *The Mountain You've Climbed: A Parent's Guide to Childhood Cancer Survivorship.*
This guide is designed to answer parents' questions regarding childhood cancer and offer suggestions on how to integrate the cancer experience into all areas of the family's life. It addresses issues beginning from the time of diagnosis through the completion of treatment and beyond. Order at: http://nationalchildrenscancersociety.com

Books

Book chapters

➤ Janes-Hodder, Honna, and Nancy Keene. 2002. *Childhood Cancer: A Parent's Guide to Solid Tumor Cancers.* 2d ed. Sebastopol, CA: O'Reilly.
This book provides a detailed overview of rhabdomyosarcoma as well as other childhood solid tumors. Chapters offer practical advice on how to cope with procedures, hospitalization, family and friends, school, social and financial issues, communications, feelings, and, if treatment is not successful, issues of grief and bereavement. The text provides stories from children and parents who have experienced childhood cancer. Appendixes include blood counts and what they mean, and an extensive resource list.

Relevant childhood cancer books

➤ Carroll, William L., and Jessica B. Reisman. 2005. *100 Questions and Answers about Your Child's Cancer.* Sudbury, MA: Jones and Bartlett.
This book presents practical answers to questions about childhood cancer, treatment options, post–treatment quality of life, and coping strategies for both patients and parents. Two child cancer experts authored this book and incorporated comments from parents of children with cancer. The book provides detailed information about diagnostic tests, supportive-care issues and side effects and complications of treatment that are common to all children treated for cancer. The text is easy to read, and definitions for key terms are provided in the sidebar.

➤ Keene, Nancy. 2003. *Educating the Child with Cancer: A Guide for Parents and Teachers.* Kensington, MD: Candlelighters Childhood Cancer Foundation.
This book was developed with the intent of promoting understanding and communication among parents, educators, and medical professionals so that together they can provide an appropriate education for children who have been treated for cancer. Learning issues that face children treated for cancer from infancy through adulthood are covered in depth, with some chapters written by experts and others by parents. Topics in-

clude gaining access to special education services, helping siblings in the classroom, physical activity in school, treatment-related late effects that may cause learning difficulties, and grief in the classroom. Each chapter ends with a list of key points.

➤ Woznick, Leigh A., and Carol D. Goodheart. 2002. *Living with Childhood Cancer: A Practical Guide to Help Parents Cope.* Washington, DC: American Psychological Association.

The focus of this book is the psychological impact of childhood cancer. It provides guidance and advice to parents on managing the emotional and practical challenges of the disease and its treatment. The book describes how adults, children, teenagers, and families may cope with illness and stress and offers strategies for successful coping. Topics include communication, stress, trauma, pain, side effects, encouraging child development, building self-esteem, dying and grieving, and long-term survivorship. Specific information is provided for different age groups and various types of families. The authors are a psychologist and her daughter who is the mother of a child with cancer.

Web Resources

Detailed sections in childhood cancer sites

➤ CureSearch. Access at: www.curesearch.org

This site has a detailed section about rhabdomyosarcoma, and the information is presented separately to parents and patients in different age groups: preschool, ages 5–10, 10–14, and 14–22. Topics covered include diagnostic tests, treatment methods, impact on the patient and family, navigating the health care system, and school issues. The interactive section of the site provides a clinical trial matching service, discussion boards, and a resource directory for national and local support groups and services. Hosted by the Children's Cancer Group and the National Childhood Cancer Foundation.

➤ Penn State Hershey Medical Center. *Home Care Guide.* Access at: www.hmc.psu.edu/hematology/homeguide/

Nurses and physicians from the children's hematology/oncology team at Penn State Hershey Medical Center developed this guide for caregivers of children with childhood cancer. It provides treatment plans for a variety of supportive-care and psychosocial issues that may occur while a child is undergoing treatment. Each plan offers caregivers the information they need in order to solve problems, including understanding the problem, when to get professional help, what caregivers can do on their own, possible obstacles, and how to carry out and adjust the plan.

Detailed sections in general cancer sites

➤ American Cancer Society. *Learn about Rhabdomyosarcoma.* Access at: www.cancer.org and select from the menu under "Choose a Cancer Topic."
A detailed guide about rhabdomyosarcoma can be printed by section or as an Adobe Acrobat (.pdf) file.

➤ Cancerbackup. *Rhabdomyosarcoma in Children.* Access at: www.cancer backup.org.uk/Home and click on "Cancer Type."

➤ National Cancer Institute. *Childhood Rhabdomyosarcoma.* Access at: www. cancer.gov and click on "Types of Cancer."
The top page of the section links to patient versions of PDQ® statements, clinical trial information, and other NCI publications on this topic.

➤ People Living with Cancer. *Rhabdomyosarcoma, Childhood Cancer.* Access at: www.plwc.org and click on "Cancer Type."
The PLWC oncologist-approved guide on rhabdomyosarcoma can be printed in its entirety, or by subtopic.

Patient-Support Organizations

➤ Candlelighters. Access at: www.candlelighters.org
Phone: 800-366-2223

➤ The National Children's Cancer Society. Access at: http://nationalchild-renscancersociety.com
Phone: 800-5-FAMILY

➤ Sarcoma Alliance. Access at: www.sarcomaalliance.org
Phone: 415-381-7236

Wilms' Tumor

Anatomical facts: The kidneys are two fist-size organs located on either side of the spine in the lower abdomen. The adrenal glands are attached to the top of each kidney. The kidneys are part of the urinary system, and their main function is to collect wastes and extra water from the blood by producing urine. Urine passes from the kidneys to the bladder through a tube called the ureter. It is stored in the bladder until it leaves the body through another tube called the urethra. It is possible to live with only one kidney.

Illustration available at the Medical Illustrations Gallery of the People Living with Cancer Web site .
Access at: www.plwc.org and click on Library on the left sidebar.

Wilms' tumor, also called nephroblastoma, is diagnosed in approximately 500 children in the United States every year. This tumor appears almost exclusively in children, and 75% of diagnoses occur before age 5. About 50 children are diagnosed with non-Wilms' cancers of the kidney. These types are treated differently than Wilms' tumor and have a different outlook. Of children who receive optimal treatment for Wilms' tumor, 85% to 90% are cured.

In most cases, the tumors are discovered when they are already very large, larger than the kidney in which they started, but before the cancer metastasized to distant organs. In about 5% of cases, the disease is "bilateral," which means it affects both kidneys. About 95% of Wilms' tumors have a "favorable" histology. The remaining 5% have an "unfavorable" appearance, with cells that are not uniform and have irregular shapes. Tumors with unfavorable histology are more difficult to treat and cure.

Treatment for Wilms' tumor consists of surgery, chemotherapy, and sometimes radiation therapy. Surgery is performed even if the primary tumor has spread to distant organs and also in cases of bilateral disease. The most common surgery to treat Wilms' tumor is radical nephrectomy, which includes the removal of cancer along with the whole kidney, the ureter, the attached adrenal gland, and the fatty tissue that surrounds the kidney. If the entire tumor is removed, the remaining kidney is capable to compensate and there is no loss in function. All children with Wilms' tumor receive chemotherapy after the surgery. Some children receive chemotherapy and/or radiation therapy before the surgery to shrink large tumors before removing them.

Information Sources
Brochures, Booklets, and Other Short Print Publications

Focusing on Wilms' tumor

➤ Kidney Cancer Association. *Wilms' Tumor: What Now?* Access at: www. curekidneycancer.org (registration required)
A practical guide for parents of children with Wilms' tumor, covering medical and psychosocial issues. Includes sections on helping the child at school and in the hospital and coping with parental stress.

Relevant childhood cancer publications

➤ National Cancer Institute. *Young People with Cancer: A Handbook for Parents.* This publication discusses the most common types of childhood cancer, treatments, and side effects, as well as issues that may arise when a child is diagnosed with cancer. Offers medical information and practical tips gathered from parents. Access at: https://cissecure.nci.nih.gov/ncipubs/

➤ National Childhood Cancer Foundation. *The Children's Oncology Group (COG) Family Handbook.*
This 80-page handbook was written by nurses, doctors, and other childhood cancer professionals. The information is relevant to all types of childhood cancer and covers medical and psychosocial issues. The publication includes illustrations and has several areas that may be customized for a specific child. Access at: www.curesearch.org.

➤ National Children's Cancer Society. *The Mountain You've Climbed: A Parent's Guide to Childhood Cancer Survivorship.*
This guide is designed to answer parents' questions regarding childhood cancer and offer suggestions on how to integrate the cancer experience into all areas of the family's life. It addresses issues beginning from the time of diagnosis through the completion of treatment and beyond. Order at: http://nationalchildrenscancersociety.com

Books

Book chapters

➤ Janes-Hodder, Honna, and Nancy Keene. 2002. *Childhood Cancer: A Parent's Guide to Solid Tumor Cancers.* 2d ed. Sebastopol, CA: O'Reilly.
This book provides a detailed overview of Wilms' tumor as well as other childhood solid tumors. Chapters offer practical advice on how to cope with procedures, hospitalization, family and friends, school, social and financial issues, communications, feelings, and, if treatment is not successful, issues of grief and bereavement. The text provides stories from children and parents who have experienced childhood cancer. Appendixes include blood counts and what they mean and an extensive resource list.

Relevant childhood cancer books

➤ Carroll, William L., and Jessica B. Reisman. 2005. *100 Questions and Answers about Your Child's Cancer.* Sudbury, MA: Jones and Bartlett.
This book presents practical answers to questions about childhood cancer, treatment options, post–treatment quality of life, and coping strategies for both patients and parents. Two child cancer experts authored this book and incorporated comments from parents of children with cancer. The book provides detailed information about diagnostic tests, supportive-care issues, and side effects and complications of treatment that are common to all children treated for cancer. The text is easy to read, and definitions for key terms are provided in the sidebar.

➤ Keene, Nancy. 2003. *Educating the Child with Cancer: A Guide for Parents and Teachers.* Kensington, MD: Candlelighters Childhood Cancer Foundation. This book was developed with the intent of promoting understanding and communication among parents, educators, and medical professionals so that together they can provide an appropriate education for children who have been treated for cancer. Learning issues that face children treated for cancer from infancy through adulthood are covered in depth, with some chapters written by experts and others by parents. Topics include gaining access to special education services, helping siblings in the classroom, physical activity in school, treatment-related late effects that may cause learning difficulties, and grief in the classroom. Each chapter ends with a list of key points.

➤ Woznick, Leigh A., and Carol D. Goodheart. 2002. *Living with Childhood Cancer: A Practical Guide to Help Parents Cope.* Washington, DC: American Psychological Association. The focus of this book is the psychological impact of childhood cancer. It provides guidance and advice to parents on managing the emotional and practical challenges of the disease and its treatment. The book describes how adults, children, teenagers, and families may cope with illness and stress and offers strategies for successful coping. Topics include communication, stress, trauma, pain, side effects, encouraging child development, building self-esteem, dying and grieving, and long-term survivorship. Specific information is provided for different age groups and various types of families. The authors are a psychologist and her daughter who is the mother of a child with cancer.

Web Resources

Sites focusing on Wilms' tumor

➤ Kidney Cancer Association. Access at: www.curekidneycancer.org
The Kidney Cancer Association addresses the needs of children and adults with kidney cancer. A free registration enables access to a wealth of information about kidney cancer, including full text of brochures and publications, detailed information about dealing with kidney cancer, video presentations by medical experts and leading researchers, and access to a clinical trial database, news, and support services offered by this organization.

➤ National Wilms' Tumor Study. Access at: www.nwtsg.org
The National Wilms' Tumor Study Group is a multi-institutional study of the treatment of patients with Wilms' tumor. The site offers information

for parents of children who are undergoing treatment for Wilms' tumor and for adult survivors of the disease.

Detailed sections in childhood cancer sites

➤ CureSearch. Access at: www.curesearch.org
This site has a detailed section about kidney and Wilms' tumor, and the information is presented separately to parents and patients in different age groups: preschool, ages 5–10, 10–14, and 14–22. Topics covered include diagnostic tests, treatment methods, impact on the patient and family, navigating the health care system, and school issues. The interactive section of the site includes a clinical trial matching service, discussion boards, and a resource directory for national and local support groups and services. Hosted by the Children's Cancer Group and the National Childhood Cancer Foundation.

➤ Penn State Hershey Medical Center. *Home Care Guide.* Access at: www. hmc.psu.edu/hematology/homeguide/
Nurses and physicians from the children's hematology/oncology team at Penn State Hershey Medical Center developed this guide for caregivers of children with childhood cancer. It provides treatment plans for a variety of supportive-care and psychosocial issues that may occur while a child is undergoing treatment. Each plan offers caregivers the information they need in order to solve problems including understanding the problem, when to get professional help, what caregivers can do on their own, possible obstacles, and how to carry out and adjust the plan.

Detailed sections in general cancer sites

➤ American Cancer Society. *Learn about Wilms' Tumor.* Access at: www. cancer. org and select from the menu under "Choose a Cancer Type or Topic."
A detailed guide about Wilms' tumor may be printed by section or as an Adobe Acrobat (.pdf) file.

➤ Cancerbackup. *Wilms' Tumour in Children.* Access at: www.cancerbackup. org.uk/Home and click on "Cancer Type."

➤ National Cancer Institute. *Wilms' Tumor and Other Childhood Kidney Tumors.* Access at: www.cancer.gov and click on "Types of Cancer."
The top page of the section links to patient versions of PDQ® statements, clinical trial information, and other NCI publications on this topic.

➤ People Living with Cancer. *Wilms' Tumor, Childhood Cancer.* Access at: www.plwc.org and click on "Cancer Type."
The PLWC oncologist-approved guide on Wilms' tumor can be printed in its entirety or by subtopic.

Patient-Support Organizations

➤ Candlelighters. Access at: www.candlelighters.org
Phone: 800-366-2223
➤ The National Children's Cancer Society. Access at: http://nationalchild-renscancersociety.com
Phone: 800-5-FAMILY

Part III

Best Information Resources about Cancer Prevention, Treatment, and Quality-of-Life Concerns

Chapter 6

Cancer Prevention

Cancer Prevention and Early Detection

This chapter explores issues that concern healthy people who are worried about their risk of developing cancer and interested in learning about ways to prevent cancer and detect it early. The first section, "Cancer Prevention and Early Detection," provides explanations and general resources about this topic. The subtopics of nutrition for cancer prevention and cancer genetics are discussed later in the chapter.

Cancer is a preventable disease. The American Cancer Society estimates that 75% of adult cancers can be linked to environmental factors, including tobacco, nutrition, infectious diseases, and exposure to chemicals and radiation. The Harvard Center for Cancer Prevention estimates that 50% of cancer cases could be avoided through lifestyle modification, such as stopping smoking, maintaining a healthy weight, increasing physical activity, and decreasing alcohol consumption. (These statistics relate only to adult cancers; childhood cancers are not caused by lifestyle factors.)

It is common knowledge that cigarette smoking is the single largest preventable cause of cancer in the United States. People are less aware that other forms of using tobacco—such as cigars, chewing tobacco, and snuff—also cause cancer. Secondhand smoke is a known risk factor for lung cancer and is responsible for approximately 3,400 lung cancer deaths each year among adult nonsmokers in the United States. Tobacco causes 90% of lung cancers, and it is a major cause of other cancers, such as larynx (voice box), oral cavity, pharynx (throat), and esophageal cancers. Tobacco use is a contributing cause in the development of cancers of the bladder, pancreas, cervix, kidney, and stomach. Of all cancer deaths in the United States, 30% are linked to tobacco use.

The second cancer cause after smoking is obesity, which may account for 25% to 30% of several major cancers: colon, breast (in postmenopausal women), endometrial, kidney, and esophagus. Some studies have also reported links between obesity and cancers of the gallbladder, ovaries, and pancreas. Overweight women (defined as weighing more the 35% above their ideal body weight) have a higher risk of developing breast, uterine, ovarian, and cervical cancer. Overweight men have a higher risk to develop colon or prostate cancer. Lack of physical activity and diet play a role in obesity, and researchers are investigating the complex interaction among diet, physical activity, and genetics and how these factors influence cancer risk.

Other preventable risk factors for cancer are exposure to sunlight and ultraviolet radiation, which is responsible for 90% of all skin cancers, including melanoma. Infectious diseases, mostly human papillomaviruses (HPV), which cause cervical cancer, are linked to 5% of cancer cases. Alcohol increases the risk for cancers of the stomach, esophagus, pharynx, larynx, liver, breast, and colon.

Regular screening of healthy people for cancer can greatly reduce the suffering and death resulting from cancer. Finding cancer in an early stage makes a huge difference in the ability to achieve a cure, prolong life, and improve the quality of life of cancer survivors. A number of screening tests have been developed to detect cancers of the breast, colon, rectum, cervix, prostate, testes (testicles), oral cavity (mouth), and skin. The prognosis of these cancers has greatly improved since the implementation of early-detection screenings. The American Cancer Society estimates that if all Americans had early-detection testing, the five-year relative survival rate for people with these cancers would increase to about 95%. Several large studies conducted around the world show that breast cancer screening with mammograms reduces the number of deaths from breast cancer for women age 40 to 69. Other very effective screening tests that save lives are colonoscopy, for detecting colorectal cancer, and Pap smear, which detects cervical cancer.

Information on ways to prevent cancer and early-detection guidelines is included in the sources listed below. Some of the information sources offer separate sections for specific cancer types. Additional prevention information on specific cancer types can be found in the type-specific resources in Chapter 5.

Information Sources

Brochures, Booklets, and Other Short Print Publications

➤ American Cancer Society. *Choices for Good Health.*
➤ American Cancer Society. *Guidelines for the Early Detection of Cancer.*
➤ American Cancer Society. *Taking Control (Take ten simple steps to reduce your cancer risk).*
➤ American Institute for Cancer Research. *Everything Doesn't Cause Cancer.* This booklet discusses major, minor, and unproven risk factors for cancer and puts them in perspective. Access at: www.aicr.org

➤ National Cancer Institute. *Cancer and the Environment: What You Need to Know, What You Can Do.*
This booklet addresses concerns about the connection between cancer and exposure to toxic substances in the environment, including tobacco, alcohol, medical drugs, fibers, pesticides, and a variety of other chemicals. The reader will learn which types of substances are known carcinogens and what can be done to reduce exposure to them. Written at a high reading level, this booklet is appropriate for the sophisticated patron looking for in-depth information in lay language. Includes a glossary and illustrations. Access at: https://cissecure.nci.nih.gov/ncipubs/

Books

➤ American Cancer Society. 2003. *Cancer: What Causes It, What Doesn't.* Atlanta: American Cancer Society.
Experts from the American Cancer Society explain the scientific evidence with regard to the causes of cancer. Opening chapters explain the biological process of cancer and how to make sense of scientific studies. Further chapters detail proven risks and dispel myths concerning materials in the environment and lifestyle choices. The text is rich with text boxes, photographs, and tables.

➤ American Cancer Society. 2002. *Good for You!: Reducing Your Risk of Developing Cancer.* Atlanta: American Cancer Society.
This handbook gives practical, manageable tips to help people stay focused on healthy habits. The authors offer advice on healthy food choices, exercise, and screening tests. The text includes many fun facts, quotes, tips, and quizzes to help readers make healthy lifestyle choices.

➤ Daniel, Rosy, with Rachel Ellis. 2001. *The Cancer Prevention Book: The Holistic Plan to Reduce Your Risk of Cancer and Revolutionize Your Life.* London: Simon & Schuster.
The author is a British physician specializing in holistic care for cancer patients. The book provides thorough explanations on cancer-causing lifestyle factors and covers self-examinations, screening tests, and early detection. It also includes a "self-help" chapter, which explains the mind/body/spirit connection and advises how to strengthen the mind and improve emotional and physical health.

➤ Runowicz, Carolyn D., Sheldon H. Cherry, and Dianne Lange. 2004. *The Answer to Cancer.* Emmaus, PA: Rodale.
This book was written for people who want to avoid ever getting cancer, arrest precancerous changes, or prevent a recurrence. The authors are two physicians, one of them a cancer survivor herself, who explain the latest

scientific findings concerning the various drugs, vitamins, therapies, and treatments that can keep cancer from showing up—or help defeat it if it does. The intent is to help readers understand the importance of taking some control of the risk factors, such as diet, exercise, lifestyle habits, and even genetic background.

➤ Stephens, Fr. 2002. *The Cancer Prevention Manual: Simple Rules to Reduce the Risks*. New York: Oxford University Press.

This is a small-size book that covers the topic in a straightforward, concise, yet detailed manner. It explains how cancer starts to develop, the lifestyle practices to avoid, and the changes to adapt. It also describes causes and risk factors for specific cancers and the measures individuals can take in order to reduce risk. Each topic includes practical recommendations, and the book provides many illustrations, photographs, and cartoons.

Audiovisual Materials

➤ *Cancer Self-Defense*. Directed by Bernanke, Jaime, Melissa Gray, and Pangolin Pictures, et al. Films for the Humanities & Sciences, 2004–2002.

This Discovery Health Channel Production presents a comprehensive screening and prevention program, focusing on breast, lung, prostate, colon, and skin. Smoking cessation and diet and nutrition are reviewed, with insightful comments by Dr. Moshe Shike, director of the Memorial Sloan-Kettering Cancer Prevention and Wellness Center, and other specialists. (51 minutes). Available in VHS and DVD format.

Web Resources

Sites focusing on cancer prevention and early detection

➤ Cancer Research and Prevention Foundation. Access at: www.preventcancer. org

This site focuses on lifestyle changes that may help reduce cancer risk. It has sections on diet, exercise, smoking, self-exams, and teaching healthy habits to children. Downloadable fact sheets on specific cancers detail risk factors, steps to reduce risk, early-detection guidelines, and symptoms of the disease.

➤ Harvard Center for Cancer Prevention. Access at: www.hsph.harvard.edu/ cancer

The Center for Cancer Prevention at the Harvard School of Public Health offers detailed information presented in a variety of formats, including podcasts, Webcasts, and audio files of the center's experts explaining new research developments. The site is integrated with an interactive tool called "Your Disease Risk," which provides personal assessment of cancer risk. The "Risk Factors" section has detailed information on lifestyle factors (like diet and activity level), exposures (such as air pollution), and personal characteristics (for instance, family history and age) that influence a person's risk to develop cancer.

➤ National Cancer Institute Division of Cancer Prevention. Access at: www. cancer.gov/prevention/
   This site provides a central access point to National Cancer Institute information and publications about cancer prevention and early detection. It links to PDQ® statements on cancer prevention, early detection, and lifestyle choices and provides news summaries of clinical trials investigating cancer prevention and early detection.

Detailed sections in general cancer sites

➤ American Cancer Society. *Prevention & Early Detection*. Access at: www. cancer.org and type "Prevention & Early Detection" in the search box.

➤ Cancerbackup. *About Cancer*. Access at: www.cancerbackup.org.uk/Home and click on the link to "About Cancer."
   This page links to information on causes, screenings, and precancerous conditions.

➤ People Living with Cancer. *Learning about Cancer*. Access at: www.plwc. org and click on "Learning about Cancer" on the left sidebar.
   This page has links to information about risk factors, genetics, prevention, and early detection.

Nutrition for Cancer Prevention

Thirty percent of all cancer deaths can be linked to diet in adult life. Despite thousands of research studies investigating the link between diet and cancer, no specific food or nutrient has been shown to be either a direct cause of, or a cure for a specific cancer. The ability of certain foods or nutrients to protect against specific cancers is still being investigated, but evidence is not yet sufficient to issue explicit recommendations. The picture emerging from the research so far is that a diet rich in vegetables and fruits and low in fat helps reduce cancer risk. The American Cancer Society recommends that individuals follow the following principles when making food choices:

➤ Eat a variety of healthful foods, with an emphasis on plant sources
➤ Eat five or more servings of a variety of vegetables and fruits each day
➤ Choose whole grains in preference to processed (refined) grains and sugars

➤ Limit consumption of red meats, especially those processed and high in fat
➤ Choose foods that help maintain healthy weight
➤ Drink alcohol only in moderation, if at all.

Public and hospital librarians may get questions about nutrition for cancer prevention from the general public, from people at high risk for cancer, and from cancer survivors in remission. The sources listed below can help provide answers to questions regarding specific foods and nutrients as well as general guidelines of nutrition suitable for people who want to reduce cancer risk or avoid recurrence. Information about herbs and supplements used by cancer patients is covered in the "Complementary and Alternative Therapies" section on page 245.

Information Sources

Brochures, Booklets, and Other Short Print Publications

➤ American Institute for Cancer Research. *Nutrition of the Cancer Survivor.* This booklet has been specifically tailored to cancer survivors. It summarizes the state of the research about nutrition for cancer prevention and provides tips for making small, everyday adjustments that may help prevent secondary tumors and recurrence. Access at: www.aicr.org
➤ American Institute for Cancer Research. *Simple Steps to Prevent Cancer.* This brochure introduces a set of simple and practical guidelines to help make food choices that may lower cancer risk. Access at: www.aicr.org.
➤ Additional brochures on various aspects of nutrition for cancer prevention are available at the American Institute for Cancer Research Web site at: www.aicr.org, including:
  ➤ *Nutrition After Fifty*
  ➤ *Moving Toward a Plant-Based Diet*
  ➤ *A Healthy Weight For Life*
  ➤ *Getting Active, Staying Active*
  ➤ *Questions and Answers about Breast Health and Breast Cancer*
  ➤ *Reducing Your Risk of Breast Cancer*
  ➤ *Reducing Your Risk of Prostate Cancer*
  ➤ *Reducing Your Risk of Colorectal Cancer*
  ➤ *Reducing Your Risk of Skin Cancer*

Books

➤ American Cancer Society. 2005. *The American Cancer Society's Healthy Eating Cookbook: A Celebration of Food, Friends, and Healthy Living.* 3d ed. Atlanta: American Cancer Society.

In addition to providing over 300 recipes from chefs, amateur cooks, and celebrities, this book also includes the latest research and updated recommendations for healthy eating. Also offered are tips for smart shopping, simple tips in the kitchen, and quick tips for judging portion sizes and substitutions.

➤ American Institute for Cancer Research. 2002. *Nutrition after Cancer: Presentations from the First Two Conferences on the Role of Diet in Cancer Survivorship, Held May 8, 2001 and October 18, 2001.* Washington, DC: American Institute for Cancer Research.

This book contains selected presentations from an American Institute for Cancer Research conference for cancer survivors. Covered topics include soy, flaxseed, vegetables, exercise, obesity, and general dietary patterns. This book can help guide survivors to make daily choices about diet and exercise that can reduce the risk of recurrence and of secondary cancers.

➤ American Institute for Cancer Research. 2005. *The New American Plate Cookbook: Recipes for a Healthy Weight and a Healthy Life.* Berkeley, CA: University of California Press.

A collection of recipes, developed by a team of AICR nutritionists, that promote healthy weight and the right proportion of food groups. The recipes utilize mainly plant foods: vegetables, fruits, and whole grains. Over 200 recipes for vegetables, grains, fish, poultry, and meat dishes are included, as well as one-pot meals and dessert recipes.

➤ Bloch, Abby S., et al., eds. 2004. *Eating Well, Staying Well during and after Cancer.* Atlanta: American Cancer Society.

A comprehensive book written by highly credentialed nutrition experts providing detailed information on diet and cancer. The sections discussing the evidence regarding foods and dietary supplements that have been promoted as fighting cancer or improving the immune system are especially interesting.

➤ Dyer, Diana. 2002. *A Dietitian's Cancer Story: Information and Inspiration for Recovery and Healing from a 3-Time Cancer Survivor.* Ann Arbor, MI: Swan Press.

This book was authored by a registered dietitian who is also a cancer survivor. Its strength is in the specific, detailed advice and suggestions about topics such as selecting dishes in restaurants, avoiding hidden fats, travel tips, and improving endurance. It includes recipes, and the author explains how to evaluate alternative and complementary nutritional therapies, herbs, and supplements. The nutrition principles are suitable for cancer survivors during and after treatment.

➤ Osbourne, Michael, et al. 2004. *The Strang Cancer Prevention Center Cookbook: A Complete Nutrition and Lifestyle Plan to Dramatically Lower Your Cancer Risk.* Updated ed. New York: McGraw-Hill.
This book is the result of collaboration between cancer prevention experts from the Strang Cancer Prevention Center and well-known professional chefs. Readers will learn how to determine the quality of their current diet and how to improve it by utilizing phytochemicals and implementing lifestyle modifications. Includes more than 100 recipes.

➤ Weldon, Glen, ed. and American Institute for Cancer Research. 2002. *Dietary Options for Cancer Survivors: A Guide to Research on Foods, Food Substances, Herbals, and Dietary Regimens That May Influence Cancer.* Washington, DC: American Institute for Cancer Research.
This book discusses and summarizes the research concerning the effectiveness of foods, food substances, herbal supplements, and dietary regimens in preventing cancer. The goal is to enable cancer survivors to check the scientific evidence before making dietary changes or taking supplements to maintain their health. Includes references to articles and reports in scientific journals.

Audiovisual Resources

➤ *Nutrition for Prevention and Adjuvant Therapy of Cancer.* 1997. Directed by Health Science Institute. (15 minutes.) The Institute. Available in VHS and CD-ROM formats.
This program covers the principles of good nutrition for cancer prevention. It describes the major food groups and nutrients and explains how antioxidant vitamins, minerals, fiber, and certain oils can prevent the growth of cancer cells. Also included are tips on reducing fat and calories and increasing fruits and vegetables in the diet. Includes a teacher's guide. Order at: http://healthscienceinstitute.com/.

Web Resources

Sites focusing on nutrition and cancer

➤ The American Institute for Cancer Research. Access at: www.aicr.org
The mission of American Institute for Cancer Research is to support research on diet and cancer prevention and educate the public about the results. Food and lifestyle choices that may reduce cancer risk and the roles of certain foods, such as soy, flaxseed, and green tea, in protecting health are discussed at length. AICR publications that address various aspects of diet and cancer prevention, including guidelines for specific cancers, are

available in print format. The site also provides an extensive recipe database.

➤ Cancer Nutrition Info. Access at: www.cancernutritioninfo.com
The author is a registered dietitian who worked with cancer patients at the University of Michigan Comprehensive Cancer Center. The core of the site are reviews of articles published in the scientific medical literature that explain in lay language what the evidence shows with regard to specific products. The section "Complementary & Alternative Medicine" focuses on supplements, vitamins, minerals, and herbs. Users also can find recipes, tips, and answers to commonly asked questions. Some of the content requires a $15 annual subscription fee.

Sections about nutrition for cancer prevention are also available at the following sites

➤ American Cancer Society. Access at: www.cancer.org
➤ Harvard Center for Cancer Prevention at the Harvard School of Public Health. Access at: www.hsph.harvard.edu/cancer

Cancer Genetics

Only 5% to 10% of cancer cases are linked to inherited genetic mutations that run in families. The presence of a cancer-causing gene or condition does not mean the affected person will automatically get cancer. Rather, this person is thought to be "predisposed" to a type of cancer, or has a higher risk than the general population in getting this cancer. Children of people who carry a genetic mutation have a likelihood of up to 50% of inheriting the mutation.

Several rare hereditary syndromes and conditions are associated with an increased risk for cancer. For example, neurofibromatosis is a genetic disorder that increases the risk for rhabdomyosarcoma, fibrosarcoma, and other cancers. Children with Down's syndrome have an increased risk to develop leukemia. Bloom syndrome is a rare inherited disorder associated with an increased risk to develop lymphoma, leukemia, and other types of carcinomas.

In recent years several inherited genetic mutations that increase the risk for specific types of cancer have been discovered. Tests to discover these mutations have been developed for a few of these mutations affecting mostly breast, ovarian, and colon cancer. Mutations in BRCA1 and BRCA2 genes increase the risk for breast and ovarian cancers and are most common in the Ashkenazi Jewish population. Women with an altered BRCA1 or BRCA2 gene are three to seven times more likely to develop breast cancer than women without alterations in those genes. They are also more likely to be diagnosed at an earlier age than the general population. The lifetime risk of developing ovarian cancer is increased as well: from 1.7% in the general population to 16–60% for women with BRCA1 or BRCA2 mutations. Men with an altered BRCA1 or BRCA2 gene also have an increased risk of breast cancer (primarily if the alteration is in BRCA2) and possibly prostate cancer. BRCA2 gene mutations also have been linked to an increased risk of lymphoma, melanoma, and cancers of the pancreas, gallbladder, bile duct, and stomach in some men and women. Women who carry the BRCA mutations can substantially reduce their risk to develop cancer by having preventive surgery to remove their breasts and ovaries.

Genetic tests can also discover two inherited conditions that increase the risk for colon cancer. People with familial adenomatous polyposis (FAP) develop hundreds and even thousands of polyps very early in life and have an almost 100% lifetime risk to develop colon cancer. Hereditary nonpolyposis colon cancer (HNPCC), also known as Lynch syndrome, is another condition that increases the risk of developing colon cancer, as well as cancers of the endometrium, ovaries, stomach, and other organs. Persons with HNPCC also develop polyps, but not as many and not at as young an age as people with FAP. They have an 80% lifetime risk to develop colon cancer, and the average age of diagnosis is 44, as opposed to 65 in the general population. People with FAP or HNPCC can substantially reduce their risk for developing colon cancer by having preventive surgery to remove the colon.

The decision to be tested for a genetic disposition for cancer is very complex. Genetic counselors are trained professionals who help people understand and navigate the process. Counselors meet with people who are considering testing to make certain that the person is psychologically prepared to cope with the possibility of a positive test. They also provide information to help the person contemplate and weigh the potential benefits and risks. If the individual decides to proceed with testing, counselors help him or her and the family adjust to the test results and assist them in arranging appropriate prevention and screening measures. Genetic counselors are well versed in the confidentiality, insurance, and job discrimination issues that may arise as a result of genetic testing. The test itself is a simple blood test.

Most information sources about cancer genetics offer separate sections for specific cancer types. It is important to include information about the role of genetic counselors when responding to questions about genetic testing.

Information Sources

Brochures, Booklets, and Other Short Print Publications

General

➤ National Cancer Institute. *Understanding Gene Testing.*
This booklet explains what genes are, how they work, and how faulty genes trigger diseases such as cancer. The benefits and limitations of gene testing and the role of genetic counselors are discussed as well. Access at: https://cissecure.nci.nih.gov/ncipubs/

Breast and ovarian cancer risk

➤ Canadian Cancer Society. *Hereditary Breast Cancer.*
This publication is designed to help those who have a family member diagnosed with breast cancer determine if they have an increased risk of getting this disease. Topics covered include breast cancer risk factors, heredity of breast cancer, prevention, screening, and treatment of breast cancer. Includes a glossary, personal notes, and a questions section. Access at: www.cancer.ca

➤ National Cancer Institute. *Genetic Testing for Breast Cancer Risk: It's Your Choice.*
This overview of genetic testing for breast and ovarian cancer risk describes testing and explains terms such as *family history, BRCA genes,* and *inherited cancer risk.* Advantages and disadvantages of genetic testing are detailed in a table, along with a list of questions to ask the doctor and/or genetic counselor. Access at: https://cissecure.nci.nih.gov/ncipubs/

Colorectal cancer risk

➤ Canadian Cancer Society. *Family History of Colorectal (Bowel) Cancer.*
This 24-page booklet is targeted to people with a family history of colorectal cancer. Covers the factors that increase the chance of getting colorectal cancer, the role of genetics in colorectal cancer, and what people can do to lower risk. A French-language version also is available. Access at: www.cancer.ca

➤ Johns Hopkins University.
➣ *Familial Adenomatous Polyposis (FAP) Guide*
➣ *Hereditary Nonpolyposis Colorectal Cancer (HNPCC) Guide*
➣ *Adenomatous Polyposis Coli (APC) Guide*
➣ *Peutz-Jeghers Syndrome Guide*
This is a series of guides for specific genetic conditions that increase the risk for colorectal cancer. The publications explain the conditions, how they affect risk, and how they are diagnosed. Follow-up guidelines for

people with these conditions are also covered. Printable Adobe Acrobat (.pdf) files are available at the Digestive Disease Library of the Johns Hopkins Medical Institutions Web site at: http://hopkins-gi.nts.jhu.edu.

Books

➤ Zimmerman, Barbara. 2004. *Understanding Breast Cancer Genetics.* Jackson, MS: University of Mississippi Press.
This book helps readers understand the genetic bases of both sporadic and inherited breast cancer. It describes how BRCA1, BRCA2, and other genes are passed on and the role they have in the development of breast cancer. The last chapter, "Issues in Prevention and Control of Breast Cancer," explains what risk is, and what is known about breast cancer prevention, and reviews the benefits and consequences of genetic testing. This book may be useful for the sophisticated reader who is interested in learning the science of breast cancer genetics. It does not give practical, specific advice or recommendations.

Web Resources

Sites focusing on breast and ovarian cancer genetics

➤ FORCE. Facing Our Risk of Cancer Empowerment. Access at: www.facing ourrisk.org
FORCE is an organization for women who have, or may be at risk for, a genetic mutation that may cause breast and ovarian cancer. The site helps women understand risk, genetic testing, and legal and ethical issues facing those with a confirmed BRCA mutation. Preventative measures that may reduce risk are discussed in detail, including prophylactic mastectomy, surgical menopause, chemoprevention, and more.

Detailed sections in genetics sites

➤ Genetic Health. Access at: www.genetichealth.com
This site provides consumers with educational information to help them understand and assess genetic risk of common diseases, including cancer. Many sections on the site are relevant to cancer information seekers, such as "Genetics 101," which provides a scientific overview of genetics in lay terms, and "Genetics Testing," which explains the testing process. The section "Ethical Issues" discusses genetic discrimination and health insurance. In addition, the site has separate sections on specific cancers, and the "Resources" section enables users to locate genetic counselors and support groups.

➤ National Library of Medicine. *Genetics Home Reference*. Access at: http:// ghr.nlm.nih.gov

Genetics Home Reference is the National Library of Medicine's Web site for consumer information about genetic conditions and the genes or chromosomes responsible for those conditions. People looking for information on cancer genetics will be interested in the condition summaries that describe the genetic causes and pattern of inheritance for specific cancer types. The *Help Me Understand Genetics Handbook* is an illustrated, basic explanation of how genes work and how mutations cause disorders. The site includes a glossary and a link library to genetics resources on the Web and organizations that provide patient support and advocacy.

Detailed sections in cancer sites

➤ National Cancer Institute. *Cancer Genetics*. Access at: www.cancer.gov and click on "Prevention, Genetics, Causes" and then on "Cancer Genetics."

This section links to PDQ® statements of genetics of specific cancers and to a cancer genetics services directory that enables users to find professionals who provide services related to cancer genetics, such as cancer risk assessment, genetic counseling, genetic susceptibility testing, and others. It also links to a talking glossary of genetics terms and an online tutorial on gene testing.

➤ People Living with Cancer. *Genetics*. Access at: www.plwc.org. Select "Learning about Cancer" in the left sidebar and then click on "Genetics."

This section has articles explaining the genetic aspects of several cancer types and discussing issues such as the pros and cons of genetic testing, sharing results with the family, and ethical, legal, and social issues of cancer genetics.

Patient-Support Organizations

➤ FORCE. Facing Our Risk of Cancer Empowerment. Access at: www.facing ourrisk.org

Phone: 866-288-7475

Chapter 7

Cancer Treatments

Bone Marrow Transplantation

Bone marrow transplantation (BMT) is a procedure that restores immature blood-forming cells called stem cells that were destroyed by high doses of chemotherapy and/or radiation therapy. Some cancers require very high doses of anticancer drugs in order to achieve cure or remission. The problem is that along with cancer cells, high doses of chemotherapy eradicate all of the stem and blood cells in the body. This is a lethal complication: without white blood cells, patients would not be able to fight infection, and without platelets, the cells responsible for clotting, patients could die from bleeding. Transplantation of stem cells right after high-dose chemotherapy enables patients to start producing new blood cells and recover from the toxic treatment.

Bone marrow transplantations have been widely used since the 1980s and have greatly improved survival and outlook statistics for people with leukemia, lymphoma, and multiple myeloma. They are also utilized to treat neuroblastoma, a type of childhood cancer, and a few other tumors.

BMT is a complex multistep procedure that requires meticulous planning and coordination. The process begins with harvesting the stem cells to be transplanted. Traditionally, stem cells were obtained from the marrow inside the pelvic bone in an invasive procedure that required general anesthesia. In recent years, a simpler procedure that retrieves stem cells from the bloodstream, as opposed to the bone marrow, has become more widespread. The procedure is called peripheral stem cells transplantation (PSCT). After the cells are harvested, the patient is given high doses of chemotherapy and sometimes radiation therapy. Lastly, the harvested stem cells are infused into the patient's vein, just like any other blood product, and find their way to the bone marrow, where they multiply and start producing healthy blood cells.

There are two main types of transplants. In autologous transplants, the patient's own marrow or stem cells are harvested before the administration of high-dose chemotherapy and infused back after treatment. In allogeneic transplants, bone marrow or peripheral stem cells from a healthy donor are transplanted. To prevent the recipient's immune system from rejecting the donated cells, the medical team searches for a donor whose white blood cells match the recipient's cells in terms of their genetic makeup. The degree of side effects and long-term complications the patient may suffer is directly related to how closely the donor's cells match the recipient's. About 30% of patients have a sibling who can be a suitable donor, and the rest may be able to find an unrelated matched donor through donor registries.

Transplant recipients experience short- and long-term side effects similar to those of standard chemotherapy, but at higher intensity and longer duration. They have to take stronger precautions against infection and bleeding than do people on standard chemotherapy. Allogeneic transplant recipients are also at risk to develop graft-versus-host disease (GVHD). This disease develops if the donor's immune cells attack certain organs, such as the skin, gastrointestinal tract, liver, and lungs. GVHD increases the risk for infection and may cause damage to the affected organs. Many patients recover from GVHD, but some symptoms may persist for a long time.

For many allogeneic transplant recipients, life after a transplant is described as "a new normal." Every patient must have a caregiver who stays beside him or her during the hospitalization and the initial recovery period at home for a total of three months. Allogeneic transplant recipients are not expected to return to work for about a year following the transplant. Many survivors experience long-term side effects that require ongoing medical care. The "new normal" may also bring about changes in emotional well-being, relationships, work, and social environment. Topics of interest for people treated with BMT or PSCT include nutrition, pain, fertility, insurance, fundraising, and employment rights.

Caregivers are a separate group with its own unique informational needs that include all the topics described above, as well as advocating for patients and caregivers' stress and burnout.

Information Sources

Brochures, Booklets, and Other Short Print Publications

> ➤ Bone Marrow Foundation. *Autologous Bone Marrow/Stem Cell Transplantation* and *Allogeneic Bone Marrow/Stem Cell Transplantation*.
> These booklets provide detailed yet easy-to-read overviews of the transplantation process starting with the basics of transplantation and including finding a donor, pre-transplantation planning, the hospital stay, post-transplant issues, and going home. Includes a glossary, a resource

guide, and a list of further reading. Available also in Spanish. Access at: www.bonemarrow.org

➤ Leukemia & Lymphoma Society. *Blood and Marrow Stem Cell Transplantation.*

This booklet is aimed at blood cancer patients facing a bone marrow or stem cell transplantation. It provides detailed explanations of different types of transplantations and a step-by-step description of the procedure. The section on allogeneic transplantations reviews side effects, infections, and graft-versus-host disease. Access at: www.leukemia-lymphoma.org

➤ National Bone Marrow Transplant Link. *Resource Guide for Stem Cell Transplant, Including Bone Marrow, Peripheral Blood, and Cord Blood: Friends Helping Friends.*

This 52-page reference booklet offers a wide range of topics providing an overview of the transplant process. Highlighted are financial and insurance concerns, and physical and practical issues. Includes a discussion of pediatric transplants and caregiving. Access at: www.nbmtlink.org

Books

➤ Carrier, Ewa, and Gracy Ledingham. 2004. *100 Questions and Answers about Bone Marrow and Stem Cell Transplantation.* Boston: Jones and Bartlett.

Detailed information about bone marrow and stem cell transplantation is presented in an easy-to-read question-and-answer format. Terms are explained in the sidebar, and the book includes lists of Web sites, organizations, literature, and resources. This book was co–authored by a physician and a bone marrow transplant survivor.

➤ Fairview-University Blood and Marrow Transplant Services. 2004. *Blood and Marrow Transplantation: A Patient's Guide to Hematopoietic Stem Cell Transplantation.* Minneapolis, MN: Fairview Press.

This book was published by a transplant center affiliated with the University of Minnesota with the purpose of educating patients and caregivers about BMT. It includes chapters on preparing for BMT (with checklists for both adults and children), the transplant process, possible complications, and living well, both physically and emotionally, after a BMT. It provides black-and-white illustrations, a glossary, and a list of resources.

➤ Jacobs, Myra, et al. 2003. *Caregivers' Guide for Bone Marrow/Stem Cell Transplant: Practical Perspectives.* Southfield, MI: National Bone Marrow Transplant Link.

This book focuses on the significant role of the BMT caregiver. Each chapter was authored by a real caregiver who provides his or her own specific perspective as a spouse, parent, health-care professional, or friend of an adult or a child going through the BMT process. The authors offer practical suggestions for coping with medical, practical, and emotional challenges. Access an Adobe Acrobat (.pdf) file at: www.nbmtlink. org

➤ Stewart, Susan K., et al. 1999. *Autologous Stem Cell Transplants: A Handbook for Patients*. Highland Park, IL: Blood & Marrow Transplant Information Network.

A patient advocate and BMT survivor wrote this handbook for patients and caregivers who face an autologous transplant. It discusses the 'nuts and bolts' of a transplant, choosing a transplant center, finding a donor, emotional and psychological considerations, practical issues, and medical topics. A special chapter addresses the unique issues of children undergoing a transplant, including stress and anxiety in the family and school reentry. The last chapters cover long-term survivors, sexuality, fertility, insurance, and fundraising.

➤ Stewart, Susan K. 2002. *Bone Marrow and Blood Stem Cell Transplants: A Guide for Patients*. Highland Park, IL: Blood & Marrow Transplant Information Network.

This is a similar book to *Autologous Stem Cell Transplants: A Handbook for Patients*, described above, except that it focuses on allogeneic transplants. In addition to the chapters mentioned above, this book discusses finding a donor and graft-versus-host disease.

➤ Stronach, Keren. 2002. *Survivors' Guide for Bone Marrow/Stem Cell Transplant: What to Expect and How to Get Through It*. Southfield, MI: National Bone Marrow Transplant Link.

The author, who is a survivor of two bone marrow transplants, provides a step-by-step description of the transplant process, while weaving in her experiences and those of 25 other bone marrow transplant survivors. The purpose of the guide is to prepare patients, caregivers, and families for a transplant by aligning their expectations with actual transplant experiences. Access an Adobe Acrobat (.pdf) file at: www.nbmtlink.org

For children undergoing bone marrow or stem cell transplantation (list arranged by age)

➤ Lilleby, Kathryn Ulberg, and Chad Chronick. 2000. *Stevie's New Blood*. Pittsburgh: Oncology Nursing Press.

The story describes bone marrow transplantation (BMT) from a child's point of view, with cartoon characters and colorful illustrations. The goal is to help children know what to expect before, during, and after transplantation. Each page features two text levels: a large-print version for kids ages 6 to 10 and a small-print version for ages 10 to 17. Younger children can follow the illustrations.

➤ Crowe, Karen. 1999. *Me and My Marrow: A Kid's Guide to Bone Marrow Transplants.* Deerfield, IL: Fugisawa Healthcare, Inc.

Humorous illustrations accompany the text in this comprehensive nonfiction overview of the bone marrow transplantation. The three main parts—before, during, and after transplantation—provide detailed explanations of medical and emotional issues. Appropriate for children between the ages of 10 and 18. Access at: www.meandmymarrow.com (It is possible to view the book as a series of Web pages, or download an Adobe Acrobat (.pdf) file for printing.)

Audiovisual Resources

➤ *The New Normal: Life after Bone Marrow/Stem Cell Transplant.* Directed by National Bone Marrow Transplant Link and Sue Marx Films. 1 videocassette (47 min.). nbmtLINK, 2001.

This 45-minute film includes interviews with survivors and BMT clinicians. Part 1 features six transplant recipients who tell how they dealt with the news that a bone marrow transplant could be their only hope for life. It also offers practical advice on how to choose the right transplant team, how to deal with financial concerns, and the reactions patients can expect from friends and family. Part 2 looks at the transplant process itself, and part 3 focuses on the recovery process and the joy experienced by patients and their families as they regain their new normal lives. The tone is hopeful yet realistic. Single copies of the film can be obtained free of charge while supplies last. Available in VHS, and the organization is planning a DVD edition once funding is secured. To order, access: www.nbmtlink. org.

➤ National Marrow Donor Program. *The Paths to Progress/Los Pasos Hacia el Progreso: Understanding Blood Stem Cell Transplants.*

This bilingual CD-ROM in English and Spanish explains the transplant process in easy-to-understand language. Includes a workbook that supports key messages heard on the CD and provides tools to help learn more about transplant. To order a free copy, access: www.marrow.org.

Audiovisual resources for children undergoing bone marrow or stem cell transplantation

➤ National Marrow Donor Program. *Discovery to Recovery: A Child's Guide to Bone Marrow Transplant.*

This is an educational, interactive DVD and booklet for children ages 5 to 9 who will be undergoing a marrow or cord blood transplant. The DVD tells the transplant story through two engaging puppets and provides interviews with children and their families who have been through the transplant process. The accompanying booklet is designed as a supportive tool to promote transplant discussion within the family. To order a free copy, access: www.marrow.org.

Web Resources

Sites focusing on BMT

➤ Bone Marrow Foundation. Access at: www.marrowfoundation.org
This Web site has information about the resources, programs, and services provided by this patient-support organization. The resource-center section includes a database of medical articles searchable by topic and keyword. The site also includes an archive of questions to experts, a comprehensive listing of organizations, and a list of transplant centers.

➤ BMTInfoNet. Access at: www.bmtinfonet.org
This organization offers help and information for persons facing or surviving a bone marrow, blood stem cell, or umbilical cord blood transplant. They published several books on the topic. The site includes a transplant-center locator, a resource directory, a drug database and information about the organization's support services. An "Archive of The Blood and Marrow Transplant Newsletter" contains the full text of articles that were published in this quarterly since 1992.

➤ National Bone Marrow Transplant Link. Access at: www.nbmtlink.org
This site is designed to help patients, caregivers, and families understand and deal with the emotional and practical aspects of transplants and post-transplant concerns. It includes a digital library that contains references to hundreds of journal articles, booklets, and reference materials, as well as comprehensive links to additional online information. The site also includes Adobe Acrobat (.pdf) files of the NBMTLink publications listed above.

➤ National Marrow Donor Program (NMDP). Access at: www.marrow.org
The NMDP is a worldwide network of more than 500 leading medical facilities in marrow and blood cell transplantation. The "Donor Resources" section has information for marrow donors and those thinking of joining the registry. "Patient Resources" is for patients and caregivers. The information is provided for adults and children who are in different stages of treatment: pre-transplant, during transplant, and post-transplant. A

step-by-step guide to financial planning and transcripts of virtual conferences also are available. The NMDP publishes several booklets and audiovisual resources that can be ordered free of charge by clicking on the link "Request Patient Materials."

Detailed overviews in general cancer sites

➤ American Cancer Society. *Bone Marrow and Peripheral Blood Stem Cell Transplants.* Access at: www.cancer.org and click on "Patients, Family, & Friends"; then click on "Preparing for Treatment."
This section has detailed overviews discussing stem cells, stem cell transplant types, allogeneic transplantations, the donor experience, and problems in the post-transplant period.

Sections about bone marrow/stem cell transplantation are also available at the following sites

➤ Cancerbackup. *Stem Cell & Bone Marrow Transplants.* Access at: www.cancerbackup.org.uk/home and click on "Treatments."
➤ CancerConsultants.com. *Stem Cell Transplant Information Center.* Access at: www.cancerconsultants.com
➤ OncoLink. *Bone Marrow Transplants.* Access at: www.oncolink.com

Patient-Support Organizations

➤ The Bone Marrow Foundation. Access at: www.bonemarrow.org
Phone: 800-365-1336
➤ National Bone Marrow Transplant Link. Access at: nbmtlink.org
Phone: 800-546-5268

Drug Therapies

For most people the term *anticancer drugs* is synonymous with the term *chemotherapy*; however, other classes of drugs are utilized in order to kill cancer cells or halt the growth of tumors. The purpose of this section is to enable librarians to provide answers to questions about drugs typically used in cancer treatment. Patients may have questions about the mechanism, efficacy, and side effects of drugs. This information may be used in decision making regarding treatment options, or as preparation before starting treatment.

Chemotherapy is a class of drugs that interacts with the cell cycle mechanism portion of DNA and RNA and destroys cells that multiply rapidly. The notorious side effects of chemotherapy, such as hair loss, nausea, and inability to fight infection, occur because these drugs affect healthy cells as well as cancer cells. Cells that multiply rapidly—such as hair follicles, blood-forming cells, and cells in the gastrointestinal tract—are most vulnerable to the effects of chemotherapy. The list of side effects is very long, and while it is true that most patients do not experience all the side effects on the list, chemotherapy treatment profoundly affects the lives of patients. Most people on chemotherapy need to make changes to their daily routine in terms of diet, activity level, employment, and social interactions. Practical and emotional support from family and friends greatly contributes to a person's ability to cope with the challenges of chemotherapy. Topics of interest for people before or during treatment include nutrition, hair loss, infection prevention, fatigue, sexuality, fertility, and practical issues such as employment rights and insurance. Most side effects of chemotherapy are reversible, but a few, such as damage to the heart or the reproductive system, may be long–term or even permanent.

Hormonal therapy is a class of drugs that blocks the production of hormones that promote some types of cancer, such as breast cancer, prostate cancer, endometrial cancer, thyroid cancer, and more. Women who have estrogen-dependent tumors take hormonal therapy either to prevent new cancers or to stop the growth of metastatic tumors. Several drugs that block estrogen are available, and in some cases surgical removal of the ovaries is performed. Premenopausal women may experience the onset of menopause as a result of hormonal therapy. This is usually reversible unless the ovaries have been removed. Postmenopausal women experience side effects that vary according to the specific drug. These may include hot flashes and loss of bone density. Men with prostate cancer take drugs to block the male hormones called androgens. Side effects may include loss of libido, impaired sexual function, hot flashes, osteoporosis, weight gain, breast tenderness, and breast enlargement. The effects of these drugs are reversible and disappear once therapy is stopped.

In recent years new classes of anticancer drugs have been developed. Immunotherapy, biological response modifiers, or biological therapy are all synonyms that refer to drugs utilizing the immune system to destroy malignant cells. Interferons, interleukins, and monoclonal antibodies are the most commonly used biological therapies. Cancer vaccines and gene therapy are still being studied in clinical trials. Side effects vary by type of therapy and may include a rash or swelling at the injection site, lowered blood pressure, and flulike symptoms such as fever, chills, nausea, vomiting, loss of appetite, fatigue, bone pain, and muscle pain.

Another new class of drugs are targeted therapies. These drugs target various proteins that exist only in malignant cells and not in healthy cells. The ability of these drugs to kill cancer cells selectively while avoiding healthy cells helps reduce side effects. A few of these drugs already have been approved by the FDA; for example, imatinib mesylate (Gleevec) has been approved to treat chronic myeloid leukemia and gastrointestinal stromal tumor. Gefitinib (Iressa) is indicated for the treatment of advanced non-small-cell lung cancer.

In addition to anticancer drugs, cancer patients are likely to use other drugs for supportive care. For example, colony-stimulating factors (CSFs) are biological response modifiers that help patients recover quickly from the effects of chemotherapy by boosting the count of white or red blood cells. Cancer patients may also use pain medications, antinausea drugs, steroids, and antiseizure drugs.

Librarians may also encounter questions regarding drug administration. Most chemotherapy drugs and many of the immunotherapy drugs are delivered by intravenous (IV) infusion. People whose treatment plan requires frequent IV drug administrations are offered the option of an implantable catheter. A catheter eliminates the pain associated with IV insertions and can also be used to draw blood and infuse fluids or blood products. Many types of catheters are available; some are permanent and may be used for many months or even years. Patients may ask for information to help them decide on the device most suitable for them.

Information Sources

Brochures, Booklets, and Other Short Print Publications

➤ CancerCare. *Understanding and Managing Chemotherapy Side Effects.*
  A concise overview of chemotherapy side effects, with a list of frequently asked questions, a glossary, and a list of resources. Access at: www.cancer care.org/reading.html

➤ Leukemia & Lymphoma Society. *Understanding Drug Therapy and Managing Side Effects.*
  This booklet is intended for people with blood cancers, but it may be useful for any person who wants to understand drug therapy in depth. It has a section about drug administration methods and reviews side effects by body system, such as the gastrointestinal tract, skin and hair, and blood cell formation. A list of potential side effects by individual drugs may be particularly helpful, although only drugs used to treat blood cancers are included. Access at: www.leukemia-lymphoma.org

➤ National Cancer Institute. *Chemotherapy and You: A Guide to Self-Help during Cancer Treatment.*

This booklet explains the principles of chemotherapy and what can be expected during treatment. It provides a detailed review of possible side effects with practical tips for management. Includes sections on nutrition during chemotherapy, getting support, complementary therapies, paying for chemotherapy, and lists of questions for doctors. Access at: https://cis secure.nci.nih.gov/ncipubs/

➤ National Cancer Institute. *Helping Yourself during Chemotherapy: 4 Steps for Patients.*

An easy-to-read booklet to help patients understand the importance of telling their doctor about any medicines they are taking, reporting any side effects, and informing him or her about any emotional problems that arise. Access at: https://cissecure.nci.nih.gov/ncipubs/

➤ National Cancer Institute. *Biological Therapy.*

This very short publication includes an explanation of the immune system, cancer vaccines, and a few terms. Access at: https://cissecure. nci.nih.gov/ncipubs/

Books

➤ Cukier, Daniel, et al. 2005. *Coping with Chemotherapy and Radiation.* New York: McGraw-Hill.

This book is written by oncologists with the goal of helping people prepare and manage their cancer treatment. It reviews the basics of chemotherapy and radiation therapy and provides guidance with regard to diet and lifestyle adjustment that may ease discomfort. Side effects of chemotherapy are reviewed by body system and by disease. Chapter 5 covers metastatic cancer, with a description of treatment for different body areas where metastases have been found. This is a comprehensive book that discusses many supportive-care concerns such as pain control, sexuality, and end-of-life issues.

➤ Dodd, Marylin J. 2001. *Managing the Side Effects of Chemotherapy and Radiation Therapy.* New ed. San Francisco: UCSF Nursing Press.

An oncology nurse who provides practical suggestions for managing the side effects of chemotherapy and radiation therapy wrote this book. Part 1 of the book is dedicated to chemotherapy and lists the drugs alphabetically with their specific signs, symptoms, and possible side effects. In addition, it reviews each side effect with a description, information concerning duration, self-care measures, and guidance as to when to consult with a clinician.

➤ Fromer, Margot Joan. 2001. *The Journey to Recovery: A Complete Guide to Cancer Chemotherapy.* Holbrook, MA: Adams Media Corp.

The book starts with a detailed explanation of the science behind chemo-therapy, biological therapy, and other cancer therapies. It has chapters on side effects, nutrition, and pain control. The chapter on nontraditional cancer therapies provides the reader with some tools to evaluate which therapies may be harmful or useful during therapy. Includes a list of oncology drugs and their indications and side effects.

➤ Joyner, Brenda L. 2002. *Chemo Sabe: A Guide to Being a Personal Advocate for a Chemotherapy Patient.* Battery Park, VA: Polonius Press.

This book was written for caregivers of people undergoing cancer therapy. It includes advice on the logistics of planning appointments and treatments, understanding blood test results, monitoring the drugs, optimizing insurance benefits and minimizing hassles, cooking for the person with cancer and the family, and using the Internet to find information and support. Included is advice on coping with caregiver's stress and creating a positive environment.

➤ Lyss, Alan P., Humberto Fagundes, and Patricia Corrigan. 2005. *Chemotherapy and Radiation for Dummies.* Hoboken, NJ: Wiley.

The purpose of this guide is to walk cancer patients through the entire process of chemotherapy and radiation therapy. The authors are cancer specialists who explain what people can expect during treatment and what choices they can make in order to make therapy easier. Many practical tips about managing symptoms and side effects are described, as well as effective ways to work with health care professionals and several complementary therapies that may be helpful during treatment. This comprehensive and detailed book is rich in graphical elements, such as bold headings, bullet points, icons, illustrations, and tables, that may help comprehension.

➤ Wilkes, Gail M., and Terri B. Ades. 2004. *Consumers Guide to Cancer Drugs.* Boston: Jones and Bartlett.

Easy-to-read short monographs describing over 200 cancer treatment and symptom-management drugs. Each drug entry includes information on the drug's action, how to take the drug, precautions, side effects, and other important facts. Has an index for generic and trade names.

Audiovisual Resources

➤ Nessim-Keeney, Susan, Bruce Postman, and Cancervive. *The Road Ahead Coping with Chemotherapy: For Patients and Families.* Cancervive, 2004.

This is a two-program set with one video addressing cancer patients and the other designed especially for family members. Presents practical advice from cancer specialists and personal insights from people who have gone through chemotherapy. Total running time is 32 minutes. Available in DVD and VHS formats. To order, access: www.cancervive.org

➤ Information Television Network. *Revolutionizing Chemo*. Boca Raton, FL: Information Television Network. (30 min.). [2005]. Available in DVD and VHS formats. To order, access at: http://www.itvisus.com or Amazon.com. Part of the public television series *Healthy Body/Healthy Mind*, this episode features cancer specialists explaining advances in chemotherapy that make treatments more effective with fewer side effects and enable patients to work and be active during their treatment. The program also features cancer patients discussing their experience with chemotherapy. Color graphics and animations illustrate the scientific content.

➤ Information Television Network. *Targeted Cancer Therapy*. Boca Raton, FL: Information Television Network. (30 min.). [2005]. Available in DVD and VHS formats. To order, access at: http://www.itvisus.com or Amazon.com Part of the public television series *Healthy Body/Healthy Mind*, this program features cancer specialists explaining how targeted therapies work and introduces patients and families describing their experience with targeted therapies. Color graphics and animations illustrate the scientific content.

➤ Patient Education Institute. *Chemotherapy Interactive Tutorial*. Access at: www.medlineplus.gov, click on "Interactive Tutorials" and select from a list. This slideshow utilizes illustrations, sound, and animations to provide basic, easy-to-understand explanations of chemotherapy and its more common side effects. It is possible to turn on a voice-over or print a text version.

Web Resources

Sites focusing on drug therapy in cancer

➤ Food and Drug Administration (FDA). *Approved Oncology Drugs*. Access at: www.fda.gov/cder/cancer/approved.htm
The Food and Drug Administration provides access to a database of approved oncology drugs. Each entry links to an approval summary, clinical studies that were done on the drug, and a product label. Includes information on drugs in the approval process and on how to access drugs that have not yet been approved by the FDA.

➤ Chemocare.com. Access at: www.chemocare.com
Scott Hamilton and the Cleveland Clinic present this comprehensive site of detailed information on chemotherapy. It includes detailed explanations about the science behind chemotherapy, as well as guidance on

coping with and managing chemotherapy side effects. This well-organized site also offers an opportunity for users to tell their cancer story and interact with other chemotherapy patients.

➤ MedlinePlus. *Drugs, Supplements, and Herbal Information*. Access at: http://medlineplus.gov and click on "Drug and Supplements."

Drug information monographs for prescription and over-the-counter medication from MedMaster™, a product of the American Society of Health-System Pharmacists (ASHP). Information on herbs and supplements is from Natural Standard©.

Detailed overviews in general cancer sites

➤ American Cancer Society. *Chemotherapy: What It Is, How It Helps; Chemotherapy Principles* and *Understanding Chemotherapy: A Guide for Patients and Families*. Access at: www.cancer.org, click on "Paients, Family, & Friends" and then on "Preparing for Treatment."

➤ National Cancer Institute. *Treatment*. Access at: www.cancer.gov and click on "Treatment," under "Cancer Topics."

The top section of the site links to information about various drug therapies, drugs in development, and drug information.

➤ OncoLink. *Cancer Treatment Information*. Access at: www.oncolink.com and click on "Cancer Treatment Information" in the left sidebar.

This section has overviews of chemotherapy and biologic, hormonal, and other drug therapies.

Sections about drug therapy are also available at the following sites

➤ Cancerbackup. *Chemotherapy*. Access at: www.cancerbackup.org.uk/home and click on "Treatments."

➤ CancerConsultants.com. *Chemotherapy Information Center*. Access at: www.cancerconsultants.com

Radiation Therapy

More than half of the people with cancer receive radiation therapy, also called radiotherapy or irradiation, as part of their treatment protocol. Radiation therapy consists of aiming penetrating high-energy beams of radiation at tumors in order to destroy cancer cells. The source for the radiation comes from X-rays, gamma rays, neutrons, and other radioactive materials.

Radiation is given as a curative treatment as well as palliative treatment in advanced disease. Administration of radiation therapy can be done in several ways. The most common technique is external radiation, which is administered utilizing a machine called a linear accelerator. The accelerator directs the radiation beams at the tumor and a small margin around it. This type of treatment requires multiple short outpatient visits. In most cases, radiation is given every day (Monday–Friday) for a specific period of time that can range from a few days to six or eight weeks. There are several methods to deliver external radiation to treat specific types of tumors

- ➤ Three-dimensional conformal radiation therapy utilizes a computer simulation to produce an accurate image of the tumor and surrounding organs so that multiple radiation beams can be shaped exactly to the contour of the treatment area. Because the radiation beams are precisely focused, nearby normal tissue is spared.
- ➤ Intensity-modulated radiation therapy (IMRT) is a form of 3-dimensional conformal radiotherapy. It uses sophisticated software and hardware to vary the shape and intensity of radiation delivered to different parts of the treatment area in order to reduce the dose of radiation to the surrounding healthy tissue.
- ➤ Stereotactic radiosurgery is used to treat brain tumors. With this technique, many radiation beams are delivered through a special helmet that focuses the beams and aims them at the target tissue from many directions.
- ➤ CyberKnife and the Peacock system also are used to treat brain tumors. These systems use special machinery that moves around the patient's head while delivering small doses of radiation from hundreds of directions. The beams continuously change shape and size to conform to the shape and size of the tumor while avoiding vital structures in the brain.

People who receive external beam radiation do not have radiation in their bodies, are not radioactive, and can come in contact with everyone.

Internal radiation therapy is administered by implanting the source of radiation inside the body. This method is called brachytherapy. A radioactive material is sealed in a small device such as a thin wire, plastic tube, capsule, or metal seed. The device is placed in close proximity to the tumor or directly in it. It is also possible to give radiation using unsealed radioactive materials, which may be taken by mouth in a pill form or injected into the body. This type of treatment requires a short hospitalization. Patients who receive internal radiation therapy may give off a small amount of radiation for a short time after treatment. Several precautions can be taken to protect those coming in contact with the patient. These include staying in a private room in the hospital and/or limiting visitors, especially pregnant women and children less than 18 years of age.

A new method of internal radiation is combining it with immunotherapy by attaching radioactive molecules to monoclonal antibodies that are injected into the body. This therapy is termed "radioimmunotherapy."

Radiation therapy is painless but has side effects. When providing information about radiation therapy side effects, it is important to find out which body part is irradiated, because symptoms vary according to the area that was treated. Most side effects are reversible and can be managed effectively with medications and diet. Common short-term side effects include fatigue and skin irritation. Long-term effects include loss of fertility for people who received radiation therapy in the pelvic area and loss of saliva for people who were irradiated in the head and neck area. People who received radiation therapy have a small risk of developing secondary cancers as a result of radiation. The younger the person the higher the risk, but in most cases the benefits of radiation outweigh the risk.

Information Sources

Brochures, Booklets, and Other Short Print Publications

➤ American Society for Therapeutic Radiology and Oncology (ASTRO). *Radiation Therapy for Cancer.*
This overview describes different types of radiation therapy; the members of the treatment team; what happens before, during, and after treatment; side effects; and self-care during radiation treatment. Other brochures focusing on radiation therapy for specific cancer types are also available on this site in Adobe Acrobat (.pdf) and HTML formats. Access at: www.astro.org/patient/treatment_information/

➤ National Cancer Institute. *Radiation Therapy and You: A Guide to Self-Help during Cancer Treatment.*
This introduction to radiation therapy reviews external and internal radiation therapy, including what to expect, managing side effects, and follow-up care. Access at: https://cissecure.nci.nih.gov/ncipubs/

Books

➤ Cukier, Daniel, et al. 2005. *Coping with Chemotherapy and Radiation.* New York: McGraw-Hill.
This book is written by radiation-oncology physicians with the goal of helping people prepare and manage their cancer treatment. It reviews the basics of chemotherapy and radiation therapy and provides guidance with regards to diet and lifestyle adjustment that may ease discomfort. Side effects of radiation therapy are reviewed by body part and by disease.

Chapter 5 covers metastatic cancer, with a description of treatment for different body areas where metastases have been found. This is a comprehensive book that discusses many supportive-care concerns such as pain control, sexuality, and end-of-life issues.

➤ Dodd, Marylin J. 2001. *Managing the Side Effects of Chemotherapy and Radiation Therapy*. New ed. San Francisco: UCSF Nursing Press.

An oncology nurse who provides practical suggestions for managing the side effects of chemotherapy and radiation therapy wrote this book. Part 2 of the book is dedicated to radiation therapy. It is arranged alphabetically by side effect. Each entry includes a description, duration, self-care measures, and when to consult with a clinician.

➤ Kornmehl, Carol L. 2003. *The Best News about Radiation Therapy: How to Cope and Survive*. Howell, NJ: Academic Radiation Oncology Press.

A detailed and comprehensive overview of radiation therapy written by a radiation oncologist. The book provides a detailed description of the whole process, including the simulation and treatment-planning phases. The author reviews side effects and complications for specific body parts, as well as special radiation therapy methods.

➤ Lyss, Alan P., Humberto Fagundes, and Patricia Corrigan. 2005. *Chemotherapy and Radiation for Dummies*. Hoboken, NJ: Wiley.

The purpose of this guide is to walk cancer patients through the entire process of chemotherapy and radiation therapy. The authors are cancer specialists who explain what people can expect during treatment and what choices they can make in order to make therapy easier. Many practical tips about managing symptoms and side effects are described, as well as effective ways to work with health care professionals and several complementary therapies that may be helpful during treatment. This comprehensive and detailed book is rich in graphical elements, such as bold headings, bullet points, icons, illustrations, and tables, that may help comprehension.

Audiovisual Resources

➤ Patient Education Institute. *Radiation Therapy—Introduction, an Interactive Tutorial*. Access at: www.medlineplus.gov, click on "Interactive Tutorials" and select from a list.

This slideshow utilizes illustrations, sound, and animations to provide basic, easy-to-understand explanations of radiation therapy and its more common side effects. It is possible to turn on a voice-over or print a text version.

Web Resources

Sites focusing on radiation therapy

➤ American Society for Therapeutic Radiology and Oncology (ASTRO). *Answers to Your Radiation Therapy Questions.* Access at: www.rtanswers.org Easy-to-read, basic information about external and internal radiation therapy methods, including sections on specific cancer types. Useful features are the list of questions for doctors and a doctor-finder database that enables searching by location and subspecialty.

➤ Jeffrey Long, M.D. *Radiation Oncology Online Journal.* Access at: www.rooj.com/Patient_Info.htm.
The "Patient Information" section of this site provides a detailed explanation of the radiation therapy process and lists side effects by body part, such as the breast, head, and pelvic area. This site also discusses self-care issues such as skin care and fatigue management.

Detailed overviews in general cancer sites

➤ American Cancer Society. *Radiation Therapy Principles and Understanding Radiation Therapy: A Guide for Patients and Families.* Access at: www.cancer.org, click on "Patients, Family, & Friends" and then on "Preparing for Treatment."

➤ OncoLink. *Radiation Oncology.* Access at: www.oncolink.com and click on "Cancer Treatment Information" on the left sidebar; then select "Radiation Oncology." Includes a detailed overview of the radiation process and how radiation works.

Sections about radiation therapy are also available at the following sites

➤ Cancerbackup. *Radiotherapy.* Access at: www.cancerbackup.org.uk/home and click on "Treatments."

➤ CancerConsultants.com. *Radiation Therapy Information Center.* Access at: www.cancerconsultants.com

Complementary and Alternative Therapies

The National Center for Complementary and Alternative Medicine (NCCAM) at the National Institutes of Health (NIH) estimates that 62% of the American public utilize complementary and alternative medicine (CAM): a group of diverse medical and health-care systems, practices, and products that are not presently considered to be part of conventional medicine. Among cancer patients, studies indicate that 60% to 70% of patients use CAM, but some experts estimate that this figure may be higher.

It is important to make a distinction between complementary and alternative treatments.

➤ Alternative therapies are promoted as replacements for conventional cancer treatment, often with promises of a cure. Unlike conventional medicine, claims regarding the effectiveness of alternative therapies have not been proven in quality scientific studies and/or published in peer-reviewed journals.

➤ Complementary treatments are used together with conventional treatments with the aim of improving the patient's well-being and quality of life. Practitioners of complementary therapies do not claim to cure cancer but rather to improve symptoms and help patients cope better with the physical and emotional problems associated with cancer and its treatment. Quality scientific studies have established that some of these therapies are indeed capable of improving nausea, stress, and other cancer-related symptoms.

➤ Integrative medicine is a term used by many conventional medicine centers to describe a total approach to care that involves the patient's mind, body, and spirit. It combines conventional medicine with CAM practices that have been shown to be safe and effective in quality scientific research.

CAM therapies are divided into five main categories:

➤ Mind-body medicines are based on the belief that the mind is able to affect the body. Psychotherapy, meditation, prayer, guided imagery, and creative therapies such as art, music, and dance therapy are included in this group.

➤ Biologically based therapies use substances found in nature, such as vitamins, herbs, foods, and special diets. Examples for biologically based therapies include Essiac tea, shark cartilage, and antineoplastons. It is important to note that although these products are promoted as "natural," they are not harmless and may have severe side effects and interactions with other drugs and supplements.

➤ Manipulative and body-based methods are manipulation and/or movement of one or more parts of the body. Some examples include chiropractic or osteopathic manipulation, massage, and reflexology.

➤ Energy therapies involve the use of energy fields that are believed to surround and penetrate the human body. Examples include tai chi, qigong, reiki, and therapeutic touch.

➤ Whole medical systems are healing systems and beliefs that have evolved over time in various cultures and parts of the world. Some examples are Chinese medicine, homeopathy, and acupuncture.

Most CAM therapies, including biologically based therapies, are not typically tested in the formal process of clinical trials, in the way conventional drugs are tested and evaluated. For this reason medical professionals describe these therapies as "unproven," meaning that the claims about their effectiveness have not been proven in a scientific methodological process.

The biggest problem in providing quality information about CAM therapies is locating unbiased information. The manufacturers and sellers of these therapies distribute a lot of misleading and erroneous information that is easily accessible on the Internet. Librarians should evaluate information sources very carefully according to the criteria in Chapter 1 and educate patrons about health information evaluation. The first thing to check is if the information provider has a financial stake in the product. Promises of a "cure," claims that are based on testimonials rather than citations to peer-reviewed medical journals, or phrases like "secret formula" or "suppressed by government" should all serve as red flags that the information is dubious. The information sources listed below are good starting points for information seeking about CAM.

Librarians should encourage patients to talk to their clinicians about any CAM therapies they want to use. A study published in the 2005 American Society of Therapeutic Radiology and Oncology meeting found that 75% of the patients who used CAM therapies did not discuss this with their physicians. Keeping this information secret may be harmful. Biologically based therapies may cause devastating side effects, interact with other drugs, and even reduce the efficacy of conventional cancer therapy. Even vitamins, which many people view as safe and harmless, can interfere with chemotherapy and radiation therapy when taken in high doses. It is a good practice to give the National Cancer Institute booklet, *Thinking about Complementary and Alternative Medicine: A Guide for People with Cancer*, to any cancer patient inquiring about CAM therapies. This short booklet, which is available full-text online, emphasizes the importance of talking to the doctor about CAM and explains how to obtain quality, unbiased information about these therapies.

Information Sources

Brochures, Booklets, and Other Short Print Publications

➤ National Cancer Institute. *Thinking about Complementary and Alternative Medicine—A Guide for People with Cancer.*
  An easy-to-read booklet that describes how to make informed choices when looking for complementary and alternative medicine (CAM). Provides an overview and examples of the six domains of CAM. Access at: https://cissecure.nci.nih.gov/ncipubs/

➤ National Center for Complementary and Alternative Medicine.
  ➤ *What Is Complementary and Alternative Medicine*
  ➤ *Are You Considering Using Complementary and Alternative Medicine (CAM)?*
  ➤ *Selecting a Complementary and Alternative Medicine (CAM) Practitioner*
  ➤ *What's in the Bottle? An Introduction to Dietary Supplements*
  These and other fact sheets on the NCCAM site provide key points for people to consider before starting treatment with CAM therapies. They discuss the differences between complementary, alternative, and integrative medicine, how to evaluate claims about the effectiveness of CAM therapies, and how to locate practitioners. Also available in Spanish. Access at: http://nccam.nih.gov/

Books

➤ American Cancer Society. 2002. *American Cancer Society's Complementary and Alternative Cancer Methods Handbook*. Atlanta: American Cancer Society. This is a quick-and-easy guide about complementary and alternative therapies most commonly used by cancer patients. It contains over 200 entries on specific herbs, vitamins, minerals, mind/body, and biological therapies. Each entry describes the method and what effects may occur.

➤ American Cancer Society. 2002. *American Cancer Society's Guide to Complementary and Alternative Cancer Methods*. Atlanta: American Cancer Society. This reference tool helps patients evaluate methods of CAM therapies that have been promoted as effective for conditions related to cancer. Each entry describes the therapy and its history and provides a review of the scientific evidence in peer-reviewed medical literature. General chapters address issues of safety, doctor-patient relationship, and insurance coverage. A broad range of topics are covered, including herbs, vitamins, minerals, diet, manual healing, and alternative treatment methods.

➤ Kumar, Nagi B. 2002. *Integrative Nutritional Therapies for Cancer: A Scientific Guide to Natural Products Used to Treat and Prevent Cancer*. St. Louis, MO: Facts and Comparisons Publishing Group. Specialists from the H. Lee Moffitt Cancer Center & Research Institute provide current information on the most common complementary nutritional therapies for prevention and treatment of cancer. Arranged alphabetically, each of the 36 entries covers the background, chemistry, potential uses, safety/toxicity and recommendations based on scientific consensus and references. The appendices include a U.S. Food and Drug Administration (FDA) list of unsafe herbs, supplements associated with injury and illness, and a table of drug, nutrient, and supplement interactions.

➤ Labriola, Dan. 2002. *Complementary Cancer Therapies: Combining Traditional and Alternative Approaches for the Best Possible Outcome.* Roseville, CA: Prima Health.

This book was written for people looking to integrate complementary therapies with conventional cancer treatment in order to minimize side effects resulting from treatment. Its author is a naturopathic physician who emphasizes the importance of communication with clinicians and careful planning and evaluation before utilization of complementary treatments. The book provides advice about selecting health care providers and includes information about important interactions between conventional and unconventional therapies.

➤ O'Toole, Carole. 2002. *Healing outside the Margins: The Survivor's Guide to Integrative Cancer Care.* Washington, DC: Lifeline Press.

The author is a cancer survivor who integrated complementary therapies into her cancer treatment. She explains how to evaluate therapies and practitioners, how to discuss the issue with physicians, and how to identify quackery. The book includes detailed explanations of 25 healing techniques that may help reduce side effects and increase energy. It also includes interviews with complementary therapy practitioners and additional sources for further information. The text was reviewed by a medical oncologist.

Audiovisual Resources

➤ M. D. Anderson Cancer Center. *Patients Talk about . . . Complementary Therapies and Cancer.*

This program features six cancer patients discussing their experiences with alternative and/or complementary therapies during treatment. Also available as a CD-ROM. Can be viewed online at: www.mdanderson.org/departments/cimer.

Web Resources

Sites focusing on complementary and alternative therapies in cancer care

➤ M. D. Anderson Cancer Center. *Complementary/Integrative Medicine Education Resources (CIMER).* Access at: www.mdanderson.org/departments/cimer/

This is an extensive educational resource designed to help patients and physicians decide how best to integrate such therapies into cancer care. It includes evidence-based reviews of published research studies on many types of CAM therapies from a variety of credible sources, including the

Cochrane Review Organization, National Institutes of Health, Natural Standards, and University of Texas M. D. Anderson Cancer Center. Additional information provides a list of drug interactions and FDA advisories, news, videos, and an extensive list of other resources. Some of the information is also available in Spanish.

➤ National Cancer Institute. *Office of Cancer Complementary and Alternative Medicine (OCCAM)*. Access at: www.cancer.gov/cam/
The section "Health Information" includes links to a number of information sources on CAM therapies. Of special interest are the links to PDQ® complementary and alternative medicine summaries that present evidence-based, peer-reviewed overviews of specific therapies. The site also includes links to government information on nutritional supplements and a listing of FDA alerts.

Detailed sections in general cancer sites

➤ American Cancer Society. *Complementary and Alternative Therapies*. Access at: www.cancer.org, click on "Patients, Family, & Friends" and then on "Preparing for Treatment."
This section has overviews of specific therapies of all types of CAM therapies, including biological and pharmaceutical therapies, mind/body therapies, touch therapies, and nutritional therapies.

➤ BC Cancer Agency and Cancer Information Centre. *Unconventional Cancer Therapies*. Access at: www.bccancer.bc.ca and click on "Patient/Public Info."
This site offers overviews of specific biologically based therapies that have been promoted as cures for cancer. Each section includes direct quotations from the medical, peer-reviewed book and journal literature discussing efficacy and risk of these therapies.

➤ Memorial Sloan-Kettering Cancer Center. *About Herbs, Botanicals & Other Products*. Access at: www.mskcc.org/mskcc/html/11570.cfm.
This database of herbs and supplements has clinical summaries for each agent, with details about constituents, adverse effects, interactions, and potential benefits or problems.

➤ National Center for Complementary and Alternative Medicine (NCCAM). Access at: http://nccam.nih.gov/ and click on "Health Information."
This site offers advice on becoming an educated consumer of CAM therapies. Has information on specific therapies, drug interactions, harmful side effects, and public-health advisories.

➤ People Living with Cancer. *Complementary and Alternative Medicine (CAM)*. Access at: www.plwc.org and click on "Diagnosis and Treatment" and then on "Treating Cancer."

This section provides general advice about the safety and risks of CAM and points to consider regarding herbs and dietary supplements.

➤ Quackwatch. Access at: www.quackwatch.org and click on "Cancer: Questionable Therapies."

This site has reviews of "Dubious Treatments" as well as information on questionable tests, quackery in health care, and reports from quackery victims.

Clinical Trials

Clinical trials, also called research or treatment studies, test new treatments for people with cancer. By enrolling in a clinical trial, patients can use an experimental treatment before the U.S. Food and Drug Administration (FDA) approves it. The experimental treatment may or may not be better than the standard treatment, and enrolling in a clinical trial is not appropriate for every cancer patient. The patient and his or her doctor should evaluate the patient's circumstances, possibility of cure with standard treatment, and potential risks and benefits of the experimental treatment before enrolling in a clinical trial.

The National Cancer Institute (NCI) online database for cancer clinical trials is a good starting point for searching trials. Cancer patient organizations, cancer treatment centers, pharmaceutical companies, and other sites offer searchable databases that may list trials not listed on the NCI site. Instructions on searching the NCI database and on how to find other trial databases are listed below.

After the initial retrieval patients can start evaluating the results to see which trials may be suitable for them. One criterion to look at is the trial phase.

➤ Phase 1 trials look only at safety data. These trials attempt to establish the highest dose a person can tolerate without harmful side effects. Because the risks and benefits of the new treatment are not fully known at this point, phase 1 trials are limited to a small group of patients who cannot be helped by other treatments.

➤ Phase 2 trials look at the efficacy of the new treatment by measuring the effect the treatment had on the cancer. As in phase 1, only a small group of people takes part in phase 2 trials, because the risks are still not completely known.

➤ Phase 3 trials compare the results of people taking the new treatment with results of people taking the standard treatment. Trial participants are assigned at random to either the treatment group, which gets the new treatment, or the control group, which is given the standard treatment. Both groups are followed to see which group has a better outcome and fewer side effects. Only treatments that have shown promise in phase 1 and 2 are tested in phase 3 studies, which may include hundreds of people around the country and the world.

Each trial has very specific eligibility criteria that form a list of characteristics that participants must have in order to be in the study. These may include age, gender, type and stage of cancer, and other characteristics. The eligibility criteria enable researchers to compare patient groups and report reliable results.

Before agreeing to enroll in a clinical trial, potential participants go through an informed consent process, which requires the trial investigators to disclose all the facts about the study, including possible benefits, potential risks, and details about the treatment and tests participants will undergo. Even after signing the consent form, participants may leave the trial at any time. The NCI site has an extensive section about the rights and protections of clinical trial participants.

Another way to gain access to experimental or investigational drugs before the FDA has approved them is to apply for "compassionate use" status with the drug manufacturer. Compassionate use programs are designed for people who lack effective treatment but are not able to enroll in a clinical trial because they do not meet eligibility criteria or the trial has been filled to capacity. There is no central database for compassionate use programs, and information can be obtained only by contacting the pharmaceutical company who produced the drug the patient is interested in.

Searching and locating clinical trials is a tedious process. The largest cancer clinical trials database is the NCI database accessible at: www. Cancer.gov. This database, however, is not all-inclusive. Some investigators do not submit their trial to cancer.gov, and some trials may only be found on pharmaceutical companies databases, comprehensive cancer centers listings, or disease-specific Web sites. For a comprehensive search, it is advisable to search TrialsCentral.org, which is a database of clinical trials databases. TrialsCentral may help locate additional registries and databases to supplement a search on the NCI trials database.

Information Sources

Brochures, Booklets, and Other Short Print Publications

➤ Coalition of Cancer Cooperative Groups. *Myths and Facts about Cancer Clinical Trials.*
  This six-page brochure reviews several important facts for people considering participating in a clinical trial, including insurance and Medicare coverage. It also reviews the phases of clinical trials. Access at: www.cancertrialshelp.org

➤ National Cancer Institute. *Taking Part in Clinical Trials: What Cancer Patients Need To Know.*
This short booklet defines clinical trials, discusses what patients might expect if they participate in a trial, and lists points to consider when deciding to participate in one. Access at: https://cissecure.nci.nih.gov/ncipubs/

➤ National Cancer Institute. *Taking Part in Clinical Trials: Cancer Prevention Studies: What Participants Need To Know.*
This short booklet discusses cancer and clinical trials and helps people decide if participation in a chemoprevention trial is right for them. Access at: https://cissecure.nci.nih.gov/ncipubs/

Books

➤ Finn, Robert. 1999. *Cancer Clinical Trials: Experimental Treatments and How They Can Help You.* Cambridge, MA: O'Reilly.
A medical journalist, Finn details the structure, administration, and laws affecting clinical trials. The purpose of this book is to help people with cancer evaluate if they should consider participating in a clinical trial. The author explains the administration of trials (and the interests and involvement of players such as the FDA, pharmaceutical companies, and the National Cancer Institute), the inclusion and exclusion criteria for joining a trial, and how to read the informed consent document and the trial protocol.

➤ Mulay, Marilyn. 2002. *Making the Decision: The Cancer Patient's Guide to Clinical Trials.* Boston: Jones and Bartlett.
This book provides a practical approach to understanding the different aspects of clinical trials, from the patient's perspective. The book reviews the process of drug development, the business of clinical research, and the structure of clinical trials. It also discusses the rights of patients, the care of the research subject, and financial considerations.

Audiovisual Materials

➤ Dana-Farber Cancer Institute. *Entering a Clinical Trial: Is it Right for You?* (22 minutes.) Dana-Farber Cancer Institute, Boston. 2004. Available in VHS and DVD formats.
The goal of this audiovisual program and accompanying educational booklet is to dispel misconceptions about clinical trials. Using their own words, patients and clinicians explain what clinical trials are and offer suggestions to help patients decide whether to enroll in a study. View online or order access at: www.dana-farber.org/res/clinical/trials-info/

➤ Newsweek Productions. *Test of Hope: Cancer Clinical Trials.* 2002.

This 30-minute public television documentary looks inside the world of research studies testing experimental therapies on cancer patients. Hosted by veteran journalist Cokie Roberts, who lost her sister, Barbara, to cancer, the program puts a human face on the promise and problems of cancer clinical trials. The issues explored are told through the stories of several cancer patients—some of whom are currently in the midst of participation in a clinical trial and some of whom have completed treatment, with very different results. Order a free VHS copy from the Coalition of Cancer Cooperative Groups at: www.cancertrialshelp.org

➤ Patient Education Institute. *Clinical Trials Interactive Tutorial.* Access at: www.medlineplus.gov and click on "Interactive Tutorials," then select from a list.

This slideshow utilizes illustrations, sound, and animations to provide basic, easy-to-understand explanations of the process and structure of clinical trials. It covers informed consent, protections for participants, and how to locate clinical trials. It is possible to turn on a voice-over or print a text version.

Web Resources

➤ National Cancer Institute. *Clinical Trials.* Access at: http://www.cancer.gov/clinicaltrials

This section of Cancer.gov has information about the phase structure of clinical trials, the rights of participants, costs, and informed consent, but its main purpose is searching the National Cancer Institute (NCI) clinical trials database. Basic and advanced search forms are available, and the user selects various parameters from such menus as cancer type, stage, location of trial, phase of trial, treatments methods, and so forth. While it is possible to narrow down the retrieval by selecting numerous parameters, this search interface does not allow keyword searching. The same database can be searched through ClinicalTrials.gov, which is the National Library of Medicine gateway to all of the National Institutes of Health trials, including those in the NCI database. The ClinicalTrials.gov search form permits keyword searching, and in some cases the search results obtained through this site may be more precise and relevant than searching the Cancer.gov interface.

➤ Coalition of Cancer Cooperative Groups. Access at: www.cancertrialshelp.org

The Coalition of Cancer Cooperative Groups is a network of cancer cooperative groups, cancer centers, academic medical centers, community hospitals, physician practices, and patient-advocate groups. One of its purposes is to facilitate enrollment in clinical trials by informing patients about clinical trials and creating an easy-to-use interface for searching trials. The information section discusses misconceptions about clinical trials, informed consent, insurance considerations, and questions to ask the doctor. The user-friendly search tool is designed for the unsophisticated user. It consists of nine simple questions, such as zip code, gender, ethnicity, cancer type, and so on. After answering some or all of the questions, users receive a list of trials in which they may be eligible to enroll. The site also includes the full text of the coalition's brochures and a fact sheet, frequently asked questions, and a glossary.

➤ TrialsCentral. Access at: www.trialscentral.org

This site, from Brown University Medical School, has a database of clinical trial registers. Searchable by condition and location, this site offers links to clinical trial registers in hospitals, government agencies, pharmaceutical companies, and other Web sites. It also includes frequently asked questions and other resources.

Chapter 8

Cancer Quality-of-Life Issues

Overview of Cancer Supportive Care

C ancer is a broad term that includes over 100 different diseases that are very different from one another. The previous chapters in this book have focused on obtaining information according to specific diseases, but there are many topics that are relevant to all cancer patients and survivors. These topics encompass the physical, emotional, economic, and spiritual dimensions of life.

Physically, cancer patients and survivors may suffer from nutritional disorders, pain, sexuality and fertility problems, fatigue, and other short- and long-term effects of treatment that may require medical care. This type of care is termed "supportive care" because its goal is not to treat or cure the cancer, but rather to lessen the severity of symptoms and enable patients to have the best possible quality of life during and after treatment.

Beyond the physical and medical concerns, cancer patients and survivors are troubled with emotional, economic, and spiritual issues. Examples of emotional issues include depression and anxiety, relationship problems, parenting concerns, body-image changes, grief, and loss. On the practical side of living, survivors may be worried about financial problems, insurance denials, geographic dislocation, and transportation concerns. Survivors may also struggle with such spiritual issues as mortality, self-actualization, and existential concerns. Interestingly, many survivors feel that the physical, medical aspects are the easiest parts of the cancer experience. A study published by Lance Armstrong Foundation in 2004 reported that more than half (53%) of respondents said the practical and emotional consequences of dealing with cancer are often harder than the medical issues. One of the reasons for this finding may be that the medical problems are well taken care of by expert professionals but patients and families are often left to fend for themselves when it comes to resolving problems in other realms of living with cancer.

Optimal cancer care programs are the ones that address the full breadth of cancer distress. Comprehensive cancer programs utilize multidisciplinary care teams that capitalize on the strength of collaboration among professionals from many fields. These programs bring together the expertise of physicians and nurses, social workers, dietitians, physical and occupational therapists, music and art therapists, financial counselors, and other dedicated professionals. Librarians are becoming an integral part of the team in many cancer care programs. Providing patients and families with current and accurate information in patient-friendly language empowers people to make informed decisions and become active partners in their health care.

Despite the progress in establishing comprehensive cancer care programs, many people with cancer receive care in hospitals and clinics that do not offer these services. The lack of an organized, coordinated professional support system for the nonmedical aspects of life with cancer makes this population vulnerable to individuals and organizations that offer unprofessional and even bogus solutions to problems. It is important to ensure the authoritativeness of information about supportive-care topics.

Information about cancer supportive-care issues can be found in the general resources listed below. These are good starting points for all questions about emotional and physical problems that occur as a result of cancer and its treatment. Several topics have a number of dedicated information sources and warrant separate sections. Sections on nutrition, sexuality, fertility, pain, lymphedema, appearance, emotional distress, practical issues of cancer survivorship, end of life, and parenting through cancer appear after the general supportive-care sources. There are two strategies for locating information about conditions that do not have a separate section, such as fatigue and anemia, nausea and vomiting, neuropathy, colostomies, and incontinence.

➤ Searching the general supportive-care information sources listed below.
➤ If the condition is typical to a specific cancer population, it is wise to check information sources that are specific to the cancer type; for example, it would be possible to find information about colostomies in information sources that discuss colorectal cancer.

Information Sources

Brochures, Booklets, and Other Short Print Publications

➤ American Cancer Society. *After Diagnosis.*
This booklet covers some of the quality-of-life issues faced by cancer patients and their families. Starting with the emotional reactions to the illness, communication with family, friends, and health care providers, it

also touches on pain, sexuality, and employment during treatment. This booklet is not available online. To order, contact the American Cancer Society at 800-ACS-2345 (or 866-228-4327 for TTY).

➤ American Cancer Society. *Caring for the Patient with Cancer at Home: A Guide for Patients and Families.*
This is an A–Z list of cancer symptoms and side effects. Each topic includes a short description and bulleted lists of "What to Do," "Do Not . . .," and "Call the Doctor." It is a good basic reference for any family caring for a patient with cancer. This booklet is not available online. To order contact the American Cancer Society at: 800-ACS-2345 (or 866-228-4327 for TTY).

Books

➤ Finegan, Wesley C. 2004. *Trust Me, I'm a ~~Doctor~~ Cancer Patient.* Abingdon, England: Radcliffe Medical.
This book is written from the perspective of a palliative care physician who is also a cancer survivor. Presented in a conversational style, the author encourages patients to communicate with clinicians about problems. The book offers practical advice on dealing with many side effects and symptoms that may occur during cancer treatment, including pain management, loss of appetite, breathlessness, poor sleep, and more. The part on personal, social, and spiritual problems includes topics such as receiving bad news, body image, employment, and spiritual needs.

➤ Kelvin, Joanne Frankel, and Leslie B. Tyson. 2005. *100 Questions and Answers about Cancer Symptoms and Cancer Treatment Side Effects.* Sudbury, MA: Jones and Bartlett.
Two oncology nurses answer questions about relieving symptoms and side effects commonly experienced by cancer patients. Practical suggestions and comments from patients address many problems, including low blood counts, appearance, energy level, shortness of breath, and more. A special chapter discusses getting and evaluating information. Emotional and social concerns are covered as well. This is a user-friendly book with key points and terms explained in the sidebar. Includes a list of relevant resources, organizations, and literature.

➤ Moore, Katen, and Libby Schmais. 2001. *Living Well with Cancer: A Nurse Tells You Everything You Need to Know about Managing the Side Effects of Your Treatment.* New York: Putnam's.
This is an A–Z reference guidebook to cancer–related side effects and symptoms was written by an oncology nurse practitioner and a medical

writer. Each entry describes the problem, how it is diagnosed, and how it may be prevented. The remedies section includes conventional and complementary approaches and a list of what is not recommended. In addition to physical symptoms, the book also provides suggestions and solutions for some of the practical and emotional issues including death and dying.

➤ Rosenbaum, Ernest H., and Isadora R. Rosenbaum. 2005. *Everyone's Guide to Cancer Supportive Care: A Comprehensive Handbook for Patients and Their Families.* Kansas City, MO: Andrews & McMeel.

This thick volume includes more than 50 chapters with in-depth discussions of quality-of-life issues affecting people with cancer. The chapters are written by well-known professionals, and the entire book was edited by Ernest Rosenbaum, M.D. and Isadora Rosenbaum, both from the University of California–San Francisco Comprehensive Cancer Center. This book is appropriate for patients and caregivers looking for comprehensive information regarding physical, emotional, and spiritual needs of the patient.

Books for caregivers

➤ Houts, Peter S., Julia A. Bucher, and American Cancer Society. 2003. *Caregiving: A Step-by-Step Resource for Caring for the Person with Cancer at Home.* Rev. ed. Atlanta, GA: American Cancer Society.

This book was written for lay caregivers of cancer patients. It offers a six-step approach to solving all kinds of problems a caregiver may face. Physical, emotional, and practical challenges are discussed in chapters such as talking with children, coordinating care from one treatment setting to another, getting help from community agencies, and getting information from medical staff. Specific emotional and physical conditions are also covered including skin and vein conditions, mobility, ostomies and prostheses, sexual conditions, tiredness, and fatigue.

➤ Rose, Susannah, and Richard Hara. 2004. *100 Questions and Answers about Caring for Family Or Friends with Cancer.* Sudbury, MA: Jones and Bartlett.

This book provides answers to questions that friends and family members caring for the person with cancer may have. Topics covered include medical treatment and care, relationships and family issues, home care, medical equipment, insurance issues, emotional reactions, and practical concerns about death and dying. Terms are explained in the sidebar, and the book includes a list of Web sites, organizations, literature, and resources on general and specific topic related to lung cancer. The authors are oncology social workers from Memorial Sloan-Kettering Cancer Center.

Audiovisual Resources

➤ *Cancer Survival Toolbox*. National Coalition for Cancer Survivorship, 2004.
The *Cancer Survival Toolbox* is a free, self-learning audio program that has been developed by leading cancer organizations to help people develop important skills for better meeting and understanding the challenges of their illness. While created primarily for people who have been recently diagnosed with cancer, the *Toolbox* can help anyone who is facing hard decisions and changes in life owing to cancer. Family members and care-givers also can use the it on behalf of a child or anyone else affected by cancer. Topics covered include communication, finding information, making decisions, solving problems, negotiating, and standing up for your rights. The program is available online at: www.cancersurvivaltool-box.org and also as a compact disc that can be ordered free from the Web site. Available in English, Spanish, and Chinese.

Web Resources

Sites focusing on cancer supportive care

➤ National Coalition for Cancer Survivorship. *Palliative Care & Symptom Management*. Access at: www.canceradvocacy.org/resources/essential/
This site includes detailed information about many supportive-care issues in people with cancer including coping with the side effects of cancer and cancer treatment, such as anemia, bowel obstruction, cognitive issues, di-arrhea, fatigue, fighting infection, hair loss, loss of appetite, mouth sore-ness, nausea and vomiting, neuropathy, and sleep problems. Special sections about pain, nutrition, end-of-life, and issues of the heart and mind are also available. Has a special section on relieving side effects in children.

➤ Cancer Supportive Care. Access at: www.cancersupportivecare.com
This Web site is from the authors of the book *Everyone's Guide to Cancer Supportive Care: A Comprehensive Handbook for Patients and Their Fami-lies* described in the "Books" section a few pages back. It includes compre-hensive articles about many supportive-care topics written by cancer specialists, mostly from the University of California–San Francisco Com-prehensive Cancer Center. The site is organized using Library of Congress classification, with descriptions similar to the old library card catalog

model. It is somewhat cumbersome to navigate and search but covers some difficult-to-find topics very comprehensively.

➤ CancerSymptoms.org. Access at: www. cancersymptoms.org
The Oncology Nursing Society provides this Web site, which includes practical and very detailed information about managing cancer-related side effects and symptoms. The "Learn" section of each symptom tab provides information that explains the causes and effects of each treatment-related symptom. The "Manage" section of each symptom tab provides helpful ideas on how to control or minimize the effects of that symptom.

Detailed sections in general cancer sites

➤ American Cancer Society. *Coping with Treatment.* Access at: www.cancer. org and click on the link to "Patients, Family, & Friends" and then on "Coping with Treatment."
This site has information on coping with physical and emotional changes, as well as the logistics of cancer treatment.

➤ Cancerbackup. *Resources & Support.* Access at: www.cancerbackup.org. uk/Home and click on the link.
This section covers physical and emotional issues.

➤ Cancer.ca. *Living with Cancer.* Access at: www.cancer.ca and click on "Support/Services" and then "Living with Cancer."
This section covers nutrition, side effects management, coping with cancer, and stress management.

➤ CancerConsultants.com. *Management or Prevention of Side Effects.* Access at: www.cancerconsultants.com and click on the link on the left sidebar.

➤ CancerSource.com. *Cope with Cancer.* Access at: http://cancersource.com/ and click on the link to "Patients."

➤ National Cancer Institute. *Coping with Cancer.* Access at: www.cancer.gov and click on "Cancer Topics" and then on "Coping with Cancer."
This page links to many PDQ® statements on supportive-care issues.

➤ People Living with Cancer. *Coping.* Access at: www.plwc.org and click on "Coping" on the left sidebar.
This section covers emotional and physical challenges, relationships, end-of-life issues, and caregiving.

➤ The Wellness Community. *Frankly Speaking About Cancer: Take Control of Side Effects with Medicine, Mind and Body.* Access at: www.thewellness community.org and click on "Cancer Information" on the left sidebar.
This section covers emotional, physical, and practical issues of cancer survivorship.

Appearance and Body Image

Body image is composed of the thoughts, attitudes, and perceptions people have about the way their body looks and how it functions. Body image is closely related to self-esteem, one's entire sense of identity and value as a human being. Negative perceptions of body image lower a person's self-esteem, and positive feelings about body image elevate it. People often have conflicting feelings about their body image. During an illness that significantly alters appearance, these feelings may become even more intense. Loss of a body part or function brings about changes in body image and self-esteem that may lead to deep feelings of sadness, grief, and even depression. Changes in body image resonate in other areas of social and emotional well-being, such as sexuality, relationships, employment, and more.

A national survey conducted in 2002 by "Look Good . . . Feel Better," an American Cancer Society support program that helps women address the appearance-related side effects of cancer treatment, revealed that 78% of women with cancer experience changes in their appearance associated with treatment; 66% of women feel that their quality of life in the area of their appearance was negatively impacted by their cancer experience.

Appearance changes are not limited to hair loss, which is the appearance change most commonly associated with cancer. Treatment may also cause weight loss or gain and impair the looks of nails, eyebrows, eyelashes, and skin complexion. A study among breast cancer patients revealed that despite the fact the hair loss is a temporary side effect and has no medical significance, it is often the most difficult side effect women experience during cancer. The author of the study, Tovia G. Freedman, offers a few reasons to explain the difficulty in coping with hair loss (Freedman, 1994). Freedman suggests that together with the hair, some of a woman's sense of self and identity is lost as well because hair has such a significant symbolic value in our society as an indicator of personality, attractiveness, sexuality, and femininity. Hair loss is public and announces to the world that a person has cancer. While it is easy to conceal the loss of a breast, the public nature of hair loss forces one to confront his or her reality as a person with cancer.

Most appearance changes are temporary and disappear after treatment ends. Some people may experience permanent changes such as scars, colostomies, loss of a breast or another body part, and lasting changes in weight and hair. The information sources listed below provide excellent tips and advice on how to deal with appearance changes. Frequently, just finding effective solutions for cosmetic problems helps individuals boost body image and self-esteem and adjust to living with cancer.

Information Sources

Brochures, Booklets, and Other Short Print Publications

➤ American Cancer Society. *"TLC"—Tender Loving Care.*
This is a catalog of products for hair loss and post-mastectomy products that includes narratives on how to wear makeup, hats and scarves and how to choose, care for, and wear wigs. Access at: www.tlcdirect.org.

➤ Shop Well with You (SWY). *Shop Well with You Guide to Body Image and Cancer.*
This pamphlet focuses on clothing and helps women select clothes that will help them feel comfortable as well as attractive during cancer treatment. Images of clothing with tips on how they can be helpful are featured, and the guide offers different looks and styles such as classic, elegant, sophisticated, eclectic, tailored, and relaxed. Access at: www.shop wellwithyou.org/guide.cfm

➤ The WHO (Women Helping Others) Foundation. *Well Beauty: A Woman's Guide to Looking and Feeling Better through Cancer Diagnosis, Treatment and Recovery.*
This publication provides tips and information to enhance a patient's well-being through positive thinking, image solutions, and resource tools that educate and inform. The text focuses on makeup, skincare, and hair solutions and includes photographs and illustrations. To order access: www.whofoundation.org

Audiovisual Materials

➤ *Look Good . . . Feel Better Just for You.* Directed by Smith, Robin, Jennifer Crescenzo, and American Cancer Society et al. 1 videocassette (30 min.). American Cancer Society, 2001.
The videotape features cancer survivors and volunteers discussing appearance-related side effects of cancer treatment, as well as detailed skincare information, "how to" makeup tips, wig information, and pointers on head coverings. The companion booklet covers nail care. To order contact the Look Good . . . Feel Better program at 800-395-LOOK. This and other appearance-related videos are available for viewing online at: www.lookgoodfeelbetter.org.

➤ *Scarves: A Fashionable Alternative.* Phi Mu Foundation.
This program features a breast cancer survivor modeling and explaining how to select, tie, and wear scarves after chemotherapy induces hair loss. The topics of makeup and skin care also are covered. VHS format available

in English and Spanish. To order, contact the Phi Mu Foundation at 770-632-2090. A DVD edition is forthcoming.

Books

➤ Gafni, Ramy. 2005. *Ramy Gafni's Beauty Therapy: The Ultimate Guide to Looking and Feeling Great While Living with Cancer.* New York: M. Evans and Co.
Celebrity makeup artist and cancer survivor Ramy Gafni views improving physical appearance as therapy that helps restore self-esteem and overall well-being. Practical solutions and step-by-step instructions instruct readers on how to find stylish head coverings, thicken thinning eyebrows and eyelashes, and camouflage damaged skin. This book is written for both men and women and includes color photographs.

➤ Noyes, Diane Doan, and Peggy Mellody. 1992. *Beauty and Cancer: Looking and Feeling Your Best.* Updated ed. Dallas: Taylor.
This book is a guide designed to help women improve their appearance and comfort both during and after treatment. It discusses hair alternatives for complete and partial hair loss and offers step-by-step techniques for reconstructing eyebrows and eyelashes. Includes chapters on skin care, makeup, and clothing to accommodate above- and below-the-waist surgeries. The book provides many illustrations, a guide on choosing post-mastectomy products, and a resource guide.

➤ Ovitz, Lori, and Joanne Kabak. 2004. *Facing the Mirror with Cancer.* Chicago: Belle Press.
A professional makeup artist who has worked with cancer patients authored this beautifully produced book. Its focus is makeup and skin care for women, but it also covers wigs and nail care and addresses the special needs of men, children, and teens. This is an excellent, thorough tutorial that includes step-by-step instructions and color photographs to help explain technique and how to use makeup tools and products.

Web Resources

Sites focusing on appearance issues

➤ Look Good . . . Feel Better. Access at: www.lookgoodfeelbetter.org
Look Good . . . Feel Better is a free, non-medical, brand-neutral, national public service program to help cancer survivors offset appearance-related changes from cancer treatment. The site includes information about makeup, hair, and coping with changes. It also provides separate sections for men, teens, family members, and friends. The program finder helps

users locate local Look Good Feel Better programs in the United States. The International section has a listing of "sister" programs in other countries.

➤ Shop Well With You. Access at: www.shopwellwithyou.org

Shop Well with You (SWY) is a not-for-profit organization and body-image resource for women surviving cancer, their caregivers, and health care providers. The Web site offers guidance on how to use clothing and accessories to maintain a positive body image during and after treatment, including customized clothing tips arranged by cancer-related treatments and side effects and articles and books focused on body image, clothing, cancer, and wellness. A directory of cancer-specific products such as swimsuits and head coverings helps users locate Web sites that offer these products.

Patient-Support Organizations

➤ Look Good . . . Feel Better. Access at: www.lookgoodfeelbetter.org
Phone: 800-395-LOOK

Emotional Distress

The discovery that one is diagnosed with cancer brings about a significant emotional response. Most individuals go through three stages, with the initial response being disbelief. Denial is a common emotional response when people are hit with a difficult new reality. After denial lifts, it is usually replaced by anxiety, anger, and/or fear—about a week after the diagnosis it is common to experience overwhelming feelings of sadness, hopelessness, anxiety, fear, and despair. This temporary depression typically lasts a few weeks, after which most individuals start the process of adjustment to living with cancer. At this third stage people are better able to confront the challenges presented by the disease and, at least partially, resume activities with family, friends, and work. The majority of newly diagnosed patients move on to the adjustment stage, but for many, a long-lasting severe depression may set in. The National Cancer Institute estimates that 15% to 25% of cancer patients in the United States suffer from clinical depression, as opposed to 10% of adults in the general population. Clinical depression may appear at any stage of the illness: after diagnosis, a recurrence, a setback in treatment, or other changes.

Depression can be treated very effectively with medication; therefore, it important to recognize that a person with cancer is suffering from clinical depression. Symptoms of clinical depression include having a depressed mood most of the day, significant diminished interest or pleasure, substantial weight or appetite changes, inability to sleep or oversleeping, agitation, significant fatigue, and more. Having a few of these symptoms may indicate that a person should be referred to a psychiatrist for assessment and possible treatment. Information sources for patients and families include self-assessment tools that help people measure the level of depression to see if it is beyond the normal distress level.

Even people who are not clinically depressed may need help coping with the psychological aspects of cancer. Social workers specializing in oncology can make suggestions and help solve some of the practical problems that may be adding to the distress. Social workers also provide counseling, screen for depression, and make suggestions for therapies that can help alleviate distress. Psychotherapy in a group or individual setting teaches people methods of lowering distress with behavior techniques, problem solving, and communication skills. Cancer support groups have been shown to improve the mood and coping skills of participants. Complementary therapies such as art, music, and dance therapy; journaling; and meditation help many people with cancer achieve an emotional balance and a positive attitude despite the illness. Others find comfort in spiritual and religious practices and beliefs. The information sources listed below have many suggestions, advice, and resources for emotional healing during cancer.

Information Sources

Brochures, Booklets, and Other Short Print Publications

➤ CancerCare. *Coping with Cancer: Tools to Help You Live.*
This booklet offers tips for dealing with the emotional impact of cancer, strengthening the spirit, and finding one's inner strength. Includes frequently asked questions, a glossary, and resources. Access at: www.cancer care.org/reading.html

➤ National Cancer Institute. *Taking Time: Support for People with Cancer.*
A sensitively written booklet for people with cancer and their families focusing on feelings, communication, and relationship changes that affect people with cancer and their loved ones. Touches on self-image issues and daily routines. Access at https://cissecure.nci.nih.gov/ncipubs/

➤ National Cancer Institute. *When Someone You Love Is Being Treated for Cancer.*
The focus of the booklet is to provide caregivers with coping strategies to help them deal with the stress and anxiety associated with caring for cancer patients. Discusses communication skills, ways to get support, feelings, helping with medical care, and the need for self-care. Access at: https://cissecure.nci.nih.gov/ncipubs/

➤ National Coalition for Cancer Survivorship. *You Have the Right to Be Hopeful.* This 58-page publication defines the many ways that hope can be present in a survivor's life and suggests means to maintain hope through the cancer journey. "Hope worksheets" at the end of the booklet offer a place for survivors to chronicle and reflect on their cancer journey. Access at: www.canceradvocacy.org

➤ National Comprehensive Cancer Network (NCCN). *Distress: Treatment Guidelines for Patients.*
This publication includes an explanation of cancer-related emotional distress as well as treatment decision "trees" explaining the treatment choices for mild, moderate, or severe distress. It was developed from the NCCN Clinical Practice Guidelines in Oncology—the standard for clinical policy in cancer care. It includes a self-assessment questionnaire to help patients decide if they need professional help to relieve their stress. A Spanish-language version also is available. Access at: www.nccn.org/patients/

Books

➤ Babcock, Elise NeeDell. 2002. *When Life Becomes Precious: The Essential Guide for Patients, Loved Ones, and Friends of Those Facing Serious Illnesses.* 2d ed. New York: Bantam.
This is a guidebook for people facing cancer, with a focus on the emotional side. Chapters explore common emotional reactions to the diagnosis, overcoming fear, communication, making holidays meaningful, and sources of support for the patient and caregiver.

➤ Buchholz, William M., and Susan W. Buchholz. 2001. *Live Longer, Live Larger: A Holistic Approach for Cancer Patients and Their Families.* Sebastopol, CA: O'Reilly.
This handbook is a supportive companion for people with cancer and other serious diseases. It covers topics such as conquering fear, finding hope, increasing quality and meaning of life, receiving support, and living comfortably with uncertainty. Part 4 of the book offers a plan for people with advanced disease who want to live fully until they die. Patient comments are woven throughout the text.

➤ Granet, Roger. 2001. *Surviving Cancer Emotionally: Learning How to Heal.* New York: Wiley.
The central focus of this book is the emotional toll of cancer. The author is a psychiatrist who believes that the patient's emotional well-being impacts quality of life and recommends various strategies for coping after diagnosis and during and after treatment. Topics covered include finding the right coping style, handling the many demands of treatment, knowing

when to ask for help and how to find it, coming to terms with changes, and handling the fear of recurrence.

➤ Harpham, Wendy Schlessel. 2005. *Happiness in a Storm: Facing Illness and Embracing Life as a Healthy Survivor.* New York: Norton.
Written by a physician and cancer survivor, this book describes how a serious illness impacts people, relationships, perspectives, thinking, and feelings. It outlines a program for getting good care and finding happiness while a person is ill.

➤ Holland, Jimmie C., and Sheldon Lewis. 2000. *The Human Side of Cancer: Living with Hope, Coping with Uncertainty.* New York: HarperCollins.
The authors are leading physicians in the field of psycho-oncology and the chairman of the department of psychiatry and behavioral sciences at the Memorial Sloan-Kettering Cancer Center. This book covers coping strategies, psychological effects of different treatments, psychosocial issues related to specific forms of cancer, and the "emotional baggage" of surviving. Advice and explanations are combined with quotes and anecdotes of cancer patients, research summaries, self-help tips, and checklists. It is intended for both the cancer survivor and family members.

Audiovisual Resources

➤ Spiegel, David, and Stanford Hospital and Clinics. *Feeling and Healing: Effects of Stress and Support on Cancer Patients.* Stanford, CA: Stanford Video, 2004, 100 min.
Dr. David Spiegel from Stanford University reviews recent research on the most effective ways to handle the inevitable stress of cancer: learning to express rather than suppress the emotions that accompany the illness, finding good social support, improving communication with loved ones and doctors, and facing fears directly. Available in DVD format. To order, go to: www.customflix.com

Web Resources

Detailed sections in a general cancer site

➤ CancerSource.com. *Emotional Support.* Access at: http://cancersource.com/, click on the link to "Cope with Cancer" and then on "Emotional Support." This section has comprehensive information about emotional wellness and spiritual care.

➤ CancerSymptoms.org. *Depression.* Access at: www.cancersymptoms.org and click on "Depression" in the left sidebar.
This section explains key points and provides tips for managing depression.

➤ National Coalition for Cancer Survivorship. *Palliative Care & Symptom Management: Issues of the Heart and Mind.* Access at: www.canceradvocacy. org/resources/essential/ and click on "Issues of the Heart and Mind." Information about effective ways to cope with anxiety and depression, finding support, and ways to communicate effectively with physicians.

Information about psychological issues of cancer patients is available at all major cancer sites including

➤ American Cancer Society. Access at: www.cancer.org
➤ Cancerbackup. Access at: www.cancerbackup.org.uk/Home
➤ Cancer.ca. Access at: www.cancer.ca
➤ CancerCare. Access at: www.cancercare.gov
➤ Cancer Supportive Care. Access at: www.cancersupportivecare.com
➤ National Cancer Institute. Access at: www.cancer.gov
➤ People Living with Cancer. Access at: www.plwc.org

Patient-Support Organizations

➤ Gilda's Club. Access at: www.gildasclub.org
  Phone: 917-305-1200
➤ The Wellness Community. Access at: www.thewellnesscommunity.org
  Phone: 888-793-9355

End of Life

Planning for a good death should ideally start when people are healthy. It is recommended that every adult have a living will and a medical power-of-attorney form choosing a health proxy, a person who has the authority to make medical decisions for one who is unable to express one's wishes. Making decisions in advance on issues such as artificial nutrition and hydration, resuscitation, machine-assisted breathing, and pain management can greatly help loved ones in having to deal with difficult issues at the end of life. In many hospitals, patients are routinely advised to prepare advance directive documents when they are diagnosed with any illness.

End-of-life care in cancer starts when treatment is no longer effective in stopping the spread of the disease and in prolonging life. As cancer progresses and invades vital organs, the focus of care shifts to alleviating symptoms, easing pain, and relieving suffering. This type of care is termed "palliative care." Palliative care is given to patients at all stages of cancer to improve symptoms and quality of life, but as cancer advances and treatment options become limited, palliative care becomes the main form of care. The goal is to improve quality of life as much as possible and enable patients to live with dignity, without pain, and close to family and friends. In many cases, the patient transitions to a hospice provider to receive medical services either in the home or as an inpatient in a medical facility or hospital.

Hospice programs use a multidisciplinary team approach utilizing professionals specializing in palliative care. Nurses, physicians, dietitians, occupational and physical therapists, speech therapists, and medical equipment and supply companies provide medical care. Social workers play a vital role and help families with practical and emotional concerns, often enlisting the help of volunteers, members of the clergy, psychotherapists, and art, music, and other therapists. Special hospice programs for children include pediatric medical professionals and child life specialists.

There are many misconceptions about hospice care and who is eligible to receive it. Information that explains what hospice and palliative care are and how to locate and choose a hospice provider can greatly help patients and families transition to palliative care at the right moment. Librarians also can help families with questions about burial and funeral planning, Medicare and insurance eligibility guidelines, talking with children about death and grief, and bereavement.

Information Sources

Brochures, Booklets, and Other Short Print Publications

➤ National Cancer Institute. *Coping with Advanced Cancer.*
This is a booklet for patients with end-stage cancer. It discusses treatment options such as palliative care, clinical trials, hospice care, and home care, as well as symptom control. It also addresses emotional concerns including feelings, communicating with friends and family, and living the rest of life to its fullest and with meaning. Access at: https://cissecure.nci.nih. gov/ncipubs/

➤ National Cancer Institute. *When Someone You Love Has Advanced Cancer.*
This booklet is for the family and friends of cancer patients who have advanced cancer that is no longer responding to treatment. It explores many of the questions and crossroads that face caregivers when remission or recovery is no longer possible. Access at: https://cissecure.nci.nih.gov/ncipubs/

➤ National Comprehensive Cancer Network (NCCN). *Advanced Cancer and Palliative Care Treatment Guidelines for Patients.*
This publication provides a narrative section that explains what palliative care is and covers topics such as hospice care, advanced directives, facing death, and grieving the loss of a loved one. It also includes treatment decision "trees" for screening for and assessing palliative care needs. This

resource was developed from the NCCN Clinical Practice Guidelines in Oncology—the standard for clinical policy in cancer care. A Spanish-language version also is available. Access at: www.nccn.org/patients/

Audiovisual Materials

➤ Family Experiences Productions. *Facing Death.* Austin TX: Family Experiences Productions, 1997.
This is a series of two programs. Tape 1 (33 minutes) is titled "Providing Physical, Emotional & Spiritual Comfort to Loved Ones." It features patients, caregivers, hospice professionals, physicians, and social workers who share their thoughts, experiences, and specific suggestions to help terminally ill patients and their loved ones comfort each other. Tape 2 (17 minutes) is titled "Practical Planning & Legal Issues" and features a nurse-attorney, hospice professionals, and physicians discussing how to help terminally ill patients express their wishes at the end of life. Order at: www.fepi.com. Available in VHS format. A DVD edition is forthcoming.

Books

Books focusing on palliative care in cancer

➤ Dahm, Nancy Hassett. 2000. *Mind, Body, and Soul: A Guide to Living with Cancer.* Garden City, NY: Taylor Hill.
This book offers a holistic plan for living with advanced cancer. It covers psychological as well as practical issues, including managing symptoms, pain, giving and receiving quality care, and overcoming stress and fear. There also are chapters on new advances in cancer treatment and answered prayers, visions, and miracles. An extensive resource appendix includes sources for free hospitalizations, low-cost prescriptions, free medication, and free travel to treatment centers. The author is a cancer nurse.
➤ Foley, Kathleen M., ed. 2005. *When the Focus Is on Care: Palliative Care and Cancer.* Atlanta: American Cancer Society.
This book answers many questions people with cancer have about progressive illness, including where to obtain quality end-of-life care and how to manage symptoms and side effects. The book also discusses coping strategies, performing a life review, and leaving a legacy. Authored by a team of oncologists and social workers.

Relevant books on end of life

➤ Lynn, Joanne, Joan K. Harrold, and the Center to Improve Care of the Dying, George Washington University. 1999. *Handbook for Mortals: Guidance for People Facing Serious Illness.* New York: Oxford.

This book addresses practical, physical, and emotional issues facing people with terminal illness. Chapters discuss coping with the uncertainty of serious illness; obtaining support from family caregivers, social workers, nurses, and doctors; getting the most out of conversations with physicians; managing symptoms; controlling pain; and what to expect as the disease progresses. The authors, both physicians, attempt to help readers make difficult decisions with regard to forgoing medical treatment such as artificial feeding, ventilators, and resuscitation. Special situations such as the death of a child and sudden death also are covered. Read the book online at: www.abcd-caring.org.

➤ Sendor, Virginia F., and Patrice M. O'Connor. 1997. *Hospice and Palliative Care: Questions and Answers*. Lanham, MD: Scarecrow Press.

This book is in question-and-answer format and offers detailed answers, supported by references, to questions about hospice and palliative care. The authors describe hospice and palliative care services and explain admission requirements, reimbursement issues, and how to locate resources in the United States. Authored by two health professionals specializing in end-of-life care.

Web Resources

Detailed sections in general cancer sites

➤ American Cancer Society. *Hospice Care*. Access at: www.cancer.org and type "hospice care" in the search box.

The section includes documents discussing what is hospice care, questions to ask when interviewing care providers, who pays for hospice care, and how to find hospice care. Other relevant sections on this site include *Advance Directives* and *Coping with Grief and Loss*.

➤ Cancerbackup. *Coping with Advanced Cancer*. Access at: www.cancer backup.org.uk/Home and click on the link "Resources & Support."

This section covers emotional issues and symptom control. The information on practical matters is relevant to people living in the United Kingdom.

➤ National Coalition for Cancer Survivorship. *Palliative Care & Symptom Management: End-of-Life Issues*. Access at: www.canceradvocacy.org/resources/essential/ and click on "End-of-Life Issues."

Covers key end-of-life concerns, including medical, emotional and practical issues.

➤ People Living with Cancer. *End-of-Life Care*. Access at: www.plwc.org, select "Coping" on the left sidebar and then click on "End-of-Life Care."

This section provides detailed information on palliative care, preparing for the end-of-life, advanced directives, cardiopulmonary resuscitation

(CPR), and do not resuscitate (DNR) orders. Also covers care during the final days and caring for the terminally ill child.

Relevant end-of-life Web sites

➤ Caring Connections. Access at: www.caringinfo.org
Provided by the National Hospice and Palliative Care Organization and National Hospice Foundation, this site provides a variety of free resources on topics such as advance care planning, caregiving, pain, financial issues, hospice and palliative care, and grief and loss. Printable versions of state-specific advance directive documents and instructions are available free on the site.

➤ Caring for the End of Life. Access at: www.caringtotheend.ca/
Provided by Princess Margaret Hospital in Toronto Canada, the purpose of this site is to give patients, caregivers, and health care professionals information about palliative care and tools to help manage care. The tips and advice on dealing with pain, symptom management, and emotional issues are relevant to all users. The resources are mostly relevant to users in the greater Toronto area.

➤ Hospice Foundation of America. Access at: www.hospicefoundation.org
This site offers extensive information for caregivers and people facing death on topics such as signs of approaching death, pain, patient comfort, and paperwork and logistics after a death in the family. The "Caregiver's Corner" includes an extensive library of articles about caring for a dying loved one and grief and loss issues. Users also can find local hospice providers and support organizations on the site.

➤ Hospice Net. Access at: www.hospicenet.org
This site provides information about hospice care and other end-of-life issues, including locating local services, communication at the end of life, pain control, and caregiving for the dying person. It also offers information on grief and bereavement.

Fertility

Each year, approximately 120,000 men and women under the age of 45 are diagnosed with cancer. It is estimated that 10% of the 10 million cancer survivors living in the United States were diagnosed during their reproductive years. Loss of fertility is a common side effect of cancer treatment, yet only 57% of patients recall receiving information from a health care provider about fertility side effects. Disclosing fertility risks and preservation options before treatment starts is crucial because certain options are available only before treatment starts. Sperm banking, for example, should be done before treatment is initiated. Unfortunately, about 40% to 50% of men go into treatment unaware of fertility risks and sperm preservation options. (These statistics are provided by Fertile Hope, an organization dedicated to helping cancer survivors facing infertility.)

All major forms of cancer treatment have the potential to cause permanent infertility. Certain types of chemotherapy may cause damage to hormone, sperm, and egg production. Radiation therapy to the pelvic area may injure the ovaries or testes, and surgery in this region may also damage components of the reproductive system. While it is difficult to predict fertility for any specific individual, data show that 40% to 80% of women who undergo chemotherapy or receive radiation to the pelvic area suffer permanent infertility. In women receiving chemotherapy, the likelihood of suffering fertility problems is dependent on the specific drug used, the dose, and the woman's age at the time of treatment. In recent years, doctors have begun to consider these factors when deciding on a treatment protocol.

Several techniques to preserve fertility in men and women are available. For men, sperm banking has been used successfully by cancer patients for decades. Testicular tissue freezing is in its very early days of study. For women, the only proven method is freezing embryos. This option is available for postpubertal women who have a partner or are willing to use donor sperm. Freezing embryos is a complex process that involves taking fertility hormones for a period of time before eggs can be harvested and fertilized in a laboratory. For many women this long process is not advisable because delaying treatment or taking fertility drugs may hurt their chances of curing cancer. Freezing unfertilized eggs is feasible, but the process of achieving a successful pregnancy from unfertilized eggs is still in its infancy. Freezing ovarian tissue is highly experimental at this point, with very few live births reported at the time of this book's publication. Another experimental option is injecting women with hormones that temporarily put the ovaries into a pseudomenopausal state during chemotherapy. The idea behind this method is that by suppressing ovarian function, fewer eggs would be exposed to chemotherapy. This method is still being evaluated in clinical trials. Other options for achieving parenthood are use of donor eggs or donor sperm, surrogacy, and adoption.

Although fertility issues are mostly associated with people diagnosed during their reproductive years, children and adolescents with cancer are also at high risk for infertility as a result of treatment. Parents of children with cancer should be made aware of fertility related side effects before treatment starts. Boys who reached puberty can preserve fertility by sperm banking before treatment begins.

Information Sources

Brochures, Booklets, and Other Short Print Publications

➤ American Society of Clinical Oncology. *ASCO Patient Guide: Fertility Preservation.*
This publication explains ASCO's clinical practice guidelines about fertility preservation in people treated for cancer. It focuses on fertility preservation options that are available before cancer treatment. Access online at: www.plwc.org

➤ Fertile Hope.
  ➤ *Breast Cancer and Fertility*
  ➤ *Cancer and Fertility: A Guide for Young Adults*
  ➤ *Cancer and Fertility*
  ➤ *Childhood Cancer and Fertility: A Guide for Parents*
  ➤ *Gynecologic Cancers and Fertility*
  Short brochures describing the challenges and possible solutions to fertility problems. Access at: www.fertilehope.org

Books

➤ Beck, Lindsay and Oktay, Kutluk H. Publication expected in 2007. *100 Questions and Answers about Cancer and Fertility.* Sudbury, MA: Jones and Bartlett.
This text provides both the doctor's and patient's perspectives by weaving comments from patients into the text that discusses the medical and practical issues faced by cancer survivors and families who want to preserve their fertility. Written by an ObGyn/reproductive medicine specialist and the founder and executive director of Fertile Hope.

➤ Fertile Hope. *Cancer and Fertility Resource Guide.* 2006–2007. New York: Fertile Hope.
This 318-page publication has information about services and resources for people experiencing cancer-related infertility. Includes introductions to specific issues and listings of clinics, specialists, tissue-freezing banks professionals, agencies, and organizations that help people with cancer become parents. Access online at: www.fertilehope.org

Web Resources

Sites focused on cancer fertility issues

➤ Fertile Hope. Access at: www.fertilehope.org
Fertile Hope is a national nonprofit organization dedicated to providing reproductive information, support, and hope to cancer patients whose

medical treatments present the risk of infertility. The Web site offers information about fertility risks, parenthood options, questions to ask before starting cancer treatment, and news about development in treatment of infertility. The site also has a "Find a Doctor" feature and Adobe Acrobat (.pdf) files of the organization's publications.

Sections about fertility are also available at the following sites:

➤ Cancerbackup. *Cancer and Fertility.* Access at: www.cancerbackup.org.uk/home and click on "Resources and Support."

➤ LIVESTRONG SurvivorCare. *Female Infertility* and *Male Infertility.* Access at: www.livestrong.org and click on "Take Control" and then on "Physical Topics."

➤ People Living with Cancer. *Sexual and Reproductive Health.* Access at: www.plwc.org and click on "Diagnosis and Treatment" and then on "Treating Cancer."

Patient-Support Organizations

➤ Fertile Hope. Access at: www.fertilehope.org
   Phone: 888-994-HOPE

Lymphedema

Anatomical Notes: *The lymphatic system is a network of vessels, similar to blood vessels, which carry the lymph fluid to different parts of the body. Lymph is a colorless fluid that contains infection-fighting white blood cells called lymphocytes. Lymph is slowly moved through larger and larger lymphatic vessels and passes through small bean-shaped structures called lymph nodes. Eventually, lymph flows into one of two large veins in the chest area.*

Illustration of the lymphatic system is available at the Medical Illustrations Gallery of the People Living with Cancer Web site under the lymphoma topics.

Access at: www.plwc.org and click on "Library" on the left sidebar.

Lymphedema is a condition in which excess fluid collects in tissue and causes swelling. The fluid buildup may cause pain and discomfort, and the affected area is more prone to infection. People with cancer have a risk of developing lymphedema because cancer treatment such as surgery or radiation therapy may damage the lymphatic vessels and nodes and disrupt the normal flow of lymph. Any person treated for cancer may develop lymphedema, but breast cancer survivors are the most susceptible to this condition; it is estimated that 15% to 30% of breast cancer survivors develop lymphedema to some degree. Other diagnoses at higher risk for lymphedema are prostate cancer, melanoma, pelvic area cancer, and lymphoma.

Most often, lymphedema occurs in the arms or legs, but it can occur in other areas as well. If lymphedema occurs after breast cancer treatment, it can affect the breast area, underarm area, and the arm on the side of surgery. If lymphedema occurs after cancer treatment to the abdomen, the swelling affects the abdomen, genitals, and one or both legs.

Lymphedema may be a temporary short-term side effect, but in many cancer survivors it becomes a chronic condition and may be permanent. It may occur right after surgery or years after treatment has been completed. Lymphedema may bring about significant emotional distress because it may cause disfigurement and is a daily reminder of the cancer. The severity of the condition varies from person to person.

Being overweight, having surgery that removes lymph nodes, and receiving radiation therapy increases a person's risk to develop lymphedema. Having another medical condition such as diabetes, high blood pressure, kidney disease, or heart disease also increases the risk for lymphedema. For people with high-risk for lymphedema, specialists recommend taking preventative steps that may reduce the risk, delay the onset of the condition, and prevent it altogether.

Lymphedema should be treated by a physical therapist or another health care professional that has gone through special training in a therapeutic method called complex decongestive therapy (CDT). This therapy consists of meticulous skin care to prevent infection, manual lymphatic massage, special compressive bandaging and garments, and decongestive exercise. This treatment is effective in reducing the swelling, preventing it from getting worse, preventing infection, and improving the use and appearance of the affected organ.

It is very important to ensure the authoritativeness of information sources when providing information about lymphedema. Several treatment approaches, including diuretics or drugs called benzopyrones, as well as surgery, are controversial and may in fact make the condition worse. The FDA has not approved several drugs and therapies that are utilized in Europe.

Information sources listed below contain authoritative information about lymphedema and explain how to locate certified trained professionals and community resources for patients and families. Information on arm lymphedema that is associated with breast cancer also may be found in the breast cancer information sources.

Information Sources

Brochures, Booklets, and Other Short Print Publications

➤ Oncology Section of the American Physical Therapy Association. *Lymphedema Fact Sheet.*
This is a three-page fact sheet with information about risk factors, symptoms, and how physical therapist can help. Access at: www.oncologypt.org

➤ National Lymphedema Network. *Lymphedema: An Information Booklet.*
This 16-page booklet covers the lymphatic system, causes of lymphedema, symptoms, lymphangitis (infection), lymphedema risk reduction, treatments, contraindications, diagnostic studies, special warnings, and reimbursement issues. Booklets are available for a fee. To order, go to: www.lymphnet.org

Books

➤ American Cancer Society. 2006. *Lymphedema: Understanding and Managing Lymphedema after Cancer Treatment.* Atlanta: American Cancer Society.
This comprehensive guide to understanding and the management of lymphedema provides information about prevention, detection, and treatment options for lymphedema. It explains how to control swelling and discomfort, and how to cope with emotional stresses and changes in body image. Practical challenges such as treatment cost, finding certified treatment providers, and insurance issues also are discussed, as well as new areas of research and experimental, unproven, and ineffective treatments.

➤ Ehrlich, Ann, Alma Vinje-Harrewijn, and Elizabeth McMahon. 2005. *Living Well with Lymphedema.* San Francisco: Lymph Notes.
This is a guide for people who suffer from lymphedema and those who have a risk of developing this condition. The patient-friendly, illustrated text explains what lymphedema is, what causes it, and how it is treated. The book offers self-management steps to control the condition, practical suggestions on coping with the emotional challenges, and information about insurance and reimbursement issues. Includes an illustrated guide to understanding the lymphatic system.

➤ McMahon, Elizabeth. 2005. *Overcoming the Emotional Challenges of Lymphedema.* San Francisco: Lymph Notes.
This book offers advice on overcoming the emotional challenges of lymphedema and avoiding common pitfalls. It explains how to recognize problems and where to go for help. It also covers communication with family, friends, coworkers, and health care professionals.

Web Resources

Sites focusing on lymphedema

➤ National Lymphedema Network. Access at: www.lymphnet.org
This organization provides education and guidance to lymphedema patients, health care professionals, and the general public by disseminating information on the prevention and management of primary and secondary lymphedema. The site includes position papers and other documents about different topics such as exercise, air travel, risk reduction, and management of lymphedema. The "Patients" section has lists of treatment centers and certified therapists as well as local support groups and other support services.

Detailed sections in general cancer sites

➤ Cancerbackup. *Lymphedema*. Access at: www.cancerbackup.org.uk/Home and click on the link to "Resources & Support."
This section has detailed information about lymphedema treatment.
➤ *Cancer Supportive Care*. Access at: www.cancersupportivecare.com and type "Lymphedema" in the search box.
This site has several documents on the topic including lower body lymphedema and living with lymphedema.
➤ National Cancer Institute. *Lymphedema PDQ®*.
This patient summary is adapted from the summary on lymphedema written by cancer experts for health professionals. It covers the different types of lymphedema that may affect people with cancer, management, and complications.

Patient-Support Organization

➤ National Lymphedema Network. Access at: www.lymphnet.org
Phone: 510-208-3200

Nutrition during Cancer Treatment

This section covers the topic of nutrition for people undergoing cancer treatment. Relevant information for survivors after treatment and in remission can be found under the section "Nutrition for Cancer Prevention" in Chapter 6. People in treatment have unique concerns about their diet and nutrition that may be due to side effects of cancer treatment. Nutritional problems are common in people undergoing cancer treatment and can include loss of appetite, sore mouth or throat, dry mouth, changes in taste or smell, nausea/vomiting, diarrhea, constipation, and changes in weight.

Staying well-nourished despite these difficulties is a challenge for patients and caregivers, but maintaining a healthy weight is crucial for several reasons. Most importantly, well-nourished patients are able to tolerate therapy better, while malnourished patients may not be able to stick with the treatment regimen and may have worse outcomes. A good diet can prevent the breakdown of body tissues and help rebuild tissues that cancer treatment can harm. Good nutrition can also improve stamina and quality of life.

Diet recommendations for people during treatment can be very different and even contradictory to the usual guidelines for healthy living. The goal is to build up strength and prevent weight loss. Patients who are starting to lose weight may be advised to eat high-protein, high-calorie, and high-fat foods. Some patients may be advised to eat less of high-fiber foods because these foods can aggravate problems such as diarrhea. Those who suffer from mouth sores may be advised to eat soft and cool food items having low acidity and smooth texture.

People on chemotherapy should pay special attention to preventing food-borne illnesses. Chemotherapy may decrease an individual's ability to fight infection because it lowers the number of white blood cells in the body. People are especially vulnerable after a stem cell or bone marrow transplantation and should follow strict guidelines to ensure food safety.

Eating problems that may bring about severe weight loss tend to affect people with certain types of cancer. These include cancers that involve the organs necessary for swallowing and digesting, such as head and neck, esophageal, and pancreatic. Registered dietitians who specialize in oncology can provide personalized expert advice to people at risk. Commercial meal replacements in liquid and powder form may help supplement nutrition and provide patients with essential nutrients. Some patients may need artificial feeding through a tube inserted into the stomach or small intestine or infused in a vein.

Nutrition-related problems have a social aspect as well, since many gatherings and celebrations are centered around food. Numerous information sources offer tips for patients and caregivers on how to cope with these challenges and stay connected with friends and family despite the difficulties.

Information Sources

Brochures, Booklets, and Other Short Print Publications

➤ American Cancer Society. *Nutrition for the Person with Cancer.*
This is an 84-page booklet for people before, during, and after cancer treatment. It offers practical tips and advice for managing eating problems

during treatment and discusses herbs, vitamins, minerals, antioxidants, and other dietary supplements. Includes recipes. This publication is not available online. To order, contact your local American Cancer Society or access at: www.cancer.org

➤ American Institute for Cancer Research. *Nutrition of the Cancer Patient.*
This brochure provides answers for the eating challenges that can occur during treatment. It explains the effects different types of treatment may have on nutrition and offers tips for handling eating problems. Access at: www.aicr.org

➤ Canadian Cancer Society. *Good Nutrition: A Guide for People with Cancer.*
This booklet is designed to help people with cancer maintain good nutrition during cancer therapy. It explains the special nutritional needs of the person with cancer and provides ideas for managing nutrition-related side effects. Available in English, French, Chinese, and Punjabi. Access at: www.cancer.ca

➤ National Cancer Institute (NCI). *Eating Hints for Cancer Patients: Before, During and After Treatment.*
This publication provides information and recipes to help patients meet their needs for good nutrition during treatment. It presents tips for managing many nutrition symptoms, including weight loss and gain, dry mouth, changes in taste or smell, and more. Includes a section for caregivers. Access at: https://cissecure.nci.nih.gov/ncipubs/

Books

➤ Bloch, Abby S. 2004. *Eating Well, Staying Well during and after Cancer.* Atlanta: American Cancer Society.
A comprehensive book written by a highly credentialed nutrition expert and providing detailed information on diet and cancer. The sections discussing the evidence regarding foods and dietary supplements that have been promoted as fighting cancer or improving the immune system are especially interesting. The author also provides sound advice about coping with nutrition-related side effects and ensuring food quality and safety, meal plans, and recipes.

➤ Clegg, Holly Berkowitz, and Gerald Miletello. 2001. *Eating Well through Cancer: Easy Recipes and Recommendations during and after Treatment.* Baton Rouge, LA: H. B. Clegg.
This book is a collaborative work of a cookbook writer and an oncologist. It is divided into chapters centering on specific side effects that may be experienced by people undergoing chemotherapy, such as low blood count, diarrhea, constipation, and sore mouth. Each chapter starts with

an explanation of the topic and includes recipes for dishes that may improve symptoms, with each recipe providing a professional nutritional analysis and diabetic exchange. The recipe cross-reference is a handy tool for locating recipes that may be helpful to relieve specific side effects.

➤ Crocker, Betty. 2002. *Betty Crocker's Living with Cancer Cookbook*. New York: Hungry Minds.

This is a beautifully designed cookbook with attractive color photographs accompanying 130 recipes. The introduction and special features add to the reader's understanding of how to eat well and relieve side effects during cancer treatment. Recipes are color-coded to show which ones are the most helpful for improving nausea, mouth sores, diarrhea, and constipation. The introduction provides a good overview of nutrition principles to maintain during treatment, and each recipe includes a nutritional analysis. Notes embedded in the text offer advice and tips from an oncologist and survivors.

➤ Dyer, Diana. 2002. *A Dietitian's Cancer Story: Information and Inspiration for Recovery and Healing from a 3-Time Cancer Survivor*. Ann Arbor, MI: Swan Press.

This book was authored by a registered dietitian who is also a cancer survivor. Its strength is in the specific, detailed advice and suggestions about topics such as selecting dishes in restaurants, avoiding hidden fats, travel tips, and managing fatigue. Recipes are included, and the author explains how to evaluate alternative and complementary nutritional therapies, herbs, and supplements. The nutrition principles are suitable for cancer survivors during and after treatment.

➤ Liu, Simin, et al. 2006. *Healing Gourmet, Eat to Fight Cancer*. New York: McGraw-Hill.

The authors—a physician, a dietitian and a chef—explain how to eat a balanced diet high in fruits, vegetables, and whole grains and low in saturated fat. This book discusses specific food groups and nutrients that may play a role in cancer, such as fats, carbohydrates, antioxidants, and phytochemicals. Practical tips and advice about coping with side effects, meal plans, and 50 recipes also are included.

➤ Mathai, Kimberly, and Ginny Smith. 2004. *The Cancer Lifeline Cookbook: Good Nutrition, Recipes, and Resources to Optimize the Lives of People Living with Cancer*. Seattle, WA: Sasquatch Books.

A registered dietitian and a food writer offer nutritional advice and recipes for people during and after treatment. This book provides descriptions of key components of good nutrition and practical suggestions for reducing side effects and incorporating healthy foods and nutrients into one's diet. Over 90 recipes accompanied by color photos are included.

➤ Weihofen, Donna L., and Christina Marino. 1998. *The Cancer Survival Cookbook: 200 Quick and Easy Recipes with Helpful Eating Hints*. Minneapolis, MN: Chronimed.

A registered dietitian and a cancer survivor who is also a physician wrote this recipe book that includes practical advice and nutrition-related information for people undergoing treatment. In addition to the 200 recipes, this book has many useful special features, for example, "eating hints"—specific suggestions for coping with problems such as loss of appetite, taste changes, sore mouth, and more. A detailed discussion of herbal remedies and sections on beverages, snacks, soft and pureed foods, and food-safety precautions are particularly helpful.

Audiovisual Resources

➤ *Nutrition for Prevention and Adjuvant Therapy of Cancer.* (15 minutes.) Directed by Health Science Institute. The Institute, 1997.

This program covers the principles of good nutrition for people with cancer. It describes major food groups and nutrients and provides dietary guidelines for a healthy diet. It also provides tips for people experiencing side effects such as weight loss, taste changes, taste aversions, dry mouth, and difficulty swallowing. Includes a teacher's guide. Available in VHS and CD-ROM formats. To order, access: http://healthscienceinstitute. com.

➤ M. D. Anderson Cancer Center. *Nutrition and Cancer.* (17 minutes.)

A clinical dietitian from M. D. Anderson discusses nutrition as it relates to cancer treatment and addresses patients' most frequently asked questions, including what foods may help build the immune system. In addition, patients and caregivers talk about their personal experiences. Can be viewed at: www.mdanderson.org/departments/cimer

Web Resources

Sites focusing on nutrition during cancer treatment

➤ Cancer Nutrition Info. Access at: www.cancernutritioninfo.com

The author is a registered dietitian who worked with cancer patients at the University of Michigan Comprehensive Cancer Center. This site offers detailed information about many aspects relating to diet and cancer. The section "Treatment Symptom Management" includes articles about coping with eating challenges during treatment. Another useful section,

"Complementary & Alternative Medicine," discusses supplements, vitamins, minerals, and herbs commonly used by cancer patients. The author reviews articles published in the scientific medical literature and explains in lay language what the evidence shows with regard to specific products. Users can also find recipes, tips, and answers to commonly asked questions. Some of the content requires a $15 annual subscription fee.

Detailed sections in general cancer sites

➤ American Cancer Society. *Nutrition for Cancer Patients.* Access at: www. cancer.org and type "nutrition" in the search box.
The section includes documents discussing treatment side effects, eating problems, and dietary supplements.
➤ Cancerbackup. *Eating Well.* Access at: www.cancerbackup.org.uk/Home and click on the link to "Resources & Support."
Information on diet during treatment, nutritional support, and alternative diets can be found here.
➤ National Coalition for Cancer Survivorship. *Palliative Care & Symptom Management > Nutrition.* Access at: www.canceradvocacy.org/resources/essential/ and click on "Nutrition."
Extensive information about the special nutritional needs of people undergoing cancer treatment, and dealing with specific problems.

Sections about nutrition during cancer treatment are also available at the following sites

➤ Cancer Supportive Care. Access at: www.cancersupportivecare.com
➤ National Cancer Institute. Access at: www.cancer.gov
➤ People Living with Cancer. Access at: www.plwc.org

Pain Control

Medical science has developed many effective treatment methods to control pain, yet it remains one of the most undertreated side effects of cancer, and many people suffer needlessly. The reasons for this are two-fold: the first is poor communication between patients and their caregivers and clinicians, and the second is people's misconceptions about using opioids for pain control.

Good communication is essential to achieving optimal pain relief. Communication problems arise when patients are reluctant to discuss this issue with their clinicians and/or when clinicians fail to ask their patients if they have pain. Many people feel that they should be able to tolerate pain and not complain about it; others fear what the presence of pain may mean. Another communication problem is that pain cannot be seen and is difficult to describe with words. To help people discuss this issue, the American Pain Society created the phrase "Pain: The 5th Vital Sign" and recommends that clinicians assess patients for pain every time they check for pulse, blood pressure, core temperature, and respiration. Clinicians ask people to rate their pain intensity on a scale and offer words to help people articulate what they are feeling. A good assessment of the type and intensity of the pain is the first step in establishing a comprehensive pain-control plan for each individual.

One of the reasons that people are hesitant to complain about pain is the widespread reluctance to use opioids, which are narcotic-like medications. There are many misconceptions about these drugs, one of the most prevalent being that opioids are addictive and people who use narcotics become dependent on them. Many people believe that opioids should be taken only as a last resort for people at the end stages of cancer and nearing death. Both of these beliefs are untrue. People with cancer who use opioids do not get "high" on these medications and do not turn into drug abusers with destructive behaviors. Opioids are very safe drugs when administered by physicians for the purpose of pain relief. The level of pain a person experience is not related to how advanced the cancer is, since even small tumors can cause a great deal of pain, depending of their location.

People with cancer may feel pain as result of the cancer itself. Tumors may press against bones, nerves, or organs and produce pain. Pain can also be caused by surgical procedures to diagnose or treat cancer. People may experience back and/or neck pain when tumors progress to the spine and cause spinal cord compression. Effective pain treatments are available to treat almost all types and intensities of cancer pain. In addition to narcotics, people with cancer can utilize many other drugs to relieve different types of pain. Pain-control drugs can be taken in the form of pills, patches, suspensions, injections, or infusions to address specific levels of pain intensity and/or severity. Sophisticated methods of drug delivery, such as implementation of nerve blocks or administration of drugs directly into the spine, can be very helpful. People who were not helped with drugs may benefit from radiation therapy that reduces the pressure tumors cause by shrinking them. Often only a single treatment with radiation is needed to relieve pain. Surgery to block nerve pathways for the purpose of preventing them from relaying pain messages is another option that can be performed by neurosurgeons specializing in pain management.

Non–drug treatments for pain control can be very effective and can be used alone or together with medications. Some people find that they need lower doses of drugs when they supplement medications with such non–drug techniques as guided imagery, relaxation, biofeedback, hypnosis, skin stimulation, acupuncture, or acupressure. Engaging in activities that occupy the person's attention, such as art and music therapy, can help distract the mind from pain and provide some level of relief.

Information Sources

Brochures, Booklets, and Other Short Print Publications

➤ American Alliance of Cancer Pain Initiatives. *Cancer Pain Can Be Relieved.* This is a 15-page booklet written in an easy-to-understand question-and-answer format. It guides patients and families through the issues essential to understanding and managing cancer pain. Access at: www.aacpi. wisc.edu/

➤ CancerCare. *Controlling Cancer Pain: What You Need to Know to Get Relief.* This booklet presents a detailed overview of pain control in people with cancer. It explains how to overcome barriers to pain management, pain terminology, and how to describe pain to the doctor. Also includes a review of pain-control drugs and tips for dealing with these drugs' side effects. The booklet concludes with frequently asked questions, a glossary, and resources. Access at: www.cancercare.org/reading.html

➤ Canadian Cancer Society. *Pain Relief: A Guide for People with Cancer.* This 28-page booklet contains general information about pain and pain relief, including drug and non-drug approaches. French and Punjabi versions are available. Access at: www.cancer.ca.

➤ National Cancer Institute. *Pain Control: A Guide for People with Cancer and Their Families.* This 57-page booklet provides a comprehensive review of cancer pain management. It describes the different types of pain that may be experienced by people with cancer, medicines used to relieve pain, and other medical approaches such as radiation therapy, surgery, and nerve blocks. It also reviews non-medical methods such as relaxation, guided imagery, and acupuncture. Access at https://cissecure.nci.nih.gov/ncipubs/

➤ National Cancer Institute. *Understanding Cancer Pain.* This is a short, easy-to-read publication with color illustrations that explains why cancer patients have pain, the ways pain can be treated, and what patients should do when they have pain. Access at https://cissecure. nci.nih.gov/ncipubs/

➤ National Comprehensive Cancer Network (NCCN). *Cancer Pain: Treatment Guidelines for Patients.*

This publication includes a comprehensive overview of cancer pain management as well as decision "trees" explaining treatment choices for different types and intensities of pain. This resource was developed from the NCCN Clinical Practice Guidelines in Oncology—the standard for clinical policy in cancer care. A Spanish-language version also is available. Access at: www.nccn.org/patients/

Audiovisual Materials

➤ *Controlling Cancer Pain, a Video for Patients and Families.* Directed by National Cancer Institute (U.S.). 1 videocassette (12 min.). National Cancer Institute, 2000.
A closed-captioned video that discusses why patients have pain, the ways pain can be treated, and what patients should do when they have pain. To order, contact the Cancer Information Service at 800-4-CANCER (800-422-6237).

Books

➤ American Cancer Society. 2004. *American Cancer Society's Guide to Pain Control: Understanding and Managing Cancer Pain.* Rev. ed. Atlanta: American Cancer Society.
The purpose of this book is to teach people with cancer how to achieve acceptable pain control and understand the balance between pain relief and potential side effects of medications. The text discusses common barriers to pain control and offers ways for overcoming these barriers. It provides a step-by-step guide to describing pain and communicating pain-relief needs, as well as practical tips and strategies for coping with various situations. Complementary and non-medical approaches to pain management are reviewed, including acupuncture, biofeedback, exercise, humor, guided imagery, and more.

➤ Cicala, Roger, and David van Alstine. 2001. *The Cancer Pain Sourcebook.* Los Angeles: Contemporary.
This book focuses on the medical management of pain people with cancer may suffer. Authored by pain-management specialists, it includes an in-depth discussion of the anatomy of pain and a comprehensive overview of medical approaches for treating cancer pain. The first chapter describes standard treatments including opioid and non–opioid medications, as well as different ways of drug administration. The second part details advanced treatments such as intraspinal treatments, treatments for specific situations, and pain control in hospice care.

➤ Patt, Richard B., et al. 2004. *The Complete Guide to Relieving Cancer Pain and Suffering.* New York: Oxford University Press.

The authors examine the physiology of cancer pain and explain how undertreatment of pain can get in the way of healing, because pain may stop patients from resuming active lives and having the strength to fight their disease. The barriers for effective pain control, including false myths and beliefs about narcotic drugs are discussed at length. The text explores all of the pain-relieving options available, from over-the-counter drugs and high-tech medical techniques to psychological mind/body techniques and home nursing tips. Authored by a cancer pain specialist and a science writer.

Web Resources

Detailed sections in general cancer sites

➤ American Cancer Society. *Pain.* Access at: www.cancer.org and type "pain" in the search box.
   The section includes a guide to pain control, a pain control record sheet, information for caregivers on how to manage cancer pain at home, and a list of local and national organizations dedicated to promoting cancer pain relief.
➤ Cancerbackup. *Controlling Cancer Pain.* Access at: www.cancerbackup. org.uk/Home and click on the link to "Resources & Support."
   This section explains cancer pain, painkillers, and non–drug methods for pain relief.
➤ CancerSymptoms.org. *Pain.* Access at: www.cancersymptoms.org and click on "pain" on the left sidebar.
   This section explains key points and provides tips for pain management.
➤ National Coalition for Cancer Survivorship. *Palliative Care & Symptom Management > Pain.* Access at: www.canceradvocacy.org/resources/essential/ and click on "Pain."
   Extensive information about management of cancer pain, including pain in specific populations.

Parenting through Cancer

Parenting is one of life's biggest challenges. This challenge is amplified when a parent is diagnosed with cancer. The first challenge parents face is telling their children about the diagnosis. Parents naturally want to protect children and do not want to expose them to the worry and sadness that an illness brings; however, all experts agree that children and teenagers need to be informed about a cancer diagnosis in the family. It is impossible to keep the illness a secret, even from very young children. Children eavesdrop on adult conversations and pick up on their parents' anxiety and worry. If children are not kept informed, they resort to their imagination and tend to believe the worst.

The key is to give children information at a level they can comprehend and provide an opportunity for them to discuss their feelings and concerns. They need to be reassured that in spite of the illness, their needs will be taken care of, and their lives will continue along their designated path with regard to school, sports, and social activities. Teenagers struggle with additional concerns stemming from the fact that adolescence is the time when children are starting to break away and be independent from their parents. A parent's cancer diagnosis complicates this developmental process because it makes it difficult for them to break away.

Parenting challenges continue through the illness on both the emotional and the practical level. Children need to be kept informed about any changes, such as new treatments that may bring about new side effects, a recurrence, or any change in the course or the outlook of the illness. Keeping communication lines open helps children and teenagers feel involved and important, and cope with their own feelings such as guilt, fear, and anger. Many parents are concerned about their ability to fulfill their parenting responsibilities during the illness. Sources for parents include tips and advice about managing both the practical and the emotional issues.

The list of information sources below is divided according to target audience and age level. Information sources for parents offer ways to explain cancer and treatment to children at different age groups and provide insight to the specific concerns and reactions children may have. Information sources for children should be chosen according to age level.

Information Sources for Children

Brochures, Booklets, and Other Short Print Publications (Titles arranged by age)

➤ American Cancer Society. *It Helps to Have Friends: When Mom or Dad Has Cancer.*
The text is written as the story of an elementary school–age child and the friends he meets in a support group for children who have a parent with cancer. The children discuss feelings they experienced at diagnosis and during treatment. Order through the American Cancer Society at: www.cancer org

➤ Canadian Cancer Society. *When Someone You Love Has Cancer: A Resource for Young People.*

This 26-page booklet addresses the issues of cancer in the family, what cancer is, and cancer treatment for young people. It includes short stories by children who have had a family member experience cancer. Access at: www.cancer.ca

➤ KidsCope. *Kemo Shark.*
This 14-page comic book features a shark as a superhero fighting bad cells in the body. It helps to explain chemotherapy to young children and why it causes bad side effects and changes in appearance. Access at: www.kids cope.org

➤ Cancer Family Care. *What About Me? A Booklet for Teenage Children of Cancer Patients.*
This booklet has answers to questions teenagers are likely to have when a parent is diagnosed with cancer. It discusses what cancer is and how it is treated, dealing with the stress of cancer, peer relations, handling feelings, grieving, and finding sources of support. Sections about single-parent families and drugs and alcohol also are included. To order access: www. cancerfamilycare.org

➤ National Cancer Institute. *When Your Parent Has Cancer: A Guide for Teens.*
This 75-page booklet describes how teens cope when they find out their mother or father has cancer. It provides information about cancer treatments, ways teens can talk to family and friends, how to connect with other teens, and where to find other resources for information and support. Access at: https://cissecure.nci.nih.gov/ncipubs/

Coloring Books

➤ American Cancer Society. *Because . . . . Someone I Love Has Cancer: Kids' Activity Book.*
This publication offers children ages 5–10 support, encouragement, and opportunity for imaginative personal expression. The creative activities and exercises progressively teach coping skills and encourage open expression of feelings. Includes a 16-page removable guide for caregivers and five twist-up, self-sharpening crayons. To order contact your local American Cancer Society or access: www.cancer org.

➤ Oncology Nursing Society. *My Book about Cancer* (father and mother versions).
This interactive workbook is both a coloring book and a sketch pad. Children can color various animal characters that depict scenes, images, and emotions likely to be encountered during a parent's illness. Order through the Oncology Nursing Society site at: www.ons.org.

Books

For preschool and kindergarten-age children

➤ Ammary, Neyal J. 2003. *In Mommy's Garden: A Book to Help Explain Cancer to Young Children*. Illustrated by Christoper Risch. United States: Canyon Beach Visual Communications.
This book can be used to educate very young children on the concept of cancer. The text is simple, and the sentences are short. The story is told from the point of view of a little girl whose mother has cancer. She talks about how her mother explained cancer to her by comparing weeds in a garden to cancer cells in the human body.

➤ Blake, Claire, Eliza Blanchard, and Kathy Parkinson. 1998. *The Paper Chain*. Santa Fe, NM: Health Press.
A young boy tells the story of his family as his mother is being treated for cancer. Simple explanations of surgery, chemotherapy, and radiation are given in a matter-of-fact but gentle and positive tone. The text touches on hair loss, fatigue, and such feelings as sadness and anger. The book ends on a positive note, with the mother feeling stronger and her hair growing back.

➤ Carney, Karen L. 2004. *"What is Cancer Anyway?" Explaining Cancer to Children of All Ages*. Wethersfield, CT: Dragonfly.
This is one of the books in the Barklay and Eve Children's Book Series. Barklay and Eve, the two lovable main characters who are dogs, define cancer and explain radiation and chemotherapy, including the reasons for hair loss. The tone is calm, clear, and reassuring.

➤ Frahm, Amelia. 2001. *Tickles Tabitha's Cancer-Tankerous Mommy*. Illustrated by Elizabeth Schultz. Hutchinson, MN: Nutcracker.
The story is told through the eyes of Tabitha, a young girl whose mother is being treated with chemotherapy. The family deals with the changes brought on by cancer, including hair loss, anger, and fear—experienced by the parents as well as the children.

➤ Kohlenberg, Sherry, and Lauri Crow. 1994. *Sammy's Mommy Has Cancer*. Library ed. Milwaukee, WI: Gareth Stevens.
Sammy's mommy receives treatment for cancer, goes into the hospital for surgery, recovers at home, and shares her continuing love for him. Appropriate for toddlers and preschool-age children.

➤ Parkinson, Carolyn Stearns, and Elaine Verstraete. 1991. *My Mommy Has Cancer*. Rochester, NY: Park Press.
Beautiful, gentle color illustrations tell the story of Eric, whose mother is being treated for cancer. The text explains the concepts of cancer, surgery, and chemotherapy.

➤ Watters, Debbie, et al. 2005. *Where's Mom's Hair? A Family Journey through Cancer.* Toronto: Second Story Press.

This picture book describes how one family with two young children coped with their mother's hair loss. The family organized a hair-cutting party at the beginning of chemotherapy and a hair-growing-back party at the end of treatment. The content is mostly photos with text suitable for very young children.

For elementary school–age children

➤ Ackermann, Abigail, and Adrienne Ackermann. 2001. *Our Mom Has Cancer.* Atlanta: American Cancer Society.

Written and illustrated by two sisters ages 9 and 11 who describe what it was like for them when their mother was diagnosed with breast cancer and underwent surgery and chemotherapy. This book is appropriate for children between the ages of 5 and 8.

➤ Hannigan, Katherine. 2004. *Ida B:—and Her Plans to Maximize Fun, Avoid Disaster, and (Possibly) Save the World.* New York: Greenwillow Books.

This is the story of a fourth-grade home-schooled girl who has to go back to a public school after her mother is diagnosed with breast cancer. This book is told in the first person by the fictional character and won praise for the compelling and moving story. Appropriate for upper-elementary-age children and preteens.

➤ Harpham, Wendy Schlessel, and Jonas Kulikauskas. 1997. *Becky and the Worry Cup.* New York: HarperCollins.

Six-year-old Becky has many adjustments to make and new feelings to deal with when her mother is diagnosed with cancer. This book accompanies the book "When a Parent Has Cancer: A Guide to Caring for Your Children," described below.

➤ Speltz, Ann, and Kate Sternberg. 2003. *The Year My Mother Was Bald.* Washington, DC: Magination Press.

This book is presented as a journal kept by an eight-year-old girl while her mother was undergoing treatment for breast cancer. It describes the illness, diagnosis, and treatment, but the focus is the feelings experienced by the child and how the family bonds together. Includes a list of resources.

➤ Winthrop, Elizabeth, and Betsy Lewin. 2000. *Promises.* New York: Clarion Books.

Told in the first person by a young girl whose world is turned upside down after her mother gets sick. During her treatment she seems to get sicker and sicker. She's often in the hospital, and at home she needs to rest. Even though the mom gets better after a very long time, she still cannot promise that she will never get sick again. This book has beautiful illustrations and is appropriate for five- to eight-year-olds.

For preteens

➤ Clifford, Christine, and Jack Lindstrom. 1998. *Our Family Has Cancer, Too!* Minneapolis, MN: University of Minnesota Press.
When their mother is diagnosed with cancer, sixth-grader Tim and his younger brother visit her in the hospital, learn about radiation and chemotherapy, and help with the chores at home. The text is illustrated with cartoons and includes suggestions of conversation starters for parents. Contains a glossary of the words kids might hear when someone in their family has cancer.

➤ Goodman, Michelle B. 1990. *Vanishing Cookies: Doing Ok When a Parent Has Cancer.* Downsview, Ont.: Benjamin Family Foundation.
Written in a question-and-answer format, this book is intended for kids ages 9 to 14 whose parents are undergoing cancer treatment. It addresses issues such as school and friends, coping with feelings, sources of support, and worrying about a parent's death.

For teens

➤ Pennebaker, Ruth. 2000. *Both Sides Now.* New York: Holt.
Fifteen-year-old Liza tries to deal with the normal everyday crises of life in an Austin, Texas, high school, a process complicated by her mother's fight with breast cancer. The story focuses on the mother-daughter relationship and how the family reinvents itself at a time of crisis. For ages 12 and up.

Information Sources for Parents

Brochures, Booklets, and Other Short Print Publications

➤ CancerCare. *Helping Children Understand Cancer: How to Talk to Your Children about Your Cancer Diagnosis* and *Helping Teenagers When a Parent Has Cancer.*
Short, two-page handouts for parents with practical tips and suggestions for communication with children about a cancer diagnosis in the family. Access online at: www.cancercare.org

Books

➤ Harpham, Wendy Schlessel, et al. 2004. *When a Parent Has Cancer: A Guide to Caring for Your Children.* Rev. ed. New York: Perennial Currents.
This book includes a companion book for children, *Becky and the Worry Cup*, described above. The author is a cancer survivor who draws on her

own experience of raising young children while struggling with cancer. Chapters discuss parenting at different stages of the illness, such as right after diagnosis, beyond the first few weeks of treatment, and at recurrence. The book also addresses the issues of communicating with children about death, parenting teenagers, caring for children in single-parent families, and other special circumstances. Special features include a glossary of cancer terms for children, information about major stages of growth and development, and a list of resources.

➤ Heiney, Sue P. 2001. *Cancer in the Family: Helping Children Cope with a Parent's Illness*. Atlanta: American Cancer Society.

This book explains to parents how help children cope with a parent's diagnosis of cancer. The author offers practical suggestions for communicating with children at every step of the illness. Topics covered include children's emotional reactions to crisis and responses at different developmental levels, understanding and using psychosocial support services, talking about death, and issues for nontraditional families. The book also provides a removable illustrated workbook designed to help young children to express their feelings through art.

➤ Russell, Neil. 2001. *Can I Still Kiss You? Answering Your Children's Questions about Cancer*. Deerfield Beach, FL: Health Communications.

This book was written by a cancer survivor and offers guidance and advice to parents. Each chapter has a list of questions children are likely to ask and suggested answers to those questions. Each also concludes with a space for children and parents to write their own personal questions and express emotions.

➤ Van Dernoot, Peter, and Madelyn Case. 2002. *Helping Your Children Cope with Your Cancer: A Guide for Parents and Families*. New York: Hatherleigh Press.

At the heart of this book are real-life stories and experiences of over 20 parents who have been diagnosed with cancer. The stories focus on the impact of cancer on the family and how parents helped their children cope. Chapters written by professionals discuss the importance of communicating with children about cancer. A few stories written by children also are included.

Audiovisual Resources

➤ *Kids Tell Kids What It's Like When Their Mother or Father Has Cancer*. Los Angeles: Cancervive, 1998.

Kids do all the talking in this 15-minute video and discuss their hopes, fears, and the adult burden placed on them when cancer strikes a parent.

The film is faithful to the kid's point of view and encourages communication among family members. Available in DVD and VHS formats. To order, access: www.cancervive.org

➤ *We Can Cope When a Parent Has Cancer.* Dir. Harpham, Wendy Schlessel, Kevin Dawkins, and Innovative Training Systems et al. 3 videocassettes (95 minutes). Inflexxion, 2000.

A series of three programs—one for parents, one for teens, and one for young children—offers specific advice to parents on how to communicate with their children about illness-related issues and how to understand and attend to their children's emotional needs in an age-appropriate manner. The programs share the stories of seven unique families from a wide range of backgrounds. An accompanying guidebook explains to parents how to use the program. Available in VHS and DVD formats. To order, access: www.wecancope.com/

Web Resources

Sections in general cancer sites

➤ American Cancer Society. *Dealing with a Cancer Diagnosis in the Family.* Access at: www.cancer.org and click on the link to "Patients, Family & Friends" and then on the link to "Children and Cancer."

This page links to several detailed overviews explaining how to help children cope with specific situations during the illness.

➤ Cancerbackup. *Talking to Children about Cancer.* Access at: www.cancer backup.org.uk/Home and follow the links to "Resources & Support" and "Relationships & Communication."

This page links to a detailed guide that discusses how to talk about cancer with children between the ages of 2 and 16.

Patient-Support Organizations

➤ Kids Konnected. Access at: www.kidskonnected.org/
Phone: 949-582-5443

Practical Issues of Survivorship: Legal, Financial, Insurance, and Employment Issues

"From the moment of diagnosis and for the balance of life, an individual diagnosed with cancer is a survivor."
— National Coalition for Cancer Survivorship Charter

Being a cancer survivor entails much more than being a cancer patient. Survivorship encompasses the whole spectrum of life dimensions. Beyond the illness, treatment, and physical condition, survivorship also includes a person's emotional well-being, relationships, social environments, employment, and financial situation. These aspects are often referred to as "psychosocial" issues. Information sources focusing on coping with the psychological issues of cancer survivorship are presented in the section "Emotional Distress" on page 266. This section covers the practical side of living with cancer, mainly legal, financial, insurance, and employment issues.

One of the greatest worries of people diagnosed with cancer is how the diagnosis will affect their employment status, which may further impinge on their ability to obtain and retain health and life insurance. This issue is of utmost importance to the 3.8 million working-age adults with a history of cancer living in the United States. Cancer may restrict a person's ability to work, especially during treatment but sometimes even after treatment. Roughly 20% of people working at the time of their diagnosis face cancer-related work limitations two to three years later (Hewitt, et al., 2006), and all survivors are at risk of experiencing subtle-to-blatant discrimination in the workplace. Cancer survivors reported problems such as dismissal, failure to hire, demotion, denial of promotion, undesirable transfer, denial of benefits, and hostility (Hewitt, et al., 2006).

In the United States and other countries, people with cancer are covered by employment discrimination laws. The Americans with Disabilities Act, also known as the ADA, is the federal law that protects disabled workers in the United States. In addition, every state has a law regulating, to a certain extent, disability-based employment discrimination. Another federal law that applies to cancer survivors and their families in the United States is the Family and Medical Leave Act (FMLA). This law requires employers with 50 or more employees to provide up to 12 weeks of unpaid, job-protected leave for family members who need time off to address their own serious health condition or to care for a seriously ill child, parent, or spouse.

Health insurance (and paying medical bills) is another difficult and complicated issue with which cancer survivors struggle. During treatment, people with cancer may need assistance and information about working with their insurance company to ensure that they are receiving the coverage they are entitled to. Uninsured individuals need information about Medicaid and special insurance plans that may be available to them. Other sources of financial help are pharmaceutical companies that offer programs to help people pay for prescriptions and agencies, organizations, and foundations that provide assistance to help pay for medical and non-medical expenses caused by the illness. After treatment is over, survivors may experience difficulties obtaining health insurance. Cancer survivors have rights under federal and state laws, but these rights are not comprehensive. Federal laws regulate mostly group plans offered by large employers. Individual insurance plans or groups plans offered by small employers are regulated by the states. The level and type of protections vary depending on whether state or federal laws apply to a specific situation. Information about disability insurance and applying for social security disability benefits may also be relevant to many survivors during and after treatment.

People possessing knowledge of the legal rights of individuals with cancer may be able to avoid employment and insurance problems. Other legal issues that may pertain to cancer survivors include custody and guardianship of minor children, estate issues, and entitlement to and collection of government benefits.

In addition to independent information seeking, it is advisable for all cancer survivors to contact an oncology social worker in their area. Social workers can be a great resource for information and referrals on all practical aspects, including the ones listed above, as well as transportation and accommodations for people who need to travel for their medical care.

Other practical matters of cancer survivorship include locating and evaluating medical providers and facilities, communicating with the medical team, and finding quality information about cancer in lay language. Many of the information sources listed below provide instructions on how to locate reliable cancer information on the Internet. Because information on health is widely accessible on the Internet, many professionals feel it is imperative to educate cancer survivors about finding authoritative and trustworthy information on the Internet and avoiding erroneous, biased, and misleading information. The evaluation checklist in Chapter 1 (p. 20) can be used by librarians and the public to evaluate health information on the Internet.

Information Sources

Brochures, Booklets, and Other Short Print Publications

➤ National Cancer Institute. *Facing Forward Series: Life after Cancer Treatment.* This 125-page spiral-bound booklet covers post–treatment issues such as follow-up medical care, physical and emotional changes, changes in social relationships, and practical matters. Includes a comprehensive resource list and worksheets. Access at: https://cissecure.nci.nih.gov/ncipubs/

➤ National Coalition for Cancer Survivorship. *Teamwork: The Cancer Patient's Guide to Talking with Your Doctor.*

Developed by cancer survivors and health care professionals, this booklet addresses the need for good communication and provides a list of sound, practical questions that patients can use when talking with their doctor. Access at: www.canceradvocacy.org

➤ National Coalition for Cancer Survivorship. *What Cancer Survivors Need to Know about Health Insurance.*
This booklet sorts through the insurance maze by explaining the many types of insurance, exploring ways cancer survivors can get the most out of their insurance coverage, and discussing laws that provide some protection for cancer survivors who are changing jobs. Access at: www.cancer advocacy.org

➤ National Coalition for Cancer Survivorship. *Working It Out: Your Employment Rights as a Cancer Survivor.*
This booklet addresses the employment challenges that many survivors face and offers advice and resources to address those challenges. It provides an overview of employment discrimination laws that protect cancer survivors, what one can do to avoid discrimination, and how to enforce legal rights. Access at: www.canceradvocacy.org

➤ National Coalition for Cancer Survivorship. *Self-Advocacy: A Cancer Survivor's Handbook.*
The purpose of this booklet is to help readers become informed and knowledgeable health care consumers who know how to communicate their needs to those who can be helpful to them as they experience cancer. This handbook focuses on self-training steps and tools to assist and empower individuals dealing with cancer. Access at: www.canceradvocacy.org

Books

Cancer guidebooks with information on practical matters

➤ Feuerstein, Michael, and Patricia Findley. 2006. *The Cancer Survivor's Guide: The Essential Handbook to Life after Cancer.* New York: Marlowe.
The authors present practical strategies for managing the complex and challenging tasks confronting persons diagnosed with cancer. It covers practical as well as emotional aspects of living with cancer, with chapters on navigating the health care system, communicating with health care providers, researching the illness and treatment options, handling finances, and improving overall health.

➤ Hoffman, Barbara, ed., and National Coalition for Cancer Survivorship (U.S.). 2004. *A Cancer Survivor's Almanac: Charting Your Journey.* 3d ed. Hoboken, NJ: Wiley.

This book provides practical information on health insurance, communicating with family and friends, dealing with loss, advocating for yourself, and job discrimination. It also includes information on medical diagnosis, treatment, pain control, long-term and late effects of cancer treatment, and coping with the personal and social impact of cancer. The resource directory lists hundreds of organizations and agencies that offer help with specific cancer-related issues and explains how to find cancer information through the Internet.

➤ Nessim, Susan, et al. 2000. *Can Survive: Reclaiming Your Life after Cancer.* Rev. and updated ed. Boston: Houghton Mifflin.
This book focuses on the needs of cancer survivors after treatment. It provides strategies for coping with many practical problems, from fear of recurrence to job and insurance discrimination, altered relationships, and the long-term effects of chemotherapy and radiation. Includes tips from survivors, doctors, and other experts.

Relevant general books

➤ Landay, David S. 2000. *Be Prepared: The Complete Financial, Legal, and Practical Guide to Living with Cancer, HIV, and other Life-Challenging Conditions.* New York: St. Martin's Press.
Authored by an attorney, this book offers practical advice on managing the complex financial, legal, employment, and insurance issues facing people with a life-threatening illness. Medical issues such as second opinions, communicating with the doctor, obtaining drugs, and navigating the health care system also are covered. The section on estate planning, living wills, and advance directives is very detailed. Other topics include support resources, necessary professionals, travel, and other practical matters relevant to people with a serious diagnosis.

Web Resources

Sites focusing on practical matters of cancer survivorship

➤ Cancer and Careers. Access at: www.cancerandcareers.org
Although this site focuses on working women with cancer, much of the information is relevant to all cancer survivors who have questions about maintaining a job during and after cancer treatment. It offers separate sections for survivors, employers, and coworkers, with detailed information about employment law and communication about the illness. Other topics include health insurance, appearance, stress management, and disability.

➤ Lance Armstrong Foundation. *LIVESTRONG SurvivorCare.* Access at: www.laf.org
The "Help & Support" section of this site contains information on many topics of interest to cancer survivors, including physical, emotional, and practical issues. Each topic has detailed information, suggestions of what to do, and a list of resources. The site also offers downloadable survivorship tools that can help manage the information and documents needed to maintain a healthy survivorship.

➤ National Coalition for Cancer Survivorship. Access at: www.canceradvocacy. org
This site of the oldest survivor-led cancer advocacy organization in the United States has information on many survivorship topics and a resource guide of myriad organizations that provide assistance to people with cancer.

Detailed sections in general cancer sites

➤ American Cancer Society. *Managing Day to Day.* Access at: www.cancer. org and click on the link to "Patients, Family & Friends," then click on "Coping with Treatment."
This section has information about the logistics of treatment, including financial and legal issues, insurance claims, and transportation.

➤ Cancerbackup. *Practical Issues.* Access at: www.cancerbackup.org.uk/ home and click on "Resources & Support," then scroll down to the section on practical issues.
Links to information about practical topics such as pet care, travel, and daily living. Some of the information is relevant only to people living in the United Kingdom.

➤ National Cancer Institute. *Support & Resources.* Access at: www.cancer.gov, click on "Cancer Topics" and then on "Support and Resources."
The top page of this site links to documents about support organizations, finances, insurance, home care, and hospice care.

Sections about practical matters are also available at the following sites

➤ CancerConsultants.com. *Cancer Resource Center.* Access at: www.cancer consultants.com.

➤ People Living with Cancer. *Survivorship.* Access at: www.plwc.org.

General sites with relevant information

➤ Georgetown University Health Policy Institute. *healthinsuranceinfo.net.* Access at: www.healthinsuranceinfo.net

This site has state-specific consumer guides for getting and keeping health insurance. The guides summarize in lay language protections with regard to obtaining health insurance as individuals or employees. The guides can be either viewed online or printed as Adobe Acrobat (.pdf) files.

➤ Patient Advocate Foundation. Access at: www.patientadvocate.org
The Patient Advocate Foundation seeks to ensure patients' access to care, maintenance of employment, and preservation of financial stability. The site has information about many programs and services pertaining to people with cancer, as well as the full-text of the organization's publications that explain how to resolve insurance and financial problems that occur as a result of a medical condition. The *National Financial Resource Guide For Patients* is a state-by-state directory of organizations providing financial relief for a broad range of needs, including housing, utilities, food, transportation to medical treatment, and children's resources.

Patient-Support Organizations

➤ Cancer Legal Resource Center. Access at: www.disabilityrightslegalcenter. org
Phone: 866-843-2572

➤ Lance Armstrong Foundation. *LIVESTRONG SurvivorCare*. Access at: www.laf.org
Phone: 866-235-7205

➤ National Coalition for Cancer Survivorship. Access at: www.canceradvocacy. org
Phone: 877-622- 7937

➤ Patient Advocate Foundation. Access at: www.patientadvocate.org
Phone: 800-532-5274

Sexuality

Human sexuality is shaped by emotional as well as physical well-being. A person's relationships, stress level, cultural attitudes, and values—as well as perceptions of self-worth and body-image—are as important to sexual functioning as are the physical aspects. Cancer brings about drastic changes in many dimensions of life; therefore, it has a profound effect on sexuality.

Not all patients suffer from sexual difficulties, but they are quite common among cancer patients during and after treatment. Research shows that approximately one-half of women who have been treated for breast and gynecologic cancers experience long-term sexual dysfunction. Sixty to ninety percent of men treated for prostate cancer experience erectile dysfunction to varying degrees of severity and duration.

Physical sexual problems are caused mostly by treatment for cancer and not by the disease itself. Surgery and radiation therapy in the pelvic and genital areas may cause damage to the organs, glands, nerves, and blood vessels necessary for sexual functioning. Hormonal treatment used to treat hormone-sensitive cancers such as breast and prostate cancer may alter the balance of body chemicals that play an essential role in the process of sexual arousal and response. Side effects of chemotherapy and biological therapy can reduce both the physical energy and the desire for sex.

Even survivors whose sexual organs and physiology have not been damaged by therapy may experience sexual dysfunction. Emotional and psychological factors are believed to be the most common causes of sexual problems in people with cancer. Changes in body image and self-perception deeply impact intimacy and relationships. Stress, depression, anxiety, and fatigue all contribute to a decrease in sexual desire and sexual pleasure.

Female sexual problems associated with cancer therapy include vaginal dryness, which may cause painful intercourse; trouble reaching orgasm; and low sexual desire. Male problems include difficulties in achieving erection; changes in ejaculation; dry orgasm; lack of orgasm; and low libido.

In many cases, sexual difficulties disappear after treatment is over. If problems persist, it is wise to seek out medical advice. A large variety of medical and psychological therapies are available to solve the great majority of sexual difficulties. An accurate diagnosis of the exact cause of problems is primary to finding the right therapeutic approach. Medical interventions such as hormone replacement, medications, and surgery can be very effective. Psychological counseling with a certified mental health professional who received additional training in sex therapy also is helpful, especially if provided together with medical intervention. Specific therapies for men with impotence include oral erectogenic drugs such as Viagra, penile vacuum erection devices, and implanted penile prostheses. Therapies for women include vaginal dilators, creams and lubricants, and Kegel exercises to strengthen vaginal muscles.

Information Sources

Brochures, Booklets, and Other Short Print Publications

➤ American Cancer Society. *Sexuality and Cancer—For the Man Who Has Cancer and His Partner.*
This 88-page booklet provides a detailed overview of male sexuality and the problems that may arise during and after cancer treatment. It discusses

specific conditions, emotional factors, and myths about cancer and sexuality. Includes a section for single men. To order contact your local American Cancer Society or access at: www.cancer.org

➤ American Cancer Society. *Sexuality and Cancer—For the Woman Who Has Cancer and Her Partner.*

This 75-page booklet provides a detailed overview of female sexuality and the problems that may arise during and after cancer treatment. It discusses specific conditions, emotional factors, and myths about cancer and sexuality. Includes a section for single women. To order contact your local American Cancer Society or access at: www.cancer.org

➤ Canadian Cancer Society. *Sexuality and Cancer: A Guide for People with Cancer.*

This is a 44-page publication aimed at men and women. It describes healthy sexual function and problems that may arise as a result of cancer treatment. Access at: cancer.ca. Available in English and French.

Books

➤ Alterowitz, Ralph, and Barbara Alterowitz. 2004. *Intimacy with Impotence: The Couple's Guide to Better Sex after Prostate Disease.* Cambridge, MA: Da Capo Lifelong Bks.

Edited by a husband-and-wife team who experienced erectile dysfunction as a result of prostate cancer, this book provides a detailed overview of the problem and possible solutions. Chapters were contributed by several urology specialists and address topics such as talking to your partner, reviving loving, commercial therapies and medications, non–approved and off-label treatments, and putting it all together. Each chapter starts with a list of key points, and appendixes include listings of treatments for erectile dysfunction, non-FDA-approved therapies, manufacturers of erectile dysfunction products, resources and references, and further reading.

➤ Schover, Leslie R. 1997. *Sexuality and Fertility after Cancer.* New York: Wiley.

This comprehensive overview of sexuality and fertility during and after cancer was written by a psychologist and sex therapist at Cleveland Clinic. It provides a detailed overview of cancer and cancer treatments' impact on sexuality, as well as suggestions on how to become sexually active again after cancer and how to address specific problems. Chapters for gay and lesbian survivors and singles also are included.

Audiovisual Resources

➤ Health Library Online Video Collection. *Sexuality after Breast Cancer.* (35 minutes.)

A group of women discuss changes they experienced after breast cancer treatment. Topics include loss of spontaneity, body image, and communication with partners. View online at: http://healthlibrary.stanford.edu/resources/videos.html

➤ Krahn, Leona. *Not Alone. Couples Share Candidly about Prostate Cancer.* Winnipeg, CA : Krahn Communications, 1998. (44 minutes.)
This program features three couples at different stages of life who openly share their personal battles with prostate cancer, including their thoughts on the sensitive issues of incontinence and impotence. Can be ordered in VHS and DVD formats at: www.prostatecancervideo.com

➤ Medical Media Associates. *Intimacy* (Women Stories Series) 2001. (20 minutes.)
Breast cancer survivors and their spouses talk about issues of intimacy, sexuality, and love after breast cancer. To view online or order access at: www.womenstories.org

Web Resources

Detailed sections in general cancer sites

➤ American Cancer Society. *Sexuality*. Access at: www.cancer.org and click on "Patients, Family & Friends" and then on "Preparing for Treatment," "Treatment Topics and Resources," and "Staying Active during Treatment." This page links to documents about men's and women's sexual health during and after treatment.

➤ Cancerbackup. *Sexuality and Cancer*. Access at: www.cancerbackup.org. uk/Home and click on the link to "Resources & Support."
This section explains how different treatments affect sexuality and ways to resolve problems.

➤ CancerSymptoms.org. *Sexual Dysfunction*. Access at: www.cancersymptoms. org and click on "Sexual Dysfunction" on the left sidebar.
This section explains key points and provides tips for pain management.

Sections about fertility are also available at the following sites

➤ LIVESTRONG SurvivorCare. *Female Sexual Dysfunction and Male Sexual Dysfunction*. Access at: www.livestrong.org and click on "Take Control" and then on "Physical Topics."

➤ People Living with Cancer. *Sexual and Reproductive Health*. Access at: www.plwc.org and click on "Diagnosis and Treatment" and then on "Treating Cancer."

References

Medical Library Association, Consumer and Patient Health Information Section (CAPHIS/MLA). The Librarian's Role in the Provision of Consumer Health Information and Patient Education [Policy Statement]. (1996). *Bulletin of the Medical Library Association* 84, no. 2: 238–239.

Abramovitz, M. 2001. "End of Life Care: Weighing Decisions. *InTouch* 3, no. 4: 50.

Abramson, D. H., and C. Servodidio. "Parent's Guide to Understanding Retinoblastoma." (1997). Retrieved 1/12/06 from A Parent's Guide to Understanding Retinoblastoma Web site: www.retinoblastoma.com/guide.htm

American Cancer Society. "American Cancer Society." (2005). Retrieved 1/12/05 from The American Cancer Society Web site: www.cancer.org

American Cancer Society. (2005). *Cancer Facts and Figures 2005*. Atlanta: American Cancer Society.

American Cancer Society. "Cigarette Smoking." (2005). Retrieved 1/11/06 from the American Cancer Web site: www.cancer.org/docroot/PED/content/PED_10_2X_Cigarette_Smoking.asp?sitearea=PED

American Cancer Society. "Detailed Guide: Bone Cancer." (2005). Retrieved 10/21/05 from The American Cancer Web site: www.cancer.org/docroot/CRI/CRI_2_3x.asp?dt=2

American Cancer Society. "Detailed Guide: Brain/CNS Tumors in Adults." (2005). Retrieved 10/22/05 from the American Cancer Web site: www.cancer.org/docroot/CRI/CRI_2_3x.asp?dt=3

American Cancer Society. "Detailed Guide: Brain/CNS Tumors in Children." (2005). Retrieved 1/12/06 from The American Cancer Society Web site: www.cancer.org/docroot/CRI/CRI_2_3x.asp?dt=4

American Cancer Society. "Detailed Guide: Breast Cancer." (2005). Retrieved 10/10/05 from The American Cancer Society Web site: http://www.cancer.org/docroot/CRI/CRI_2_3x.asp?dt=5

American Cancer Society. "Detailed Guide: Cancer (General Information)." (2005). Retrieved 1/11/06 from The American Cancer Society Web site: www.cancer.org/docroot/CRI/CRI_2_3x.asp?dt=72

American Cancer Society. "Detailed Guide: Cervical Cancer." (2005). Retrieved 09/08/05 from The American Cancer Society Web site: www.cancer.org/docroot/CRI/CRI_2_3x.asp?dt=8

American Cancer Society. "Detailed Guide: Endometrial Cancer." (2005). Retrieved 9/3/05 from The American Cancer Society Web site: www.cancer.org/docroot/CRI/CRI_2_3x.asp?dt=11

American Cancer Society. "Detailed Guide: Esophagus Cancer." (2005). Retrieved 11/12/05 from The American Cancer Society Web site: www.cancer.org/docroot/CRI/CRI_2_3x.asp?dt=12

American Cancer Society. "Detailed Guide: Ewing's Family of Tumors." (2005). Retrieved 1/12/06 from The American Cancer Society Web site: www.cancer.org/docroot/CRI/CRI_2_3x.asp?dt=48

American Cancer Society. "Detailed Guide: Hodgkin's Disease." (2005). Retrieved 10/28/05 from The American Cancer Society Web site: www.cancer.org/docroot/CRI/CRI_2_3x.asp?dt=84

American Cancer Society. "Detailed Guide: Kidney Cancer." (2005). Retrieved 09/12/05 from The American Cancer Society Web site: www.cancer.org/docroot/CRI/CRI_2_3x.asp?dt=22

American Cancer Society. "Detailed Guide: Leukemia—Acute Lymphocytic (ALL)." (2005). Retrieved 10/10/05 from The American Cancer Society Web site: www.cancer.org/docroot/CRI/CRI_2_3x.asp?dt=57

American Cancer Society. "Detailed Guide: Leukemia—Acute Myeloid (AML)." (2005). Retrieved 10/15/05 from The American Cancer Society Web site: www.cancer.org/docroot/CRI/CRI_2_3x.asp?dt=82

American Cancer Society. "Detailed Guide: Leukemia—Chronic Lymphocytic (CLL)." (2005). Retrieved 10/1505 from The American Cancer Society Web site: www.cancer.org/docroot/CRI/CRI_2_3x. asp?dt=62

American Cancer Society. "Detailed Guide: Leukemia—Chronic Myeloid (CML)." (2005). Retrieved 10/15/05 from The American Cancer Society Web site: www.cancer.org/docroot/CRI/CRI_2_3x.asp?dt=83

American Cancer Society. "Detailed Guide: Liver Cancer." (2005). Retrieved 9/23/05 from The American Cancer Society Web site: www.cancer.org/docroot/CRI/CRI_2_3x.asp?dt=25

American Cancer Society. "Detailed Guide: Lymphoma, Non-Hodgkin's Type. (2005). Retrieved 10/28/05 from The American Cancer Society Web site: www.cancer.org/docroot/CRI/CRI_2_3x.asp?dt=32

American Cancer Society. "Detailed Guide: Male Breast Cancer." (2005). Retrieved 09/5/06 from The American Cancer Society Web site: www.cancer.org/docroot/CRI/CRI_2_3x.asp?dt=28

American Cancer Society. "Detailed Guide: Neuroblastoma." (2005). Retrieved 1/12/06 from The American Cancer Society Web site: www.cancer.org/docroot/CRI/CRI_2_3x.asp?dt=31

American Cancer Society. "Detailed Guide: Osteosarcoma." (2005). Retrieved 1/12/06 from The American Cancer Society Web site: www.cancer.org/docroot/CRI/CRI_2_3x.asp?dt=52

American Cancer Society. "Detailed Guide: Ovarian Cancer." (2005). Retrieved 09/08/05 from The American Cancer Society Web site: www.cancer.org/docroot/CRI/CRI_2_3x.asp?dt=33

American Cancer Society. "Detailed Guide: Pancreatic Cancer." (2005). Retrieved 9/20/05 from The American Cancer Society Web site: www.cancer.org/docroot/CRI/CRI_2_3x.asp?dt=34

American Cancer Society. "Detailed Guide: Prostate Cancer." (2005). Retrieved 10/18/05 from The American Cancer Society Web site: www.cancer.org/docroot/CRI/CRI_2_3x.asp?dt=36

American Cancer Society. "Detailed Guide: Retinoblastoma (An Eye Cancer)." (2005). Retrieved 1/12/06 from The American Cancer Society Web site: www.cancer.org/docroot/CRI/CRI_2_3x.asp?dt=37

American Cancer Society. "Detailed Guide: Rhabdomyosarcoma." (2005). Retrieved 1/12/06 from The American Cancer Web site: www.cancer.org/docroot/CRI/CRI_2_3x.asp?dt=53

American Cancer Society. "Detailed Guide: Sarcoma—Adult Soft Tissue Cancer. (2005). Retrieved 10/2105 from The American Cancer Web site: www.cancer.org/docroot/CRI/CRI_2_3x.asp?dt=38

American Cancer Society. "Detailed Guide: Skin Cancer—Melanoma." (2005). Retrieved 09/17/05 from The American Cancer Web site: www.cancer.org/docroot/CRI/CRI_2_3x.asp?dt=39

American Cancer Society. "Detailed Guide: Skin Cancer—Nonmelanoma." (2005). Retrieved 09/17/05 from The American Cancer Web site: www.cancer.org/docroot/CRI/CRI_2_3x.asp?dt=51

American Cancer Society. "Detailed Guide: Stomach Cancer." (2005). Retrieved 9/20/05 from The American Cancer Web site: www.cancer.org/docroot/CRI/CRI_2_3x.asp?dt=40

American Cancer Society. "Detailed Guide: Testicular Cancer." (2005). Retrieved 09/12/05 from The American Cancer Web site: www.cancer.org/docroot/CRI/CRI_2_3x.asp?dt=41

American Cancer Society. "Detailed Guide: Thyroid Cancer." (2005). Retrieved 09/08/05 from The American Cancer Web site: www.cancer.org/docroot/CRI/CRI_2_3x.asp?dt=43

American Cancer Society. "Detailed Guide: Uterine Sarcoma." (2005). Retrieved 09/03/05 from The American Cancer Web site: www.cancer. org/docroot/CRI/CRI_2_3x.asp?dt=63

American Cancer Society. "Detailed Guide: Wilms' Tumor." (2005). Retrieved 1/12/06 from The American Cancer Web site: www.cancer. org/docroot/CRI/CRI_2_3x.asp?dt=46

American Cancer Society. "Early Detection." (2005). Retrieved 1/11/06 from The American Cancer Web site: www.cancer.org/docroot/PED/content/ PED_2_3X_Early_Detection.asp?sitearea=PED

American Cancer Society. "Helping Children When a Family Member Has Cancer: Dealing with Diagnosis." (2005). Retrieved 1/27/06 from The American Cancer Web site: www.cancer.org/docroot/CRI/content/ CRI_2_6X_Dealing_With_Diagnosis.asp?sitearea=CRI

American Cancer Society. "Secondhand Smoke." (2005). Retrieved 1/11/06 from The American Cancer Web site: www.cancer.org/docroot/PED/ content/PED_10_2X_Secondhand_Smoke-Clean_Indoor_Air.asp? sitearea=PED

American Cancer Society and National Comprehensive Cancer Network (U.S.). 2004. *Advanced Cancer and Palliative Care: Treatment Guidelines for Patients.* United States: American Cancer Society, National Comprehensive Cancer Network.

American Cancer Society and National Comprehensive Cancer Network. 2005. *Distress: Treatment Guidelines for Patients* (2d ed.). United States: American Cancer Society, National Comprehensive Cancer Network.

American Pain Society. "Pain: The Fifth Vital Sign." (2006). Retrieved 2/8/06 from The American Pain Society Web sit: www.ampainsoc.org/advocacy/ fifth.htm

Boughton, B. 2003. "Facing the Future: Planning for a Good Death." *CURE: Cancer Updates, Research & Education* 2, no. 1: 50–53, 55.

Caley, B. A. 2005. "With Curative Intent at Every Turn, Patients with Hodgkin's Disease Are Successfully Getting to the Other Side." *CURE: Cancer Updates, Research & Education* 4, no. 1: 40–47.

Card, I., and National Coalition for Cancer Survivorship (U.S.). 1993. *What Cancer Survivors Need to Know about Health Insurance.* Silver Spring, MD: NCCS.

Carroll, W. L., and J. B. Reisman. 2005. *100 Questions and Answers about Your Child's Cancer.* Sudbury, MA: Jones and Bartlett.

Children's Oncology Group. "Long-Term Follow-up Guidelines for Survivors of Childhood, Adolescent, and Young Adult Cancers." (2004). Retrieved 1/12/06 from CureSearch Web site: www.survivorshipguidelines.org/

Committee on Cancer Survivorship: Improving Care and Quality of Life, National Cancer Policy Board. 2006. Employment, Insurance, and Economic Issues. *From Cancer Patient to Cancer Survivor: Lost in Transition.* Washington, DC: National Academies Press.

Dunn, C. 2003. "Finding and Fighting Ovarian Cancer: To Catch a Thief." *CURE: Cancer Updates, Research & Education* 2, no. 4: 20–24, 26–27.

Eyre, H. J., et al. 2002. *Informed Decisions: The Complete Book of Cancer Diagnosis, Treatment, and Recovery.* 2d ed. Atlanta: American Cancer Society.

Feder, D. 2004. "Testicular Cancer." *CURE: Cancer Updates, Research & Education* 3, no. 2: 48–51, 53–54.

FertileHope. "Statistics, 2006." (2006). Retrieved from www.fertilehope.org/about/statistics.cfm

Freedman, T. G. 1994. "Social and Cultural Dimensions of Hair Loss in Women Treated for Breast Cancer." *Cancer Nursing* 17, no. 4: 334–341.

Gangloff, J. M. 2004. "Special Report. Compassionate Use Offers Access to Unapproved Drugs." *CURE: Cancer Updates, Research & Education* 3, no. 3: 72–73.

Gentry, L. 2003. "Melanoma: Only Skin Deep." *CURE: Cancer Updates, Research & Education* 2, no. 1: 42–49.

Granet, R. 2002. "How to Heal Emotionally." *Coping* 16, no. 1: 16.

Grillo, C. 2002. "Into the Mainstream: Complementary Therapies." *CURE: Cancer Updates, Research & Education* 1, no. 4: 48–54.

Hammelef, K. 2006. *Breadth of Cancer Distress.* Ann Arbor, MI: Personal Communication.

Hartmann, L. C., and C. L. Loprinzi. 2005. *Mayo Clinic Guide to Women's Cancers.* Rochester, MN: Mayo Clinic.

Harvard Center for Cancer Research. "Cancer fact sheet." (2002). Retrieved 1/11/06 from the Harvard Center for Cancer Prevention Web site: http://www.hsph.harvard.edu/cancer/press/archives/cancer_fact.pdf

Haylock, P. J. 2001. *Men's Cancers : How to Prevent Them, How to Treat Them, How to Beat Them.* Alameda, CA: Hunter House.

Hoffman, Barbara, For Cancer Survivorship (U.S.). (1997). *Working It Out: Your Employment Rights as a Cancer Survivor* 3d ed. Silver Spring, MD: National Coalition for Cancer Survivorship.

Keene, N., W. Hobbie, and K. Ruccione. 2000. *Childhood Cancer Survivors: A Practical Guide to Your Future.* Cambridge, MA: O'Reilly.

Kidney Cancer Association. 2001. *We Have Kidney Cancer: A Practical Guide for Patients and Families.* Evanston: Kidney Cancer Assn.

Komaromy, M. "What Is FAP." (2002). Retrieved 1/11/06 from Genetic Health Web site: www.genetichealth.com/CRC_FAP_A_Hereditary_Syndrome.shtml

Komaromy, M. "What Is HNPCC." (2000). Retrieved 1/11/06 from Genetic Halth Web site: www.genetichealth.com/CRC_HNPCC_A_Hereditary_Syndrome.shtml

Lai, Y. Stephen, and Jennifer R. Grandis. 2005. "Treating Head and Neck Cancer." *Coping* 19, no. 2: 38.

Lance Armstrong Foundation and Livestrong. "2004 news archive." (2004.) Retrieved 2/14/06 from LiveStrong Web site: www.livestrong.org/site/apps/nl/content2.asp?c=jvKZLbMRIsG&b=738963&ct=901209

Layke, J. C., and P. P. Lopez. 2004. "Gastric Cancer: Diagnosis and Treatment Options." *American Family Physician* 69, no. 5: 1133–1140.

Leukemia & Lymphoma Society. 2002. *Understanding Drug Therapy and Managing Side Effects*. White Plains, NY: Leukemia & Lymphoma Society.

Liebermann, J. "Ethics and the Consumer Health Librarian. (2004). Retrieved 9/28/05 from Consumer Health Manual, National Network of Libraries of Medicine Web site: nnlm.gov/scr/conhlth/ethics.htm

Lymphoma Research Foundation. 2004. *Understanding Non-Hodgkin's Lymphoma: A Guide for Patients*. Los Angeles: Lymphoma Research Foundation.

McCarthy, A. 2004. "Advanced Prostate Cancer: A Focus on Therapies." *CURE: Cancer Updates, Research & Education* 3, no. 3: 32–38.

McGinn, K. A., and P. J. Haylock. 2003. *Women's Cancers : How to Prevent Them, How to Treat Them, How to Beat Them*. 3d ed., fully updated ed. Alameda, CA: Hunter House.

National Cancer Institute. "Biological Therapies For Cancer: Questions and Answers." (2005). Retrieved 9/13/05 from the National Cancer Institute Web site: www.cancer.gov/cancertopics/factsheet/Therapy/biological

National Cancer Institute. "Bone Marrow Transplantation and Peripheral Blood Stem Cell Transplantation: Questions and Answers." (2004). Retrieved 11/21/05 from the National Cancer Institute Web site: www.cancer.gov/cancertopics/factsheet/Therapy/bone-marrow-transplant

National Cancer Institute. "Complementary and Alternative Medicine in Cancer Treatment (PDQ®)." (2003). Retrieved 11/25/05 from the National Cancer Institute Web site: www.cancer.gov/cancertopics/pdq/cam/cam-cancertreatment/Patient/page2

National Cancer Institute. 2005. *Coping with Advanced Cancer*. Rev. Aug. 2005 ed. Bethesda, MD: National Institutes of Health, National Cancer Institute.

National Cancer Institute. "Depression PDQ." (2006). Retrieved 2/14/06 from the National Cancer Institute Web site: www.cancer.gov/cancertopics/PDQ/supportivecare/depression/patient

National Cancer Institute. 1998. *Eating Hints for Cancer Patients: Before, During and After Treatment.* Rev. July 1997 ed. Bethesda, MD: National Institutes of Health, National Cancer Institute.

National Cancer Institute. "Genetic Testing for BRCA1 and BRCA2: It's Your Choice." (2002). Retrieved 1/11/06 from the National Cancer Institute Web site: www.cancer.gov/cancertopics/factsheet/Risk/BRCA

National Cancer Institute. "How To Evaluate Health Information on the Internet: Questions and Answers." (2005). Retrieved 7/4/06 from the National Cancer Institute Web site: www.cancer.gov/cancertopics/factsheet/Information/internet#4

National Cancer Institute. "Human Papillomavirus Vaccines: Questions and answers." (2006). Retrieved 9//06 from the National Cancer Institute Web site: www.cancer.gov/cancertopics/factsheet/risk/HPV-vaccine

National Cancer Institute. "Obesity and Cancer." (2004). Retrieved 2/14/06 from the National Cancer Institute Web site: www.cancer.gov/newscenter/obesity1

National Cancer Institute. 2003. *Pain Control: A Guide for People with Cancer and Their Families.* Bethesda, MD: U.S. Dept. of Health and Human Services, National Institutes of Health, National Cancer Institute.

National Cancer Institute. "Sexuality and Reproductive Issues (PDQ®)." (2005). Retrieved 1/17/06 from the National Cancer Institute Web site: www.cancer.gov/cancertopics/PDQ/supportivecare/sexuality/ Patient/page2

National Cancer Institute. 1998. *Taking Part in Clinical Trials : What Cancer Patients Need to Know.* Rev. June 1998 ed. Bethesda, MD: National Institutes of Health, National Cancer Institute.

National Cancer Institute. "Targeted Cancer Therapies: Questions and answers." (2005). Retrieved 9/13/05 from the National Cancer Institute Web site: www.cancer.gov/cancertopics/factsheet/Therapy/targeted

National Cancer Institute. "Testicular Cancer: Questions and Answers." (2005). Retrieved 9/13/05 from the National Cancer Institute Web site: http://cis.nci.nih.gov/fact/6_34.htm

National Cancer Institute. 1997. *Understanding Gene Testing.* Bethesda, MD: U.S. Dept. of Health and Human Services, Public Health Service, National Institutes of Health.

National Cancer Institute. 2002. *What You Need to Know about Brain Tumors.* Rev. July 2002 ed. Bethesda, MD: National Institutes of Health, National Cancer Institute.

National Cancer Institute. 2003. *What You Need to Know about Breast Cancer*. Rev. Apr. 2003 ed. Bethesda, MD: National Cancer Institute.

National Cancer Institute. 2004. *What You Need to Know about Cancer of the Cervix*. Rev. December 2004 ed. Bethesda, MD: National Institutes of Health, Nation Cancer Institute.

National Cancer Institute. 2003. *What You Need to Know about Cancer of the Colon and Rectum*. Rev. July 2003 ed. Bethesda, MD: National Institutes of Health, Nation Cancer Institute.

National Cancer Institute. 2000. *What You Need to Know about Cancer of the Esophagus*. Rev. October 1999 ed. Bethesda, MD: National Institutes of Health, National Cancer Institute.

National Cancer Institute. 2002. *What You Need to Know about Cancer of the Thyroid*. Rev. September 2002 ed. Bethesda, MD: National Institutes of Health, Nation Cancer Institute.

National Cancer Institute. 2001. *What You Need to Know about Cancer of the Uterus*. Rev. Apr. 2001 ed. Bethesda, MD: National Institutes of Health, National Cancer Institute.

National Cancer Institute. 1999. *What You Need to Know about Hodgkin's Disease*. Rev. June 1999 ed. Bethesda, MD: National Institutes of Health, National Cancer Institute.

National Cancer Institute. 2003. *What You Need to Know about Kidney Cancer*. Rev. Apr. 2003 ed. Bethesda, MD: National Institutes of Health, National Cancer Institute.

National Cancer Institute. 2002. *What You Need to Know about Leukemia*. Rev. July 2002 ed. Bethesda, MD: National Institutes of Health, National Cancer Institute.

National Cancer Institute. 2001. *What You Need to Know about Liver Cancer*. Rev. Sep. 2001 ed. Bethesda, MD: National Cancer Institute.

National Cancer Institute. 2002. *What You Need to Know about Melanoma*. Rev. July 2002 ed. Bethesda, MD: U.S. Dept. of Health and Human Services, Public Health Service, National Institutes of Health, National Cancer Institute.

National Cancer Institute. 2005. *What You Need to Know about Non-Hodgkin's Lymphoma*. Rev. Jan. 2005 ed. Bethesda, MD: National Institutes of Health, National Cancer Institute.

National Cancer Institute. 2005. *What You Need to Know about Prostate Cancer*. Rev. May 2005 ed. Bethesda, MD: National Institutes of Health, National Cancer Institute.

National Cancer Institute. 2005. *What You Need to Know about Skin Cancer*. Rev. June 2005 ed. Bethesda, MD: National Institutes of Health, National Cancer Institute.

National Cancer Institute. 2005. *What You Need to Know about Stomach Cancer.* Rev. Aug. 2005 ed. Bethesda, MD: National Institutes of Health, National Cancer Institute.

National Cancer Institute and National Institutes of Health. 2004. *Biological Therapy: Treatments That Use Your Immune System to Fight Cancer.* Bethesda, MD: National Cancer Institute.

National Cancer Institute and National Institutes of Health. 2003. *Chemotherapy and You: A Guide to Self-Help during Cancer Treatment.* Bethesda, MD: National Cancer Institute.

National Cancer Institute and National Institutes of Health. 2003. *Radiation Therapy and You: A Guide to Self-Help During Cancer Treatment.* Bethesda, MD: National Cancer Institute.

National Cancer Institute and National Institutes of Health. 2004. *Thinking about Complementary and Alternative Medicine: A Guide for People with Cancer.* Bethesda, MD: National Cancer Institute.

National Cancer Institute and National Institutes of Health. 2001. *What You Need to Know About Cancer of the Pancreas.* Rev. July 2001 ed. Bethesda, MD: National Institutes of Health, National Cancer Institute.

National Cancer Institute and National Institutes of Health. 2004. *Young People with Cancer: A Handbook for Parents.* Rev. Jan. 2001 ed. Bethesda, MD: The Institute.

National Cancer Institute and US TOO International, Inc. 2000. *Understanding Treatment Choices for Prostate Cancer.* Bethesda, MD; Hinsdale, IL: National Cancer Institute; US TOO International, Inc.

National Comprehensive Cancer Network. Ades, T., et al., eds. *Colon and Rectal Cancer: Treatment Guidelines for Patients.* 2005. Jenkintown, PA: National Comprehensive Cancer Network.

National Institutes of Health. 2000. *What You Need to Know about Ovarian Cancer.* Rev. March 2000 ed. Bethesda, MD: National Institutes of Health, National Cancer Institute.

National Institutes of Health. Osteoporosis and Related Bone Diseases. "What Is Bone?" (2005). Retrieved 1/12/06 from the National Institute of Arthritis and Musculoskeletal and Skin Diseases Web site: www.niams. nih.gov/bone/hi/what_is_bone.htm

National Institutes of Health and National Center for Complementary and Alternative Medicine. "NCCAM National Center for Complementary and Alternative Medicine Web Site." (2005). Retrieved 11/2/05 from the National Center for Complementary and Laternative Medicine (NCCAM) Web site; nccam.nih.gov

Novari, R. M. 2005. "Treating Depression in People with Cancer. *Coping* 19, no 6: 8.

Oeffinger, K., et al. "Prevalence and Severity of Chronic Diseases in Adult Survivors of Childhood Cancer: A Report from the Childhood Cancer Survivor Study [Abstract]." (2005). Abstract retrieved 1/12/006, from the American Society of Clinical Oncology (ASCO), Abstracts & Virtual Meeting database: www.asco.com database.

Pinkwater, S. 2005. "Talking with Your Child about Cancer." *Coping* 14, no. 5: 14.

Reidenbach, F. 2002. "Conceiving Solutions: Fertility and Cancer Treatment." *CURE: Cancer Updates, Research & Education* 1, no. 4: 20–22, 24–26.

Rich, W. M. "Cancer of the Uterus." (2003). Retrieved 09/03/05 from Introduction to Gynecologic Oncology Web site: www.gyncancer.com/uterus.html

Ries, L. A. G., L. Bernstein, and National Cancer Institute. "Cancer Incidence and Survival among Children and Adolescents in United States SEER Program 1975–1995." (1999). Retrieved 11/26/05 from the Surveillance, Epidemiology, and End Results (SEER) Program of the National Cancer Institute (NCI) Web site: seer.cancer.gov.proxy.lib.umich.edu/Publications/childhood/

Ries, L. A. G., et al. "SEER Cancer Statistics Review, 1975–2003." (2004). Retrieved 3/3/07 from the Surveillance, Epidemiology, and End Result (SEER) Program of the National Cancer Institute (NCI) Web site: seer.cancer.gov/csr/1975_2003/

Rosenbaum, E. H., and I. R. Rosenbaum. 2005. *Everyone's Guide to Cancer Supportive Care: A Comprehensive Handbook for Patients and Their Families.* Kansas City, MO: Andrews & McMeel.

Sarcoma Alliance. "Sarcoma Alliance." (2005). Retrieved 10/21/05 from the Sarcoma Alliance Web site: www.sarcomaalliance.com/

Schover, L. R., and American Cancer Society. 2001. *Sexuality and Cancer: For the Man Who Has Cancer, and His Partner.* Rev. ed. Atlanta, GA: American Cancer Society.

Schover, L. R., and American Cancer Society. 2001. *Sexuality and Cancer: For the Woman Who Has Cancer, and Her Partner.* Rev. ed. Atlanta, GA: American Cancer Society.

Steen, Grant. 2000. *Childhood Cancer: A Handbook from St. Jude Children's Research Hospital.* Cambridge, MA: Perseus.

Steinberg, D. 2003. "Positives for Pancreatic Cancer." *CURE: Cancer Updates, Research & Education* 2, no. 4: 38–42, 44, 46.

Stewart, S. K. 2002. *Bone Marrow and Blood Stem Cell Transplants: A Guide for Patients.* Highland Park, IL: Blood & Marrow Transplant Information Network (BMT InfoNet).

Susman, E. 2005. "Still an Issue: Many Cancer Patients Not Telling Their Physicians about Use of Alternative Treatments." [Electronic version]. *Oncology Times* 27, no. 22: 16.

Thomas, D. A. 2005. "The Consumer Health Reference Interview." *Journal of Hospital Librarianship* 5, no. 2: 45–56.

University of Wisconsin's Comprehensive Cancer Center. "Outlook: Life Beyond Childhood Cancer." (2005). Retrieved 1/12/06 from Outlook: Life Beyond Childhood Cancer Web site: www.outlook-life.org/

Vokes, Everett E. 2005. "Weighing Your Options for Treating Head and Neck Cancer. *Coping* 19, no. 4: 28.

Wood, D. 2003. "Options for Kidney Cancer." *CURE: Cancer Updates, Research & Education* 2, no. 2: 28–35.

Wu, H. 2005. "Sexuality and Cancer." *Coping* 19, no. 3: 42–43.

Index

(Page references in **bold** indicate the main entry for that topic.)

About the Author

R uti Malis Volk, MSI, is the librarian in charge of the Patient Education Resource Center (PERC) at the University of Michigan Comprehensive Cancer Center. A graduate of the University of Michigan School of Information, Ruti has been working in the cancer field since 1999. As the PERC librarian, Ruti developed a number of innovative information tools, products, and services, as well as an automated system for ordering brochures for libraries and medical institutions. She is also involved with research regarding the information-seeking behavior of people with cancer and their families and has been published in professional library periodicals and conference proceedings.

Ruti's bachelor degree is from the Hebrew University of Jerusalem. She has been a resident of Ann Arbor, Michigan, since 1987.